**BRITISH MEDICAL BULLETIN**

2001

KW-475-395

# Ischaemic heart disease: therapeutic issues

*Scientific Editors:    A H Gershlick and S W Davies*

http://www.bmb.oupjournals.org

## Acknowledgements

The planning committee for this issue of the *British Medical Bulletin* was chaired by Professor Keith Fox and also included Anthony Gershlick, Simon Davies, Neil Moat and John Pittard.

The British Council and Oxford University Press are most grateful to them for their help and advice and for the valuable work of the Scientific Editors in completing this issue.

# BRITISH MEDICAL BULLETIN
VOLUME 59    2001

# Ischaemic heart disease:
# therapeutic issues

*Scientific Editors*

## A H Gershlick
## S W Davies

*Series Editors*
L K Borysiewicz PhD FRCP
M J Walport PhD FRCP

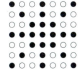

OXFORD
UNIVERSITY PRESS

PUBLISHED FOR THE BRITISH COUNCIL BY
OXFORD UNIVERSITY PRESS

OXFORD UNIVERSITY PRESS
Great Clarendon Street, Oxford OX2 6DP, UK

**British Library Cataloguing in Publication Data**
A catalogue record for this book is available from the British Library
ISBN 0–19–922485–4
ISSN 0007–1420

**Subscription information** *British Medical Bulletin* is published quarterly on behalf of The British Council. Subscription rates for 2001 are £160/$275 for four volumes, each of one issue. Prices include distribution and is distributed by surface mail within Europe, by air freight and second class post within the USA*, and by various methods of air-speeded delivery to all other countries. Subscription orders, single issue orders and enquiries for 2001 should be sent to:

Oxford University Press, Great Clarendon Street, Oxford OX2 6DP, UK
(Tel +44 (0)1865 267907; Fax +44(0)1865 267485; E-mail: jnl.orders@oup.co.uk

*Periodicals postage paid at Rahway, NJ. US Postmaster: Send address changes to *British Medical Bulletin*, c/o Mercury Airfreight International Ltd, 365 Blair Road, Avenel, NJ 07001, USA.

**Back numbers** of titles published 1996–2000 (see inside back cover) are available from The Royal Society of Medicine Press Limited, 1 Wimpole St, London W1G 0AE, UK. (Tel. +44 (0)20 7290 2921; Fax +44 (0)20 7290 2929); www.rsm.ac.uk/pub/bmb/htm).

**Pre-1996 back numbers**: Contact Jill Kettley, Subscriptions Manager, Harcourt Brace, Foots Cray, Sidcup, Kent DA14 5HP (Tel +44 (0)20 8308 5700; Fax +44 (0)20 8309 0807).

*This journal is indexed, abstracted and/or published online in the following media: Adonis, Biosis, BRS Colleague (full text), Chemical Abstracts, Colleague (Online), Current Contents/ Clinical Medicine, Current Contents/Life Sciences, Elsevier BIOBASE/Current Awareness in Biological Sciences, EMBASE/Excerpta Medica, Index Medicus/Medline, Medical Documentation Service, Reference Update, Research Alert, Science Citation Index, Scisearch, SIIC-Database Argentina, UMI (Microfilms)*

Editorial services and typesetting by BA & GM Haddock, Ford, Midlothian EH37 5RE
Printed in Great Britain by Bell & Bain Ltd, Glasgow, Scotland.

# Preface

Ischaemic heart disease is common. In the UK alone, 250,000 present each year with acute myocardial infarction and a further 250,000 with unstable angina. In 1995, 2.2 million Americans were discharged from hospital with a diagnosis of coronary artery disease. The factors leading to the point of partial or complete coronary artery occlusion are multiple and complexly interactive. They include the basic developmental pathology of early vessel wall abnormalities, consequent on the interaction between haemostatic, hormonal, and various blood constituents (such as lipid fractions and glucose), and the cellular constituents of the vessel wall. Epidemiology is important in helping us to understand how and why atheromatous coronary disease presents clinically and how we might develop strategies to prevent it. Many of the therapeutic developments that have improved outcome in patients with coronary artery disease have come from our understanding of the pathology and from strategies tested in peripheral vascular disease. Thus knowing, for example, that thrombus formation has a central role in the initiation of acute coronary syndromes has led to the development of lytic therapy and the trialing of powerful antiplatelet drugs. Concepts of ventricular remodelling have emphasised and help explain the effectiveness of ACE inhibitor therapy, while an increasing understanding about which arrhythmia to treat and with what has improved patient survival.

Managing patients to improve outcome is not only about drug treatment however. Secondary prevention through lifestyle change and improving self confidence, perception and optimising quality of life through the implementation of rehabilitation programmes are as critical as getting the initial treatment right. Managing patients with coronary artery disease also involves revascularisation. Average rates world-wide are 600 per million for both percutaneous and surgical procedures. Issues such as use of stents and more recently how to prevent in-stent re-stenosis as well as choice of by-pass conduit and operative approach are all developments designed to improve the outcome of intervention. New developments such as the use of gene therapy to promote vessel collateral growth or alternative ways of treating chest pain in those patients who cannot be managed with conventional therapies are becoming available.

Picking out the important issues to represent the various components in the development, clinical presentation, therapeutic options and interventional management of ischaemic heart disease could never be regarded as an easy task. Convincing experts in the field to give up time to summarise and provide opinion on these various aspects is always difficult. However, we believe we have collected together an outstanding group of individuals all respected in their field, who have provided in this book contemporary opinions that go a long way to summarising what happens during the pathological events that take a vessel from being normal to being diseased. They have explained how such events translate into clinical presentation and how they form the basis for therapeutic strategies that alter the natural history of the disease.

The overall aim of this volume of the *British Medical Bulletin* was to provide an up to date evidence-based overview of the issues involved in the development and management of ischaemic heart disease to provide authority for the reader to alter, if necessary, their medical practice. We hope this aim will be achieved.

*A H Gershlick*
*S W Davies*

# Asymptomatic individuals – risk stratification in the prevention of coronary heart disease

## David Wood

*Department of Cardiology, Charing Cross Hospital, London, UK*

The report of the World Health Organization Expert Committee on Prevention of Coronary Heart Disease considered that a comprehensive action for coronary heart disease (CHD) prevention has to include three components:

1. A population strategy – for altering, in the entire population, those life-style and environmental factors, and their social and economic determinants, that are the underlying causes of the mass occurrence of coronary heart disease

2. A high risk strategy – identification of high risk individuals, and action to reduce their risk factor levels

3. Prevention of recurrent coronary heart disease events and progression of the disease in patients with clinically established coronary heart disease[1].

Prevention targeted at patients with established coronary disease and the high risk strategy targeted at healthy individuals at high risk are an integral part of clinical practice. The clinical approaches and the population approaches for coronary heart disease prevention are complimentary, but the population strategy is fundamental to reducing the burden of cardiovascular disease.

While recognising the importance of the public health strategy embodied in the UK Government's *Health of the Nation* document[2], which outlines a policy seeking to reduce morbidity and mortality from CHD and other atherosclerotic disease in the population, it is essential that specialists and general practitioners also recognise their responsibilities for preventive medicine in routine clinical practice. Clinicians regularly see patients who have either presented with CHD or other atherosclerotic disease, or are found to be at high risk of developing atherosclerotic disease because of hypertension, dyslipidaemia, diabetes or a combination of these risk factors. In defining the objectives for CHD prevention in clinical practice, it is implicit that priority is given to those patients who are at highest risk of developing CHD, rather than attempting to reach every adult in the population. Therefore, risk stratification is required.

In 1998, the Joint British Societies' Recommendations on Prevention of Coronary Heart Disease in Clinical Practice[3] set an order of priority

*Correspondence to: Prof. David Wood, Department of Cardiology, Charing Cross Hospital, Fulham Palace Road, London W6 8RF, UK*

for CHD in clinical practice:

1(a)   Patients with established CHD

1(b)   Patients with other major atherosclerotic disease

2      Individuals with hypertension, dyslipidaemia, diabetes mellitus, family history of premature CHD, or a combination of these risk factors, which puts them at high risk of developing CHD or other atherosclerotic disease. Patients with diabetes mellitus are at particularly high risk of CHD.

## Concept of coronary heart disease risk

The biology of atherosclerotic disease, its determinants and complications, is a continuum of risk in the population. At one end of the spectrum are young individuals without atherosclerotic disease who have not yet been sufficiently exposed to the life-style and environmental factors responsible for this disease and its complications. Then there are an increasing number of individuals who develop asymptomatic atherosclerosis as a consequence of their exposure to smoking, an unhealthy diet and sedentary life-style which result in obesity, hypertension, dyslipidaemia, diabetes and other risk factors for atherosclerosis and its complications. Finally, at the other end of the spectrum are patients with symptomatic atherosclerosis – angina, myocardial infarction, stroke and peripheral arterial disease – whose subsequent risk of recurrent disease and death is in part driven by those factors responsible for the diseases initial manifestation. Given this continuum of risk exposure and disease, the traditional division of prevention into tertiary, secondary and primary is artificial. While patients with symptomatic atherosclerotic disease are at high absolute risk of a further event (or a new event in another arterial territory) compared to the healthy population, some individuals without any clinical manifestation of atherosclerosis, such as those with diabetes mellitus, may be at greater risk because of multiple predisposing factors which have not been addressed. For example, a man with an uncomplicated inferior myocardial infarction and well preserved ventricular function may actually be at lower risk of a further coronary event compared to a man of the same age, currently smoking, with an elevated systolic blood pressure of 156 mmHg, a total cholesterol of 6.4 mmol/l, high density lipoprotein (HDL) cholesterol of 0.8 mmol/l and impaired glucose tolerance. Therefore, it is appropriate to address life-style and other risk factors for atherosclerotic disease for patients with symptomatic atherosclerotic disease, and those at high risk of developing symptomatic disease in the same way. This view does not conflict with the clinical priorities for CHD prevention.

Patients with symptomatic atherosclerosis are the top priority for CHD prevention in clinical practice for pragmatic reasons[3]. Such patients present themselves to medical services because of symptoms and are at high risk of recurrent coronary disease or death. Risk stratification of these patients is unnecessary in relation to life-style and risk factor intervention. They all require professional intervention on smoking, diet and physical activity and appropriate management of weight, blood pressure, lipids and glycaemia. In addition, there are cardioprotective drugs – aspirin or other platelet modifying agents, β-blockers, ACE inhibitors, lipid modification therapies and anticoagulants – which reduce the risk of recurrent disease and improve survival. However, in contrast to symptomatic patients, high risk asymptomatic individuals have to be sought through population screening, whether systematic or opportunistic. Attendance in general practice or hospital is an opportunity to risk-stratify a healthy individual by assessing absolute risk of developing CHD – that is, the probability of developing non-fatal myocardial infarction or fatal CHD over a defined time period given a particular combination of risk factors – and then, depending on the degree of risk, to intervene appropriately. Taking account of all major cardiovascular risk factors avoids undue emphasis being placed on an individual risk factor at the expense of overall or absolute risk. Risk factors exert an accumulative effect on absolute CHD risk. Therefore, an individual with a number of mildly abnormal risk factors may be at a level of absolute CHD risk greater than that of someone with just one high risk factor.

For example, using the Framingham risk equation, a man of 50 years, who is a non-smoker, with a systolic blood pressure of 125 mmHg, a serum cholesterol of 8.2 mmol/l, and an HDL cholesterol of 1.0 mmol/l, has an absolute risk of developing CHD of about 15% over the next 10 years. A man of the same age who smokes cigarettes, with a systolic blood pressure of 140 mmHg, cholesterol of 6.2 mmol/l, and an HDL cholesterol of 0.8 mmol/l and is diabetic has an absolute CHD risk of about 30% over the same period. In other words, his risk of developing a CHD event compared with the first man (relative risk) is increased 2-fold, despite the fact that none of his risk factors considered individually (apart from smoking) would be thought sufficiently high to merit action. In contrast, by taking a unifactorial approach, the first man's cholesterol level may be considered sufficiently high to require treatment by diet, and possibly even drug therapy, despite his absolute CHD risk being low.

Therefore, in assessing healthy individuals' risk stratification by estimating absolute risk of developing CHD, or other atherosclerotic disease, is necessary to identify those highest risk individuals requiring the most intensive life-style intervention and, where appropriate, drug treatment. Specifically, prescribing antihypertensive and/or lipid lowering medication should reflect both absolute CHD risk as well as individual risk factor levels, and not just individual risk factor levels alone. The man of 50 years already described with an absolute CHD risk of less than 15%, and a cholesterol level of 8.2 mmol/l. would not be a candidate for lipid lowering therapy in the absence of familial dyslipidaemia. In contrast, the man with an absolute CHD risk of greater than 30%, and a cholesterol level of 6.2 mmol/l, would be given lipid lowering therapy if there was no response to diet despite his cholesterol level being lower than that of the first man. This absolute multifactorial risk approach fundamentally challenges the traditional medical model focused on single risk factors, as evidenced by hypertension[4] and dyslipidaemia[5]. Undue emphasis in the past has been placed on elevations of single risk factors rather than on overall multifactorial coronary or cardiovascular risk. In practice, physicians deal with the whole patient rather than one aspect of his or her risk. Clusters of risk factors have a multiplicative effect and thus an individual with a number of modest risk factors can be at considerably greater risk than a person with one very high risk factor (Table 1).

Because CHD risk rises with increasing age, older individuals are more likely than younger ones to qualify for intervention based on an absolute CHD risk approach. Given a proportionate reduction in risk for an intervention, the benefit will inevitably be greatest in those at highest multifactorial risk – namely the older and elderly patients. Yet, life expectancy in these older, high risk patients is shorter than younger patients and the benefits of intervention need to be considered in the context of a life-course approach. Although younger individuals are at lower absolute CHD risk, they will certainly accumulate more benefit from effective life-style and therapeutic interventions over a life-time. To take account of life-time exposure to risk factors, the European recommendations on coronary prevention[6,7] advocate estimating absolute CHD risk today and projecting that risk to say age 60 years, assuming no change in risk factor levels. In this way, accumulative exposure to risk over a life-time can be estimated and individuals tracking towards a high risk category in later life can be identified earlier and appropriately managed.

The risk stratification of asymptomatic individuals in the population identifies those at highest risk who should be targeted first. As a minimum,

**Table 1** Examples showing the impact of a single risk factor, multiple risk factors and clinically established coronary heart disease on the absolute risk of developing a coronary heart disease event over 10 years

| Sex | Age (years) | Plasma cholesterol (mmol/l) | Systolic blood pressure (mmHg) | Smoking | Clinical CHD | Minimum estimate of the 10-year risk |
|---|---|---|---|---|---|---|
| Male | 50 | 7 | 120 | − | − | 10% |
| Male | 50 | 6 | 140 | + | − | 20% |
| Male | 50 | 7 | 120 | − | + | > 20% |
| Male | 50 | 6 | 140 | + | + | > 40% |

the Joint British Societies[3] recommend that healthy individuals with a 30% or higher CHD risk over 10 years should all be identified and treated appropriately and effectively now. As the scientific evidence clearly justifies risk factor intervention in healthy individuals with a CHD risk lower than 30%, it is entirely appropriate, as the next step, for physicians to expand progressively opportunistic screening and risk factor intervention down to individuals with a 15% CHD risk over 10 years, as long as those at higher levels of risk have received effective preventive care. Taking a progressive, staged approach to coronary prevention ensures those at highest risk are targeted first, and delivery of care is commensurate with medical services being able to identify, investigate and manage patients properly over the long-term. As there is evidence from randomised control trials that, for some risk factor interventions, drugs significantly reduce the risk of CHD events, and all cause mortality, in individuals with a risk as low as 6% over the next 10 years, it would be appropriate to extend risk factor intervention to individuals with a CHD risk lower than 15% as long as there are resources to do so.

## Calculation of coronary heart disease risk

The concept of calculating absolute CHD risk as the clinical context in which decisions about the management of individual risk factors are made was first proposed for the management of hypertension in New Zealand in 1993[8]. The Joint European Societies – European Society of Cardiology, European Society of Hypertension and European Atherosclerosis Society – then proposed, in 1994, that absolute risk should be the basis for prevention of coronary heart disease in the healthy population embracing blood pressure, lipids and diabetes[6]. The Joint European Societies produced a coronary risk chart based on age, smoking, systolic blood pressure and total cholesterol. A separate coronary risk chart was produced for patients with diabetes mellitus. This was followed by the New Zealand cardiovascular risk chart which employed a combination of systolic and diastolic blood pressure values, the ratio of total cholesterol to HDL cholesterol and a 5-year rather than 10-year risk model[8]. The Sheffield Risk and Treatment Table differed from these initial risk assessment charts in that its first use was to determine whether total cholesterol and HDL cholesterol need be measured and, if so, whether the lipid ratio confers an absolute 10-year CHD risk of 30% or more in the context of other risk factors. Subsequently, a Sheffield Table was published to identify individuals at ≥ 15% CHD risk[9]. The Joint British Societies produced a coronary risk prediction chart (see <http://www.hyp.ac.uk/bhs/riskpv.htm>) and an associated computer programme *Cardiac Risk Assessor*, the latter calculating both 10-year CHD risk and cardiovascular risk (including stroke) over the same period[3]. The Joint British Societies chart is based on age, smoking, systolic blood pressure and the ratio of total cholesterol to HDL cholesterol and diabetes. The chart risk stratifies healthy individuals into three categories: those individuals at highest CHD risk (30% or higher, red band); those at the next level of CHD risk (15% or higher, orange band); and finally those whose CHD risk is less than 15% (green band).

When a physician sees a patient, an intuitive assessment of cardio-vascular risk will take place based on their age, exposure to tobacco, visible obesity including central obesity, blood pressure, a measurement of lipids (cholesterol, HDL cholesterol and triglycerides) and glycaemic response to a glucose load (impaired glucose tolerance and frank diabetes), family history of CHD, especially premature CHD, and clinical evidence of end organ damage such as retinopathy, renal impairment, micro-albuminuria, left ventricular hypertrophy on ECG or echocardiography, and so on. This intuitive risk assessment is formalised by using coronary risk charts or computer programmes and, because clinical judgement can be imprecise, it is important to estimate risk as objectively as possible. However, this does not exclude the need for clinical judgement as the risk charts do not incorporate all of the risk factors for atherosclerotic disease and it is necessary to adjust the risk obtained to take account of these other factors. For example, clinical evidence of end organ damage will increase the risk, as will a family history of premature CHD. Therefore, in making a decision about whether to introduce antihypertensive or lipid lowering medication, the absolute risk assessment from the chart or computer programme has to be interpreted in the context of other information and ultimately clinical judgement about an individual's management is required.

To identify individuals at high multifactorial risk requires screening which for the most part is undertaken in general practice, either as new patient checks or opportunistically at other consultations. Other contacts with medical services through occupational health screening or specialised hospital clinics can afford the same opportunity. Risk estimation is based on an interview and some physical measurements including blood tests.

To estimate CHD or cardiovascular risk as accurately as possible, the statistical models should be derived from prospective epidemiological data from the population to which the model is to be applied. The model should include all the important risk factors which are easily and routinely measured in clinical practice. The following variables are considered important: smoking, blood pressure, total cholesterol, HDL cholesterol, diabetes, family history of premature CHD and ECG evidence of left ventricular hypertrophy. The Framingham Study from the US is the epidemiological model used in the European, New Zealand, Sheffield and Joint British Societies charts and related computer programmes[10].

With this information, it is possible to calculate an individual's absolute risk of developing CHD – that is, the risk of a non-fatal myocardial infarction (MI) or coronary death over 10 years. As risk increases exponentially with age, the risk will be closer to the lower decennium for the first 6 years of each decade – for example, at age 45 years, the risk will be closer to that at age 40 years but at age 47 years it will be closer to that at age 50 years. Family history of premature CHD (for example, in men under 55 years or women under 65 years) increases risk by a factor of approximately 1.5-fold and should also be taken into account in assessing an individual's risk.

The Framingham risk equation is based on measurements made at baseline on a single occasion and, therefore, it is appropriate to estimate risk in clinical practice in the same way. However, the slope of the relation between the true mean risk factor level and risk of developing disease is steeper than that of a single measurement and risk because of regression dilution bias. The slope of the regression line relating CHD risk to risk factor measurements based on a series of recordings is steeper because the effects of biological variation are largely abolished. Therefore, CHD risk will be somewhat higher than the estimate based on the first blood pressure or cholesterol measurement made at an initial screening visit. Absolute risk will also be underestimated by using values of blood pressure on treatment, or cholesterol recorded after dietary intervention, because the true risk is likely to be closer to the life-long habitual levels of these risk factors. By the same token, it would be inappropriate to classify a cigarette smoker, who has recently stopped, as a non-smoker because risk will reflect life-time exposure to tobacco. Whilst it is appropriate to estimate absolute CHD risk on the basis of single risk factor measurements, a decision to treat requires a series of recordings of say blood pressure or cholesterol over a period of time. So it is important to distinguish risk assessment from the final decision to introduce antihypertensive or lipid lowering therapy. The latter is dependent on both the context provided by absolute CHD risk and the long-term levels of individual risk factors observed over time. Life-style intervention will also impact on these levels.

# Healthy individuals and management of risk

For individuals without clinical atherosclerotic disease, the absolute risk of developing CHD (non-fatal MI or coronary death), or other atherosclerotic disease, during the next 10 years should strongly influence the intensity of life-style and therapeutic intervention. As the absolute CHD risk increases, so should the intensity of intervention, thus maximising the potential benefit from risk factor reduction. In addition, as the absolute risk increases, so the threshold for drug treatment of blood pressure and dyslipidaemia should be lowered. With advancing age, the absolute risk associated with any one risk factor, or combination of risk factors, may over time become sufficiently great to justify intervention.

The concept of intervention based on absolute CHD risk is justified by evidence that a given reduction in blood pressure or serum cholesterol produces a constant proportional reduction in risk, independent of absolute risk. For example, the relative risk reduction with statin treatment is constant at 33%. Therefore, the absolute benefit is determined by an individual's absolute risk. Consider two men aged 45 years with a serum cholesterol of 6.0 mmol/l; one has no other risk factors while the other smokes cigarettes, has diabetes mellitus and hypertension complicated by left ventricular hypertrophy. Absolute risk of CHD in the next 10 years are <10% and > 30%, respectively; both would gain the same relative risk reduction from treatment with a statin, but absolute benefit is more than 3 times greater in the latter individual (>10% *versus* < 3%).

The threshold for drug treatment of blood pressure and blood lipids in terms of absolute CHD risk is a matter of judgement, and for blood pressure it is necessary to consider cardiovascular risk because of the additional benefits seen for stroke. Considerations include the following: (i) absolute CHD (or cardiovascular) risk of patients in the trials that demonstrated benefit; (ii) the number of at-risk patients at these levels of risk who must be treated for a defined period of time for one individual to benefit; and (iii) the cost of preventing a CHD event at these different levels of absolute CHD or cardiovascular risk.

When considering cost, the cost of drug therapy is only one part as there are resource implications for screening, investigation and follow-up of individuals at different levels of CHD risk, principally in general practice but also in specialised hospital clinics.

The evidence from clinical trials has unequivocally shown that individuals with an absolute CHD risk as low as 15% (equivalent to a cardiovascular risk of 20%) over 10 years do benefit from blood pressure and lipid lowering therapies that reduce coronary and cardiovascular morbidity and mortality. So the scientific evidence justifies life-style and therapeutic interventions in the population, at least down to a 15% absolute CHD risk, but the magnitude of this task and its cost for the medical services would be considerable. The costs would include those of opportunistic screening, follow-up, laboratory and other investigations, referral of some patients for a specialist opinion, *etc*, as well as the cost of drugs. In advocating an order of priorities for coronary prevention, and having started with patients with established atherosclerotic disease, it is appropriate to stage risk factor intervention in the general population, and audit the results achieved at each stage. As a minimum, all individuals with an absolute CHD risk of 30% or more over 10 years should be targeted now for comprehensive risk factor management, which will include, as appropriate, blood pressure and lipid lowering therapy. When it has been shown that those at highest risk have been effectively targeted, the scientific evidence justifies a progressive expansion of coronary prevention from 30% down to 15% absolute CHD risk, linked to NHS resources needed to deliver effective preventive care. For individuals with an absolute CHD risk less than 15% over the next 10 years, drug therapy is not normally recommended.

The exceptions to treatment in the context of absolute CHD risk are severe hypertension (systolic >160 mmHg and/or diastolic >100 mmHg), familial hypercholesterolaemia or other inherited dyslipidaemia, or patients with diabetes mellitus with associated target organ damage.

The proportions of men and women (excluding patients with reported CHD or other atherosclerotic disease) who are potentially eligible for treatment at different levels of absolute CHD risk in England and Scotland, has been estimated by applying the Framingham Risk Function to the Health Survey for England (1994) and the Scottish Health Survey (Table 2). The Health Survey for England did not measure HDL cholesterol and this has been estimated from the Scottish data. The Scottish Survey is based on people aged 30–64 years whereas in England the population 30–75 years were surveyed. For the age group 64–75 years in England, the average HDL cholesterol at age 64 years in Scotland was used: 28% of men and 9% of women in England have an absolute CHD risk of ≥15% over 10 years. The corresponding proportions in Scotland are 21% and 6% but for a younger age range which stops at 64 years.

# Blood pressure

In the management of blood pressure, assessing absolute CHD or cardiovascular risk is logical and the Joint British Societies produced an

**Table 2** Percentage of men and women in England and Scotland at different levels of CHD risk

| Absolute CHD risk (%)* | England (aged 30–74 years) | | Scotland (aged 30–64 years) | |
|---|---|---|---|---|
| | Men | Women | Men | Women |
| ≥30 | 3 | – | 2 | 0.3 |
| 25–29 | 5 | 2 | 3 | 1 |
| 20–24 | 8 | 2 | 6 | 1 |
| 15–19 | 12 | 5 | 10 | 4 |

*Framingham function: absolute risk of non-fatal myocardial infarction and coronary death over 10 years.

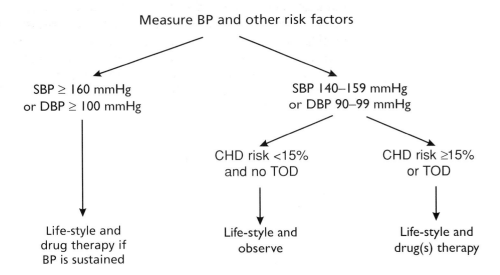

**Fig. 1** Absolute CHD risk and management of blood pressure. CHD risk = non-fatal myocardial infarction and coronary death over 10 years; TOD = target organ damage.

algorithm based on this principle.(Fig. 1). The exception to the absolute risk approach is individuals with a sustained diastolic blood pressure of 100 mmHg or greater and/or systolic blood pressure over 160 mmHg. Such individuals should always be prescribed antihypertensive drugs because of established benefit in reducing total cardiovascular risk, and stroke in particular. In those with lower levels of sustained diastolic or systolic blood pressure, 10-year cardiovascular (CHD and stroke) risk should be calculated. It is important to calculate cardiovascular and not just CHD risk in the management of hypertension because of the additional benefit of blood pressure lowering in relation to stroke. An absolute cardiovascular risk of 20% over 10 years is equivalent to an absolute CHD risk of 15% over the same time and this is the recommended threshold for antihypertensive drug treatment.

Diastolic blood pressure measurements of 110 mmHg or greater should be repeated over 1–2 weeks to confirm a sustained increase, despite life-style intervention, after which drug treatment should be started. Individuals with diastolic blood pressure in the range 100–109 mmHg, but with no evidence of target organ damage, should be given life-style advice and observed, initially weekly and thereafter monthly. If there is a downward trend in blood pressure (diastolic <100 mmHg), observation should be continued together with re-inforced life-style advice. If diastolic blood pressure is sustained at or above 100 mmHg during this 3–6 month period drug treatment should be started. The management of individuals in whom diastolic blood pressure remains between 90–99 mmHg and/or systolic blood pressure between 140–159 mmHg on repeated measurements should be considered in the context of their absolute risk of CHD and stroke, not CHD alone.

In patients with target organ damage (left ventricular hypertrophy, retinopathy – haemorrhages or exudates – renal impairment or proteinuria, for example) antihypertensive therapy is indicated.

## Lipids

To assess absolute CHD risk, a non-fasting serum cholesterol and non-fasting HDL cholesterol are adequate. A measurement of HDL cholesterol is essential to assess accurately absolute CHD risk. This is particularly true in women who frequently maintain high serum HDL cholesterol concentrations long after their menopause, which means that a raised total cholesterol can be misleading. Also, as low HDL cholesterol tends to cluster with other risk factors such as diabetes and hypertension, reliance on total cholesterol alone in such men and women will often underestimate risk. All patients who have a pronounced hyperlipidaemia, or for whom lipid lowering therapy is being considered, should have a fasting lipoprotein profile to include fasting cholesterol, triglycerides and HDL cholesterol. Figure 2 is an algorithm for cholesterol management based on absolute CHD risk. Fasting serum triglycerides are important to measure before introducing lipid lowering drug therapy because a raised cholesterol may not be caused by increased LDL cholesterol. If severe hypertriglyceridaemia is present, an increase in serum cholesterol may be caused by cholesterol transported in very low density lipoprotein (VLDL)

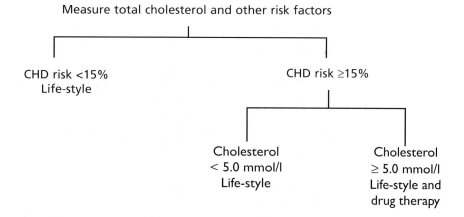

**Fig. 2** Absolute CHD risk and management of blood lipids. CHD risk = non-fatal myocardial infarction and coronary death over 10 years.

and chylomicrons (type V hyperlipoproteinaemia). Secondary causes of hyperlipidaemia should always be excluded. This includes enquiring about possible excessive alcohol consumption and screening for thyroid disorders, renal disease, liver disease, diabetes mellitus and impaired glucose tolerance.

Patients with familial hypercholesterolaemia are at especially high risk of premature coronary atherosclerosis and its complications. Typically, the patient has a cholesterol of around 9 mmol/l or greater together with clinical signs such as tendon xanthomata, early corneal arcus and the premature development of CHD. Untreated, the majority of male heterozygotes and half of the female heterozygotes will have a clinical CHD event before the age of 60 years. Once the diagnosis is made, the need to screen the immediate family is implicit in view of its autosomal dominant inheritance. Patients with familial hypercholesterolaemia do not require risk stratification using the coronary risk chart. They all require treatment with a combination of diet and drug therapy. The drug class of first choice for familial hypercholesterolaemia is a statin.

# Risk calculation

It should be emphasised that CHD risk calculation may be less accurate in certain groups of patients. Particular attention is drawn to patients with familial hypercholesterolaemia, patients with diabetes and target organ damage, and patients of Indo-Asian descent. All these groups appear to be at greater risk than that calculated from the Framingham equation and clinicians should make allowance for this.

# Diabetes mellitus

For individuals with diabetes mellitus, CHD risk is greatly increased with both type I and type II diabetes. Over 70% of patients with diabetes die from macrovascular disease, mainly coronary heart disease. Thus, implicit in the long-term management of diabetic patients is the requirement for multiple risk factor modification for coronary prevention. Hypertension is very common in type II diabetes, is strongly related to obesity and highly predictive of cardiovascular complications. Antihypertensive treatment is required for all patients with type II diabetes and blood pressure ≥ 160 mmHg, aiming for a target blood pressure of <130 mmHg systolic and <80 mmHg diastolic. For patients with type II diabetes and systolic pressure 140–159 mmHg but diastolic pressure of <90 mmHg, treatment is recommended if target organ damage or microvascular or macrovascular complications are present, or if the absolute coronary risk is ≥15% over 10 years. Many patients with type II diabetes are overweight and have high cardiovascular risk. They need intensive and sustained advice on life-style and appropriate treatment to achieve other risk factor targets as well as glycaemic control. Cholesterol lowering therapy is indicated in patients with diabetes if the absolute CHD risk exceeds 15% over 10 years and the total cholesterol is >5 mmol/l.

# Chronic renal failure

Hypertension and hyperlipidaemia are common in chronic renal disease and the co-existence of hypertension and proteinuria is a very powerful marker for CHD. Rigorous control of blood pressure is important; a target blood pressure of <130 mmHg systolic and <80 mmHg diastolic is recommended. Hypercholesterolaemia occurs in association with proteinuria, but the management of hyperlipidaemia is often complicated by the unsuitability of many lipid lowering drugs and by complex dietary and therapeutic regimens.

# Special considerations

## Gender differences

The absolute risk of CHD is lower in women at all ages up to the very elderly when disease rates almost converge. Over the age of 55 years, women have more obesity, higher total cholesterol and more diabetes than men, and over the age of 65 years have more hypertension than men. At younger ages, blood pressure and LDL cholesterol are lower among women than men and throughout life women smoke less and have higher HDL cholesterol levels. One further large difference between men and women is that levels of central obesity, as measured by waist hip ratios, are very much smaller among women. Despite these differences, absolute CHD risk estimation is as appropriate in women as in men and the same threshold of an absolute CHD risk ≥ 15% over 10 years defines those women who may be eligible for antihypertensive and/or lipid lowering therapy.

## The elderly

The absolute risk of CHD and other atherosclerotic diseases is higher in the elderly compared with any other age group. The same proportionate risk reduction will, therefore, potentially have a much more beneficial impact in the elderly compared with younger age groups.

## Ethnic minorities

Coronary mortality is significantly higher among South Asian immigrants in this country. In contrast, CHD death rates are profoundly reduced among the Afro-Caribbean population whereas stroke rates are highest among the Afro-Caribbean community. Europeans have the lowest stroke rates and the South Asians have rates between those of the Europeans and the Afro-Caribbean, which is compatible with the prevalence of hypertension among the three ethnic groups. The coronary risk chart will underestimate the absolute CHD risk in the Asian community and overestimate absolute CHD risk in the Afro-Caribbean population. Therefore, this chart should be used with caution in these ethnic minorities.

## References

1   World Health Organization. *Prevention of Coronary Heart Disease*. Report of a WHO Expert Committee; WHO Technical Report Series 678. Geneva: World Health Organization, 1982

2   Department of Health. *The Health of the Nation: A Strategy for Health in England*. London: HMSO, 1992

3   British Cardiac Society, British Hyperlipidaemia Association, British Hypertension Society, British Diabetic Association. Joint British recommendations on prevention of coronary heart disease in clinical practice. *Heart* 1998; **80 (Suppl 2)**: S1–26

4   Sever P, Veevers G, Bulpit C *et al*. Management guidelines in essential hypertension: report of the second working party of the British Hypertension Society. *BMJ* 1993; **306**: 983–7

5   Betteridge DJ, Dodson PM, Durrington PN *et al*. Management of hyperlipidaemia: guidelines of the British Hyperlipidaemia Association. *Postgrad Med J* 1993; **69**: 359–69

6   Pyorala K, De Backer G, Graham I, Poole-Wilson P, Wood D. Prevention of coronary heart disease in clinical practice. Recommendations of the Task Force of the European Society of Cardiology, European Atherosclerosis Society and European Society of Hypertension. *Eur Heart J* 1994; **15**: 1300–31 and *Atherosclerosis* 1994; **110**: 121–61

7   Wood DA, De Backer G, Faergeman O *et al*. Prevention of coronary heart disease in clinical practice. Recommendations of the second joint task force of the European Society of Cardiology, European Atherosclerosis Society and European Society of Hypertension. *Eur Heart J* 1998; **19**: 1434–503

8   Jackson R. Updated New Zealand cardiovascular disease risk-benefit prediction guide. *BMJ* 2000; **320**: 709–10.

9   Ghahramani P, Jackson PR, Rowland-Yeo K *et al*. Coronary and cardiovascular risk estimation for primary prevention: validation of a new Sheffield table in the 1995 Scottish health survey population. *BMJ* 2000; **320**: 671–76.

10  Anderson KM, Wilson PWF, Odell PM *et al*. An updated coronary risk profile: a statement for health professionals. *Circulation* 1991; **83**: 356–62.

# Clinical presentation and diagnosis of coronary artery disease: stable angina

## S W Davies

*Department of Cardiology, Royal Brompton Hospital, London, UK*

Angina pectoris is a clinical syndrome of discomfort in the chest, jaw, arm, or other sites which is associated with myocardial ischaemia. The nature of angina has many individual variations, and it is easier first to consider the typical syndrome. It is hard to better the descriptions of William Heberden[1]:

*There is a disorder of the breast, marked with strong and peculiar symptoms, considerable for the danger belonging to it.... Those who are afflicted with it are seized, while they are walking, and more particularly when they walk soon after eating, with a painful and most disagreeable sensation in the breast ... the moment they stand still all this uneasiness vanishes.... After it has continued some months, it will not cease so instantaneous upon standing still ... (most) whom I have seen, who are at least twenty, were men, and almost all above 50 years old, and most of them with a short neck, and inclining to be fat.... But the natural tendency of this illness be to kill the patients suddenly.... The os sterni is usually pointed to as the seat of this malady ... and sometimes there is with it a pain about the middle of the left arm.*

The usual cause of myocardial ischaemia is coronary atherosclerosis. Other diseases of the coronary arteries (emboli, spasm, vasculitis, Kawasaki disease, congenital anomalies), other cardiac diseases (hypertrophic cardiomyopathy, severe hypertension, severe aortic valve disease), and high output states (severe anaemia, thyrotoxicosis) are all uncommon or rare causes of angina. However, while angina is usually associated with atherosclerotic coronary artery disease, the converse is not always true. The condition of coronary atherosclerosis is very common (fatty streaks and more advanced plaques are almost universal in adults in industrialised countries) but it does not always cause myocardial ischaemia. Furthermore, myocardial ischaemia may present other than with angina – for each presentation there is a wide differential diagnosis.

*Correspondence to:*
*Dr S W Davies,*
*Department of Cardiology,*
*Royal Brompton Hospital,*
*Sydney Street,*
*London SW3 6NP, UK*

## Angina

Approximately 50% of cases are recognised because of chest pain. Cardiac ischaemic pain is thought to arise from stimulation of nerve

**Table 1** The differential diagnosis of chest pain

| | |
|---|---|
| Cardiac causes | Angina |
| | Myocardial infarction |
| | Variant angina (Prinzmetal angina) |
| | Microvascular angina (syndrome X) |
| | pericarditis, myocarditis |
| Other vascular causes | Discrete thoracic aortic aneurysm |
| | Aortic dissection |
| Respiratory causes | Pulmonary embolism, pulmonary infarction |
| | Pneumonia |
| | Viral pleurisy, *e.g.* Bornholm disease |
| | Pneumothorax, pneumomediastinum |
| | Acute asthma |
| Gastrointestinal causes | Oesophagitis, oesophageal spasm, hiatus hernia |
| | Oesophageal rupture, mediastinitis (Boerhaave's syndrome) |
| | Peptic ulcer |
| | Biliary colic, pancreatitis, splenic infarct |
| Other causes | Chest wall syndromes, costochondritis (Tietze's syndrome) |
| | Cervical spondylosis, thoracic disk problems, thoracic outlet syndrome |
| | Herpes zoster |
| | Psychogenic |

endings near the endocardium by factors such as adenosine, lactate, and H⁺. These afferent fibres run predominantly with sympathetic fibres through the stellate ganglion to thoracic roots T1 to T5. The pain is typically described as tight, squeezing, like a weight on the chest, or like indigestion; as with any visceral pain, the localisation is vague and there is considerable individual variation between patients[2].

There are many other causes of chest pain, and the differential diagnosis is summarised in Table 1. The characteristics of angina are well known, and the points of differentiation from non-cardiac pain are summarised in Table 2.

**Table 2** The characteristics of cardiac and non-cardiac chest pain

| | Cardiac pain (Usually angina) | Non-cardiac pain (Usually musculoskeletal or gastro-oesophageal) |
|---|---|---|
| Descriptors of pain | Heavy, tight, pressure, dull Band, squeezing | Sharp, stabbing, shooting, needle |
| Site | Central anterior Left arm, right arm, teeth Interscapular, epigastric | Left submammary Right submammary |
| Precipitants | Exercise, emotion Cold Post-prandial | Stress Locally tender Posture, particular movements of arms or neck Swallowing (odynophagia) |

The diagnosis of strengthened by recognition of precipitating factors (exertion, emotion, extremes of temperature), relieving factors (rest, sublingual nitrates), associated symptoms (sweating, pallor, nausea, alarm), and some special patterns (diurnal rhythm, walk-through, warm-up).

Difficulty arises because angina can cause atypical pains, for example interscapular or epigastric without any anterior chest discomfort. Individual patients often have more than one type of chest pain, and musculoskeletal and gastro-oesophageal pains commonly co-exist with angina as well as forming part of the differential diagnosis. Often, a detailed accurate history will clarify the diagnosis or diagnoses. However, the frequency and severity of angina provides only an approximate guide to the severity of the underlying coronary artery atherosclerosis and to the prognosis; some patients with myocardial ischaemia are asymptomatic.

## Acute myocardial infarction

In some patients, coronary artery disease is first diagnosed when they present with the severe pain and haemodynamic disturbance of acute infarction[3], usually as a result of sudden thrombotic occlusion of an atherosclerotic coronary artery. On close questioning, there may be a history of some chest discomfort prior to the infarct, but in some cases no warning at all.

## Dyspnoea

For some patients, dyspnoea is the only sensation experienced during myocardial ischaemia, so-called 'angina equivalent'. The mechanisms are thought to be the same as for angina, but with a different central appreciation of the afferent stimuli. More often, dyspnoea occurs together with angina – many patients experience their tightness across the chest both as a pain and as a sense of restriction in breathing. It is important to avoid asking leading questions in order to obtain an accurate description from the patient.

Dyspnoea may also arise in patients with coronary artery disease if there is ischaemic left ventricular dysfunction causing pulmonary venous congestion or pulmonary oedema, if there is papillary muscle dysfunction causing mitral regurgitation, or in a chronic low output state (see below). The mechanisms of dyspnoea in these cases may involve hypoxia, pulmonary receptors, and a sense of the effort made by the respiratory muscles[4,5].

## Cardiac failure

The triad of dyspnoea, fatigue, and dependent oedema suggests overt cardiac failure. In industrialised countries, coronary atherosclerosis is the commonest cause of cardiac failure[4,5]. This presentation suggests advanced coronary artery disease with myocardial infarction, or with diffuse myocardial fibrosis as a result of previous ischaemic episodes.

## Arrhythmias

Atrial fibrillation is seen in 20% of patients with coronary artery disease. Serious ventricular arrhythmias such as ventricular tachycardia may also occur. Atrioventricular block may result from myocardial infarction, and sometimes transiently during exercise-related ischaemia. These arrhythmias are usually detected during the investigation of a patient with chest pain or dyspnoea, and it is less common for patients to present with palpitation or dizzy spells as the primary symptom.

## Sudden death

It is now recognised that in a proportion of patients the first manifestation of coronary artery disease is sudden collapse and death, due to acute myocardial infarction and/or ventricular arrhythmias. The absence of premonitory symptoms emphasises the need for a population approach to primary prevention. A family history of sudden collapse and death is relevant when taking the history of a patient, but there are other cardiovascular causes including cardiomyopathies, long QT syndromes and cerebrovascular aneurysms and malformations.

## Other presentations

Many other symptoms can occur with coronary artery disease, but it is rare for them to be the main presentation in the absence of one of the above symptom complexes. Fatigue is common in coronary artery disease, possibly related to its psychological effects, but also when there is cardiac failure[5]. Coronary artery disease may present with peripheral arterial embolism and with embolic stroke, usually when there has been myocardial infarction and mural thrombus within the left ventricle.

## Clinical diagnosis of chest pain

*General considerations*

Given a clinical history of chest discomfort suggestive of angina, the diagnosis depends as much upon the probability that the given individual has coronary artery disease as upon the exact nature of the symptoms. The main predictors of coronary artery disease are age, male gender, family history, tobacco smoking, diabetes mellitus, and hyperlipidaemia. Thus somewhat atypical chest pain in a 60-year-old male smoker with a strong family history is more likely to represent angina than is typical exertional pain in a 20-year-old woman with no risk factors.

## Symptoms

The differing presentations of coronary artery disease have been listed above, and the differential diagnosis of chest pain is given in Table 1. The distinction of angina from other chest pains is not always as easy as one might suppose, and a good history is important, with particular regard to the characteristics of the pain outlined in Table 2.

It is also important to ask how symptoms affect the patient's daily activities including their ability to work, and the nature of their work. The level of angina (and of dyspnoea) can be graded on the NYHA or Canadian Cardiovascular Society scales, which both run from I (very mild) to IV (symptoms at rest or on minimal exertion). Although crude, these scales are useful in clinical trials and in following changes over time in a given patient.

At this stage, the clinician uses the information which he has obtained to form a judgement whether the pain is angina or not. There are a number of simple scores to assist with this[6,7], but they are not widely used in clinical practice.

## Physical examination

The physical examination is usually normal, and is most useful in providing evidence of alternative diagnoses such as chest wall pain and other musculoskeletal pains. The physical examination may give indirect clues to coronary artery disease such as evidence of severe hyperlipidaemia (xanthomas, premature corneal arcus) or evidence of left ventricular impairment (third heart sound, signs of overt cardiac failure such as dependent oedema).

## Role of investigations

Investigations may be used to confirm the diagnosis, to detect associated conditions (such as heart failure, diabetes mellitus), and for the assessment of prognosis to guide further investigation and treatment – so-called 'risk stratification'. Here we will consider the diagnostic value of investigations (risk stratification will be discussed elsewhere in this volume).

## Basic investigations

### Resting electrocardiogram

The ECG is often normal. Pathological Q waves almost always indicate myocardial infarction and other causes are uncommon. Finding Q waves, therefore, has considerable specificity but it is insensitive for the diagnosis of coronary artery disease. The ECG may also show changes suggestive of other diagnoses including pericarditis, LV hypertrophy, right heart strain, and atrial fibrillation.

### Chest X-ray

This is usually normal, but if there is cardiac failure there may be increased cardiothoracic ratio and/or pulmonary venous congestion. The aortic contour may give a clue to aortic dissection or thoracic aortic aneurysm, but is not reliable in this regard. Other causes of chest pain may be suggested by pleural shadowing, radiographic features of pulmonary hypertension, masses in the lung fields or mediastinum, and the fluid level of a hiatus hernia behind the heart.

### Blood tests

Full blood count to detect any anaemia, thyroid function tests to detect thyrotoxicosis (high output state, angina) or hypothyroidism (hyper-lipidaemia and coronary disease), and urea and electrolytes to assess renal function are usually performed. A lipid profile including HDL, LDL, triglycerides, and glucose measurement are also routine as they may require management in their own right. Additionally, a very high cholesterol or a new finding of impaired glucose tolerance would sway the diagnostic probabilities towards coronary artery disease.

## Optional cardiac and non-cardiac investigations for alternative diagnoses

Upper GI endoscopy, barium studies or abdominal ultrasound may be indicated, as may be a lateral chest X-ray of the thoracic or cervical spine. CT or MRI of the chest is useful to examine the aorta, lung fields, and mediastinum. An echocardiogram is useful: (i) if there is a murmur or other specific reason; (ii) for a general assessment of left ventricular function; and (iii) following myocardial infarction to document LV function, regional wall motion abnormalities, any mitral regurgitation, ischaemic septal defect, or LV thrombus.

## Non-invasive coronary assessment

The four most common non-invasive tests are:

### Exercise test

This focuses on abnormal ST segment depression but also offers the opportunity to assess the patient's overall exercise capacity, the symptoms limiting exertion, and heart rate and blood pressure responses to exercise.

### Radio-isotope myocardial perfusion scanning

This provides imaging of myocardial perfusion, with reversible perfusion deficits indicating ischaemia, and fixed perfusion deficits indicating infarction or sometimes attenuation by overlying tissue. Modern methods may also allow the definition of hibernating and stunned myocardium, helping the planning of revascularisation.

### Coronary calcification score

The use of fast electron-beam CT scanning allows non-invasive calculation of a coronary calcification score, much more accurately than the old method of fluoroscopy to detect coronary calcification.

### Stress echocardiography

This observes changes in regional wall motion and overall LV function during exercise and/or pharmacological stress. It may also be possible to observe dynamic LV outflow tract gradients as in hypertrophic cardiomyopathy, and ischaemic papillary muscle dysfunction causing mitral regurgitation

### Other methods

Other methods used occasionally include 24-hour ambulatory ST-segment monitoring, and PET scanning for myocardial perfusion and metabolism. MRI and MR angiography of the coronary arteries is a developing field likely to be of great value in future. Currently, available MRI technology is well able to define LV function regional wall motion abnormalities and may be more accurate than stress echocardiography.

These will be discussed in more detail elsewhere in this volume, but we should make some general points. All the above non-invasive tests are inaccurate to some degree. If we use coronary angiography as the gold standard to define the presence a stenosis of 50% or greater in a major epicardial vessel, then typically the sensitivity is 70–90% and specificity 70–90% for the above methodologies. Each method has further specific weaknesses – for example, the treadmill exercise ECG is poor at reflecting disease in the circumflex territory.

If more than one non-invasive test is performed in a given patient, one may give a result indicating normality and the other indicate coronary disease. When there are discrepant data, the clinician has to make a decision on the overall situation as to whether there is likely to be coronary artery disease or not. Performing additional tests is also of limited usefulness because 'predictive redundancy' – the incremental information offered by performing a second non-invasive test is less than would be expected if they were independently predictive[8]. Patients who have an equivocal test with one modality are more likely to have an equivocal test with another modality, and those who are false positives with one are also more likely to be false positive with another – the reasons for this are unclear, but it is of practical importance. If the most appropriate non-invasive test has been correctly selected for the individual patient, then if the result is borderline or does not fit with the clinical picture, performing a different non-invasive test in addition may not be helpful. However, all of the non-invasive tests have considerable prognostic value, aside from their ability to detect structural coronary artery disease – this will be discussed below.

# Diagnosis in special groups

## Silent ischaemia

During an episode of myocardial ischaemia, there is a sequence of events often termed the 'ischaemic cascade'. Perfusion and metabolic abnormalities are followed by abnormalities of regional wall motion, changes in global LV diastolic function, then changes in LV systolic function, about which time there are changes in the resting ECG, and finally anginal pain. It is, therefore, possible to have considerable myocardial ischaemia and changes in LV function before any pain is manifest. Indeed Herrick in 1912 described autopsies revealing myocardial infarction in patients with no history of chest pain whatever. Ambulatory ST-segment ECG monitoring in patients with extensive coronary artery disease has shown that whilst only 5–10% of these patients have no angina whatever, about 40% of all episodes of ST depression are asymptomatic. Episodes of so-called 'silent myocardial ischaemia' are more common in the elderly and in patients with diabetes mellitus.

The sequence of the ischaemic cascade may help explain why different non-invasive tests may give discrepant data, as they depend upon different disturbances in cardiac function. For example, the thallium scan detects changes in perfusion, the PET scan detects changes in metabolism, but the stress echo will only detect a later stage when there are wall motion abnormalities, and the exercise ECG may be the last to change. We should also consider the interpretation of a patient without chest pain who has abnormal non-invasive tests for coronary artery disease – possibly undertaken because of pain in the past, or as a pre-operative assessment. The possible interpretations include: (i) the test is incorrect, in other words a false positive result; or (ii) silent ischaemia, where the stress was of insufficient intensity or duration to cause pain as the last change in the ischaemic cascade.

## The elderly

The incidence of coronary artery disease rises rapidly with age in men and also in women following the menopause. It is important to exclude contributory factors such as anaemia, thyrotoxicosis, and fast atrial fibrillation or severe bradycardias. They may present a difficult challenge in knowing how far to investigate, and there may be practical difficulties with undertaking simple non-invasive tests such as treadmill or cycle exercise. The elderly are also more likely to have silent ischaemia and to suffer silent myocardial infarcts[9].

## Diabetes mellitus

Type II diabetes mellitus is of increasing prevalence in non-industrialised countries, and a major association of coronary artery disease and of a poor prognosis. These patients are more likely to have diffuse coronary artery disease, and more likely to have silent myocardial infarction and episodes of silent ischaemia.

## Patients following myocardial infarction

These patients have already declared themselves as having significant coronary artery disease and of being at increased risk unless treated vigorously. There is a strong evidence base for secondary prevention which involves more stringent targets for blood pressure and lipids than does primary prevention. There is also considerable randomised controlled trial data for the benefits of aspirin, clopidogrel, β-blockers, ACE inhibitors, and statins. In this area where the treatment guidelines are well worked out, the main problem is ensuring implementation and the provision of adequate healthcare resources.

## Patients following cardiac transplantation

Angina can occur in patients some years after transplantation, implying re-innervation of the transplanted heart. However most angina in transplant recipients is painless or atypical; hence, most transplant centres have a programme of regular non-invasive testing and, in some cases, of annual coronary arteriography starting 5 years after transplantation.

# International differences

It is estimated that cardiovascular disease is responsible for 30% of mortality world-wide, about half of which is attributable to coronary artery disease. It is much more prevalent in industrialised countries with established market economies, but there is a rapid increase in prevalence in many of the former socialist economies, the lowest prevalence being in non-industrialised countries[10]. Although the prevalence has always been low in some industrialised countries (such as Japan) and is slowly declining in others (USA, Canada, Australia, France), the prevalence of coronary artery disease world-wide is predicted to increase. This is partly because of demographic changes with increasing proportions of the elderly, overall population growth, and ethnic differences. Certain groups such as those from South Asia (India, Bangladesh, Pakistan, Sri Lanka) and from China have a very high incidence of coronary artery disease if they migrate to industrialised countries or adopt a Western lifestyle. It has been speculated that this is due to a 'thrifty gene' and impaired glucose tolerance[10].

Healthcare resources are the major determinant of the technologies for investigation, the range of treatments, and healthcare personnel numbers per head of population available locally. In some regions, it may only be practical to make a clinical diagnosis unsupported by investigation, to treat symptomatically with GTN, and to give advice on diet and other aspects of life-style. In well-funded healthcare systems such as the US the majority of patients would have at least an echocardiogram to assess LV function plus a non-invasive test for coronary artery disease, such as a myocardial perfusion scan or exercise ECG; a large number would go on to invasive angiography.

# Key points for clinical practice

- Myocardial ischaemia is usually caused by coronary artery atheroma and thrombosis – other pathologies are rare

- The most common symptom of myocardial ischaemia is angina (50% of cases); other symptoms include dyspnoea, fatigue, and arrhythmias

- In some patients with coronary artery disease, episodes of myocardial ischaemia can occur without symptoms; 'silent ischaemia' is more common in the elderly and in diabetics

- Most patients describe angina as a pressure, a tightness, or a discomfort, rather than as a pain. The perception of angina varies between individuals, and atypical pains may, nonetheless, represent angina in a patient with coronary risk factors

- The clinical diagnosis of angina depends upon an appreciation of the probability that the individual patient has coronary artery disease (age, male, family history, smoking, diabetes mellitus, hyperlipidaemia) as well as on a detailed account of the symptoms

- The physical examination is usually normal, but may give clues to coronary risk factors (signs of hyperlipidaemia) or clues to an alternative diagnosis (musculoskeletal pain)

- Simple investigation such as the chest X-ray and the resting ECG are usually normal, but are useful as a baseline in the majority of patients, and in a minority show specific abnormalities informing the diagnosis (enlarged heart, pathological Q waves)

## References

1   Heberden W. Some account of a disorder of the breast. *Med Trans R Coll Physicians (Lond)* 1772; **2**: 59–67
2   Henderson AH. Chest pain. In: Weatherall DJ, Ledingham JGG, Warrell DA. (eds) *Oxford Textbook of Medicine*, 3rd edn. Oxford: Oxford University Press, 1996; 2165–9
3   Hofgren C, Karlson BW, Herlitz J. Prodromal symptoms in subsets of patients hospitalized for suspected acute myocardial infarction. *Heart Lung* 1995; **24**: 3
4   Davies SW, Lipkin D. Breathlessness. In: Weatherall DJ, Ledingham JGG, Warrell DA. (eds) *Oxford Textbook of Medicine*, 3rd edn. Oxford: Oxford University Press, 1996; 2162–5
5   Davies SW, Lipkin D. Fatigue. In: Weatherall DJ, Ledingham JGG, Warrell DA. (eds) *Oxford Textbook of Medicine*, 3rd edn. Oxford: Oxford University Press, 1996; 2171–3
6   Diamond DA, Staniloff HM, Forrester JS *et al.* Computer-assisted diagnosis in the noninvasive evaluation of patients with suspected coronary disease. *J Am Coll Cardiol* 1983; **1**: 444–55
7   Diamond GA, Forrester JS. Analysis of probability as an aid in the clinical diagnosis of coronary-artery disease. *N Engl J Med* 1979; **300**: 1350–8
8   Weissler AM. Assessment and use of cardiovascular tests in clinical prediction. In: Giuliani ER, Holmes DR, Hayes DL *et al.* (eds) *Mayo Clinic Practice of Cardiology*, 3rd edn. St Louis, MO: Mosby-Yearbook, 1996; 400
9   Madias JE, Chintalapaly G, Choudry M *et al.* Correlates and in-hospital outcomes of painless presentation of acute myocardial infarction: a prospective study of a consecutive series of patients admitted to the coronary care unit. *J Invest Med* 1995; **43**: 567
10  Reddy KS. Global perspective on cardiovascular disease. In: Yusuf S, Cairns JA, Camm AJ, Fallen EL, Gersh BJ. (eds) *Evidence Based Cardiology*. London: BMJ Books, 1998; 147–64

## Author Query

Morise AP, Detrano R, Bobbio M, Diamond GA. Development and validation of a logistic regression-derived algorithm for estimating the incremental probability of coronary artery disease before and after exercise testing. *J Am Coll Cardiol* 1992; **20**: 1187–96. – in reference list but not cited?

# Non-invasive investigations

## C Anagnostopoulos, M Y Henein and S R Underwood

*Royal Brompton Hospital and Imperial College School of Medicine, London, UK*

The most commonly used techniques for imaging the effects of coronary artery disease (CAD) on the heart are myocardial perfusion scintigraphy (MPS) and echocardiography. Both tests have been validated during exercise and pharmacological stress and they are valuable for the diagnosis and aiding management decisions in patients with suspected or known CAD. In a proportion of these patients, repetitive episodes of myocardial ischaemia can lead to intracellular and extracellular changes so that myocytes, although viable, have insufficient energy to sustain contraction. This phenomenon is known as myocardial hibernation and it can be detected accurately by both MPS and stress echocardiography. The review that follows highlights the role of these techniques as powerful diagnostic and prognostic tools in clinical cardiology. In order to make the best use of them, attention to detail and planning are required to design the test to suit the clinical problem and to obtain the most accurate data possible.

Cardiac imaging is an important component of diagnosis and assessment in cardiology, and it is now essentially a sub-speciality of its own. The imaging techniques include echocardiography, nuclear cardiology, and magnetic resonance imaging, and there are other techniques in which cardiologists have an interest, such as electron beam computed tomography.

## Myocardial perfusion scintigraphy: basic principles

Correspondence to:
Dr C Anagnostopoulos,
Consultant Physician in
Nuclear Medicine,
Honorary Senior Lecturer,
Department of Radiology,
Chelsea and Westminster
Hospital,
369 Fulham Road,
London SW10 9NH, UK

Myocardial perfusion scintigraphy (MPS) is the only widely available and validated method of assessing myocardial perfusion and hence is an essential component of modern cardiology. The technique involves the injection of a radioactive tracer followed by imaging of its myocardial distribution using a gamma camera. The images are now almost exclusively tomographic (single photon emission computed tomography, or SPECT) using a rotating gamma camera, often with two heads. Thus, the images are truly three dimensional, albeit of relatively low resolution (10–15 mm).

There are three commercially available tracers of myocardial perfusion, thallium-201 and two thallium analogues, which are also univalent cations labelled with technetium-99m (see below). All three tracers have two requirements for myocardial uptake to be seen. First, there must be viable myocytes since they are taken up mainly passively across an active myocyte membrane that maintains a negative intracellular potential. Second, there must be adequate myocardial perfusion since the tracers are avidly taken up by the myocardium and their initial distribution is proportional to delivery. Thus, all three tracers are combined tracers of myocardial viability and perfusion.

The normal myocardial perfusion image shows relatively uniform uptake throughout the myocardium (Fig. 1). Areas with either reduced myocyte density (as after infarction) or relatively reduced perfusion (as in inducible ischaemia) show defects. If the tracer is injected during stress, the initial stress images will show a defect in either case. Subsequent rest images (see below) will show a persistent defect with infarction but recovery of uptake if the initial defect is caused by stress-induced ischaemia or perfusion heterogeneity (Fig. 2). This is the basis of defects that are commonly described as fixed or reversible.

## Forms of stress

Dynamic exercise is the most common type of stress because of the important clinical information that is provided by exercise tolerance and haemodynamic response. However, between one-third and one-half of patients in most centres are not able to exercise adequately and this seriously limits the value of dynamic exercise. In addition, many patients have already had an exercise ECG before referral for perfusion imaging and, in these circumstances, a pharmacological alternative to dynamic exercise is very valuable. The established pharmacological stressors are the coronary vasodilators adenosine and dipyridamole, and the β-agonist dobutamine.

Dipyridamole is administrated intravenously at a dose of 0.14 mg/kg/min for 4 min. The radiotracer is given 4 min after the end of the infusion, at which time vasodilation is maximal[1]. Adenosine is infused at the same dose over 4–6 min with injection of radiotracer 2 min from the end[2]. It is also possible to combine stress techniques; the commonest pairing is dynamic exercise with either adenosine or dipyridamole, which increases sensitivity for the detection of perfusion defects and also their conspicuity.[3,4]. The addition of submaximal exercise has other benefits. It reduces the side-effects caused by peripheral vasodilation, it reduces the incidence of bradyarrhythmia, and it reduces splanchnic uptake of tracer, which can interfere with interpretation of the inferior wall when using the technetium tracers[4]. Patients with left bundle branch block, bifascicular block or paced rhythm should receive adenosine or dipyridamole alone in order to reduce the likelihood of inducing septal perfusion abnormalities related to the conduction abnormality. Adenosine and dipyridamole are contra-indicated in patients with reversible airways obstruction since they can induce bronchospasm. These patients can, however, safely be stressed by dobutamine.[5]. This is normally infused into a peripheral vein starting at 5 μg/kg/min and increasing in increments of 5 μg/kg/min to a maximum of 20 or 40 μg/kg/min, with stages lasting for 2–5 min to allow stabilisation of the haemodynamic effect.

## Radiopharmaceuticals

Thallous chloride has been used routinely as a tracer of myocardial perfusion for almost 25 years. Imaging starts within 5–10 min of injection and should be completed within 30 min. During this period, the distribution of thallium within the myocardium is relatively fixed and, despite the cessation of stress, the images reflect myocardial distribution at peak stress. Because there is a dynamic exchange of thallium between the intra- and extracellular spaces, redistribution over the next 2–4 h leads to uptake of thallium in all viable myocytes, irrespective of perfusion[6]. The initial images are, therefore, a combination of viability and perfusion, the redistribution images are viability alone, and differences between the images are areas of hypoperfusion at the time of tracer injection. If a stress induced defect is profound, then redistribution is often incomplete at 4 h. In these circumstances, thallium can be injected again at rest and a third set of images acquired. These re-injection images reflect viability more reliably.

Although thallium is an excellent tracer of perfusion and viability, it has some limitations. First, because of its relatively long half-life (72 h), radiation exposure is high: 80 MBq delivers an effective dose equivalent to 18 mSv, which is more than the average exposure during coronary arteriography. Second, only 4% of the injected dose is taken up by the myocardium, which leads to images with relatively low count density. Third, the low energy emission at 80 keV leads to low resolution images with significant attenuation by soft tissues. Technetium-99m (Tc-99m) compounds do not suffer the first and third of these problems, and these include Tc-99m-2-methoxy-isobutyl-isonitrile (MIBI) and Tc-99m-1,2-bis[bis(2-ethoxyethyl) phosphino] ethane (tetrofosmin)[7,8]. The benefits of the technetium tracers include the lower radiation exposure and better quality images in obese patients and women with large breasts.

In contrast to thallium, the technetium tracers do not redistribute and separate injections have to be given in order to assess stress and rest perfusion[8,9]. The 6 h half-life of Tc-99m means that the two studies should ideally be performed on separate days to allow for the decay and clearance of activity from the first injection. The two studies can be performed on the same day if a larger dose (at least 3-fold) is given on the second occasion in order to swamp the residual activity from the first injection. The maximum dose allowed for routine use in the UK is 400 MBq each for stress and rest injections on separate days, or a total of 1000 MBq if stress and rest studies are performed on the same day: 1000 MBq corresponds to an effective dose equivalent of 10 mSv.

# Myocardial perfusion scintigraphy: clinical applications

## Diagnosis of coronary artery disease

### Chronic chest pain

MPS has an established role in the detection of perfusion abnormalities caused by coronary artery disease (CAD). Used as a diagnostic tool, it has a sensitivity of 91% and specificity 89%[10]; this is significantly better than exercise electrocardiography, which has a sensitivity of 68% and specificity 77%[11]. Several factors militate against replacing the exercise ECG entirely with MPS. The most important is the relative availability of the two techniques, but radiation burden and cost are also relevant. Although the cost of MPS (£220) is higher than that of the exercise ECG (£70), this is more than outweighed by its greater effectiveness[12]. Studies of cost-effectiveness have shown significant advantages for strategies of investigation using MPS, with savings in total diagnostic and management costs over 2 years in the region of 20% in centres routinely using scintigraphy[12].

MPS is the most appropriate diagnostic test for patients with an intermediate probability of CAD. This category includes patients with atypical chest pain or asymptomatic individuals with a positive exercise ECG, and those with equivocal ST segment changes or a normal exercise ECG despite a history of typical angina. Perfusion imaging should be the initial investigation in patients who are unlikely to exercise adequately, in women (because of the very high number of false positive ECGs), and if the exercise ECG will be uninterpretable because of resting abnormalities such as left bundle branch block, pre-excitation, left ventricular hypertrophy, or drug effects[13].

### Acute chest pain

Nuclear techniques are less commonly used in patients presenting with acute chest pain, mainly because of the logistical problems of imaging in the emergency department or coronary care unit. Nonetheless, several centres have demonstrated the value of perfusion imaging in the acute setting, especially when the resting ECG is not diagnostic of myocardial ischaemia[14]. The presence of a resting perfusion defect has a high positive predictive value for acute infarction in patients without previous infarction, particularly if it is associated with a wall motion abnormality on gated imaging, and these patients should be admitted to the coronary care unit.

Conversely, a normal perfusion scan excludes acute infarction and suggests that exercise ECG or stress perfusion imaging should be the next diagnostic step. If the perfusion tracer is injected during chest pain, a normal perfusion scan excludes a cardiac cause and allows the patient to be discharged pending further investigation.

## Prognosis of CAD

### Suspected or known CAD

Beyond diagnosis, the most valuable contribution that perfusion imaging can make to the management of known or suspected CAD is to assess the likelihood of a future coronary event such as myocardial infarction or coronary death. Prognosis is strongly influenced by the extent and severity of inducible perfusion abnormality and this can guide the need for invasive investigation and revascularisation (Figs 3 & 4). MPI is more powerful as an indicator of prognosis than clinical assessment, the exercise ECG, and coronary angiography, and it provides incremental prognostic value even once the other tests have been performed[15-17].

The most important variables that predict the likelihood of future events are the extent and depth of the inducible perfusion abnormality. The relative value of the fixed component of a stress defect is unclear, but it is likely that left ventricular function is the best indictor of prognosis in patients with predominantly fixed defects. Thus the patient with extensive ischaemia is at high risk of a coronary event irrespective of the presence of infarction, and the patient without ischaemia but with a fixed defect is only at risk if the defect leads to significantly impaired function. Additional markers of risk are increased lung uptake on stress thallium images[5] since this indicates raised pulmonary capillary pressure either at rest or in response to stress, and ventricular dilation that is greater in stress thallium images than at rest. Transient ischaemic dilation can also be seen with technetium imaging and it may the result of extensive subendocardial ischaemia giving the impression of cavity dilation (Fig. 5).

In patients with known or suspected CAD, a normal perfusion scan is very valuable because it indicates a likelihood of a coronary events of less than 1% per year, a rate that is lower than that in an asymptomatic population. Thus whether minor coronary disease is present or not, further investigation can be avoided. This negative predictive value is independent of the type of imaging agent and technique, the method of stress, the population studied, and the clinical setting.

### Management after infarction

An important aspect of clinical management after infarction is to identify patients at high risk of further events such as re-infarction or death, and hopefully to intervene in order to prevent these events. Clinical indicators of

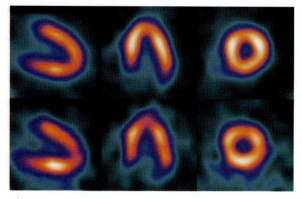

Fig. 1

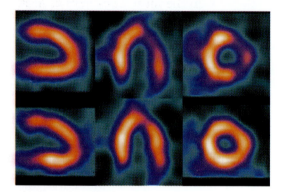

Fig. 2

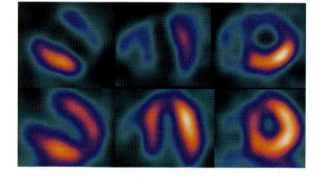

Fig. 3

Fig. 4

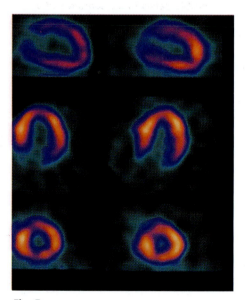

Fig. 5

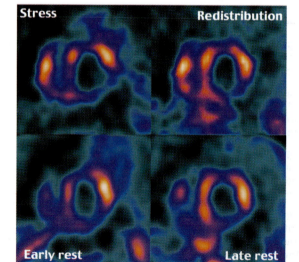

Fig. 6

high risk in the acute phase include hypotension, left ventricular failure, and malignant arrhythmias; these patients are candidates for early coronary angiography. After the acute phase, prognosis is related to the degree of left ventricular dysfunction and the extent and severity of residual ischaemia; both can be assessed objectively by radionuclide imaging[18].

Patients without high risk clinical markers or severely impaired LV function are at lower risk, but some form of stress testing is required in order to assess exercise tolerance and the presence of residual ischaemia. This is often performed by exercise electrocardiography at 6 weeks, but there is increasing evidence that very early stress testing is better since the majority of recurrent clinical events occur early. Perfusion imaging using vasodilator stress is an ideal tool since many physicians are reluctant to exercise patients very early after infarction. In the most aggressive centres, adenosine perfusion imaging will be performed at 5 days and used to guide the need for coronary angiography or discharge and medical therapy[19].

### Risk assessment before non-cardiac surgery

The aim of risk assessment before non-cardiac surgery is to identify myocardial ischaemia and to estimate the risk of peri-operative cardiac

---

*See page opposite for figures*

**Fig. 1** Normal thallium myocardial perfusion tomograms in vertical long axis (left), horizontal long axis (centre) and short axis planes (right). Stress images (top) and redistribution (bottom). There is homogeneous uptake of tracer throughout the myocardium and hence no coronary obstruction.

**Fig. 2** Short axis thallium-201 tomograms, immediately after stress (left) and following redistribution (right) in a patient with angina and previous inferior myocardial infarction. There is a reversible defect in the septum and a partially reversible defect in the anterior wall, which are both suggestive of inducible ischaemia in the left anterior descending artery. In addition there is a fixed defect in the inferior wall indicative of myocardial infarction.

**Fig. 3** Stress (top) and redistribution (bottom) thallium tomograms in the vertical long axis (left), horizontal long axis (centre) and short axis (right) planes in a patient with left circumflex stenosis. There is inducible ischaemia of moderate extent and severity in the lateral wall.

**Fig. 4** Thallium tomograms in vertical long axis (left), horizontal long axis (centre) and short axis (right) immediately after stress (top) and following reinjection of thallium at rest (bottom). There is severe and extensive inducible ischaemia in most of the myocardium sparing only the inferior wall. The appearances are characteristic of left main stem disease.

**Fig. 5** Thallium tomograms in vertical long axis (top), horizontal long axis (middle) and short axis (bottom) immediately after stress (left) and following reinjection of thallium at rest (right). There is mild-to-moderate inducible myocardial ischaemia sparing only the septum and, in addition, ventricular dilation that is greater in the stress thallium images than at rest.

**Fig. 6** Short axis thallium-201 tomograms showing stress induced perfusion abnormalities in the septum and the anterior wall and a fixed defect in the infero-lateral wall in the conventional stress and redistribution images (top row). On a separate occasion, thallium was injected at rest with immediate and delayed imaging (bottom row). These images also show reduced perfusion in the septum and a fixed infero-lateral defect. MRI showed severe hypokinesis in most of the anterior wall and septum and akinesis in the infero-lateral wall. Thus, the antero-septal region is viable but ischaemic and hypokinetic and it will recover function after revascularisation. The infero-lateral wall is infarcted and it will not recover.

---

events. Initial risk assessment is based on clinical risk factors, functional capacity and the risk of the surgery itself[20]. Patients with intermediate clinical predictors (mild angina, prior infarction, treated heart failure, or diabetes) or with minor predictors (age >70 years, abnormal resting ECG, history of stroke or hypertension) and impaired exercise tolerance need further assessment if they are to undergo moderate or high-risk surgery. Patients at high clinical risk (recent infarction or unstable angina, decompensated heart failure, or significant arrhythmias) require investigation even for low risk surgery. When further investigation is required, the first test is most commonly the exercise ECG in patients who are able to exercise. However, if maximal exercise is unlikely or if the resting ECG is uninterpretable, then MPS is the most appropriate investigation.

### Myocardial revascularisation

MPS can be valuable both before and after myocardial revascularisation, either by angioplasty or bypass surgery. Neither procedure should be undertaken without objective evidence of ischaemia, and perfusion imaging is often the most reliable way of obtaining this information and of ensuring that angioplasty is targeted at the culprit lesion. It has an excellent negative predictive value for predicting restenosis and clinical events after angioplasty, and this can be particularly helpful in patients with recurrent, but atypical, symptoms[21]. Routine perfusion imaging after angioplasty in the absence of symptoms is not common, although it can sometimes be useful as a new baseline in case symptoms recur. It can, however, be justified routinely in patients with impaired left ventricular function, proximal LAD and multivessel disease, suboptimal results of angioplasty, diabetes, and those with occupations requiring low coronary risk. If perfusion imaging is performed after angioplasty, then it should ideally be performed later than 6 weeks since perfusion abnormalities can persist even with a good anatomical result. Possible exceptions to this are patients with high-risk anatomy who can benefit from earlier imaging.

As with angioplasty, patients who are asymptomatic after bypass surgery do not routinely undergo perfusion imaging, although it can be helpful as a baseline for future management since revascularisation is frequently incomplete. More commonly, it is used for follow-up and it can be used 5 years after surgery to guard against silent progression of prognostically important disease. Patients with symptoms after surgery may benefit from perfusion imaging and the algorithms to be used are very similar to those in the diagnostic setting.

## Myocardial viability and hibernation

Perfusion and metabolic tracers play an increasing role in the detection of viable, hibernating and stunned myocardium. The term 'viable' strictly refers to myocardium that is alive, without implying any particular state of function, perfusion or metabolism. Sometimes the term is used interchangeably with 'hibernation' although it is better to avoid this potentially confusing terminology. Stunning is a state of altered metabolic and contractile function that follows an ischaemic episode and occurs despite restoration of perfusion. In hibernation, the chronic reduction in myocardial perfusion is matched by down-regulation of contractile function. However, the concept of chronic reduced resting flow is disputed, and it has been suggested that hibernation is simply repetitive stunning. In clinical practice, hibernation is assumed if viable myocardium is dysfunctional at rest, but this is only one possible explanation since other pathology such as remodelling and myopathy may present with the same pattern.

Detection of hibernating myocardium is particularly important in patients where left ventricular performance is severely compromised. A pivotal issue in this group is whether revascularisation will lead to a clinically significant improvement in ventricular function which may in turn lead to improved symptoms and survival. Studies have demonstrated that the increase of ejection fraction postoperatively is related to the amount of hibernating myocardium[22,23]. In addition, revascularisation reduces the risk of infarction and death in patients with impaired left ventricular function and hibernating myocardium demonstrated by positron emission tomography.

Thallium can also be used in several ways to identify viable and hibernating myocardium. Regional uptake of thallium identifies regional viability, and a common threshold for defining clinically significant viability is 50% of maximal uptake. An important additional criterion is the presence of inducible ischaemia before diagnosing hibernation since it is an ischaemic syndrome (Fig. 6). Care must be taken in these studies that sufficient time is allowed for redistribution, because the latter may be incomplete even after 4 h. Simple stress and redistribution imaging may, therefore, be insufficient, and alternative strategies are 24 h redistribution imaging, re-injection of thallium-201 at rest after stress and redistribution imaging and resting injection with immediate and delayed imaging. These protocols have been validated in a number of studies and reasonable agreement has been shown between thallium-201 imaging and PET[24-27].

MIBI and tetrofosmin have also been used for the detection of viable and hibernating myocardium. In theory, these tracers may underestimate viability in areas with reduced resting perfusion because they are combined tracers of viability and perfusion without the property of redistribution that allows viability to be assessed independently. Some studies have found thallium to be better for the assessment of viability, but others have found them to be similar[28-30]. It does appear though that if the tracers are given under the cover of intravenous or sublingual nitrates, then resting perfusion is improved and the technetium tracers are good markers of viability.

An important problem in studies of hibernation is that viability and function are often assessed from different techniques, and it can be difficult to be sure that the same myocardial segment is being compared in each. Thus, the ideal technique should combine information on viability, perfusion and function in a single image, and ECG-gated technetium SPECT is very helpful. This is our own initial technique in patients referred for the assessment of hibernation. Although, assessment of regional function is difficult in regions of previous infarction and significantly reduced tracer uptake, this is not a major limitation since these areas contain little myocardium and will not benefit from revascularisation.

# Echocardiography

Transthoracic echocardiography provides a simple non-invasive method of assessing ventricular function, and stress echocardiography can be used to assess the severity of ventricular dysfunction associated with exertional symptoms. Intravenous ultrasound allows the arterial wall to be studied in the catheter laboratory[31], and transoesophageal echocardiography provides a way of assessing proximal coronary flow velocity at the time of bypass surgery or in the early postoperative period, particularly in patients in whom ventricular function is slow to recover.

## Resting echocardiography

In patients with previous myocardial infarction, two dimensional transthoracic echocardiography shows obvious wall motion abnormalities. The localised loss of myocardial tissue indicates scar formation when the myocardium decreases in total thickness and the muscle is irreversibly damaged[32]. After antero-apical infarction, an aneurysm may develop that is easily diagnosed by paradoxical motion (Fig. 7). In the absence of myocardial infarction, resting left ventricular echocardiography may be entirely normal as shown by both two-dimensional images and M-mode. Segmental minor axis hypokinesis develops as the disease progresses. Long axis function is particularly sensitive to ischaemia[33], and this can easily be studied using a M-mode technique with or without tissue Doppler myocardial velocities. Long axis function is remarkably sensitive to coronary artery disease even in the absence of symptoms or ECG changes. Systolic abnormalities in the form

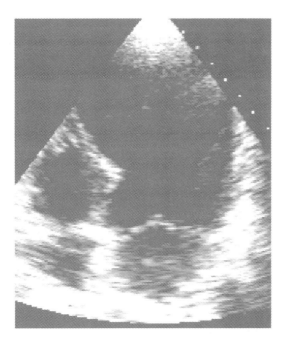

**Fig. 7** Two dimensional echocardiogram in the apical four chamber view showing a large apical aneurysm that had paradoxical motion.

of reduced amplitude of motion and post-ejection shortening are seen after myocardial infarction but, even in the absence of infarction, diastolic disturbances such as delayed onset of lengthening and slow lengthening velocity are associated with inducible ischaemia. These wall motion disturbances can be used as objective markers of disease progression or successful response to revascularisation[34]. Furthermore, these disturbances determine the pattern of mitral flow (Fig. 8), which is predominantly late diastolic[35]. As long as left ventricular function is maintained, colour and continuous wave Doppler can detect mild mitral regurgitation. In more advanced ischaemic heart disease, systolic function is reduced and filling pressures rise resulting in a well-defined restrictive filling pattern[36], that is always associated with functional mitral regurgitation of varying severity. Similar changes can affect the right ventricle.

## Stress echocardiography

Stress echocardiography can be used to identify inducible wall motion disturbances in patients with coronary insufficiency[37], but it is difficult to acquire clear images during dynamic exercise. Pharmacological stress overcomes this problem and agents such as adenosine[38], dipyridamole[39], and dobutamine[40] are used. Dobutamine echocardiography has become a common investigation and it is more sensitive than the exercise ECG for the diagnosis of CAD[41]. Standard stress echocardiography involves semi-quantitative analysis of two dimensional echocardiographic images

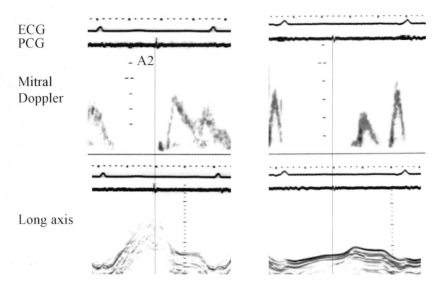

ECG
PCG

Mitral
Doppler

Long axis

**Fig. 8** Long axis M-mode recording of left ventricular free wall from a normal subject (left) and from a patient with ischaemic heart disease (right). There is abnormal ventricular filling in the patient caused by the incoordinate long axis relaxation.

of the left ventricular short and long axes (Fig. 9). A summed segmental wall motion score is used to assess the extent and severity of stress induced wall motion disturbances. An akinetic segment at rest that does not change with stress represents infarcted myocardium[42].

Patients who develop severe ventricular dysfunction are at high risk of future cardiovascular events. The prognostic accuracy of the wall motion score increases when more than one ventricular segment is involved. Also, the diagnostic accuracy of the score index is significantly

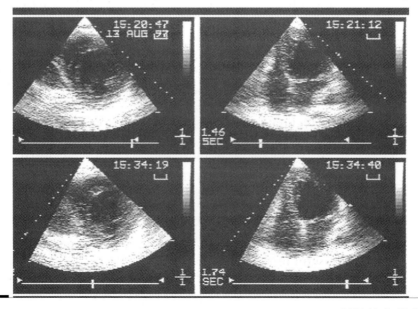

**Fig. 9** Stress echo-cardiography showing left ventricular minor and long axis images at rest (top) and during peak dobutamine stress (bottom).

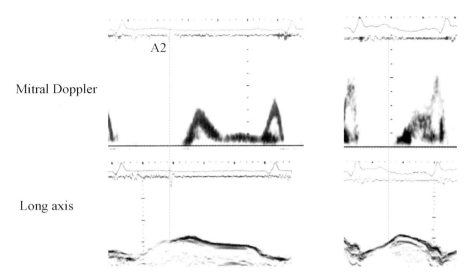

**Fig. 10** Long axis recordings from the left ventricular free wall in a patient with coronary artery disease (bottom), and transmitral Doppler recordings (top) at rest (left) and during dobutamine stress (right). There is uncoordinated long axis relaxation during stress that compromises early diastolic filling.

higher in patients with multivessel coronary disease compared with single vessel[43]. As a marker of global ventricular function, stress ejection fraction can also be used to stratify cardiac risk after myocardial infarction and before non-cardiac surgery[44]. Although stress-related wall motion abnormalities are obviously different in essence from those of myocardial perfusion, the diagnostic accuracy of the two techniques is similar[45]. The sensitivity of stress echocardiography has improved with the advent of harmonic imaging[46] and the use of contrast agents[47].

## Myocardial viability and hibernation

Both resting and stress echocardiography have been used for the assessment of myocardial viability. Resting diastolic wall thickness of 6 mm is commonly used as a sign of viable myocardium[48]. Hibernation has a biphasic response to dobutamine infusion with contractile reserve at low dose, but deterioration at higher dose[49]. Hibernation in at least 5 of the 16 conventional segments predicts good recovery of left ventricular function after revascularisation[50,51].

## Long axis function during stress

Ventricular long axis function studied during dobutamine stress is also useful in the diagnosis of CAD (Fig. 10)[52]. Systolic disturbances such as a decrease in excursion amplitude, correlate with stress induced QRS broadening. Diastolic disturbances such as slow lengthening velocity correlate with delayed repolarisation (prolonged QTc interval). This close association between electrical and mechanical function is not surprising. Uncoordinated long axis function during stress compromises ejection and filling times[53], and this relationship is independent of inotropic state. Abnormalities are also seen in patients with rate-related left bundle branch block but normal coronary arteries[54]. In this condition, the diastolic incoordination itself can compromise subendocardial perfusion and lead to angina. Right ventricular ischaemia also leads to abnormalities[55].

## References

1 Beller GA, Holzgrefe HH, Watson DD. Effects of dipyridamole induced vasodilation on myocardial uptake and clearance kinetics of thallium-201. *Circulation* 1983; **68**: 1328–38

2 Verani MS, Mahmarian JJ, Hixson JB, Boyce TM, Staudacher RA. Diagnosis of coronary artery disease by controlled coronary vasodilation with adenosine and thallium-201 scintigraphy in patients unable to exercise. *Circulation* 1990; **82**: 80–97

3 Walker PR, James MA, Wilde RPH, Wood CH, Russell RJ. Dipyridamole combined with exercise for thallium myocardial imaging. *Br Heart J* 1986; **55**: 321–9

4 Pennell DJ, Mavrogeni SI, Forbat SM, Karwatowski SP, Underwood SR. Adenosine combined with dynamic exercise for myocardial perfusion imaging. *J Am Coll Cardiol* 1995; **25**: 1300–9

5 Iscandrian AE. State of the art of pharmacological stress imaging. In: Zaret BL, Beller GA. (eds) *Nuclear Cardiology, State of the Art and Future Direction*, 2nd edn. St Louis: Mosby, 1999; 312

6 Grunwald AM, Watson DD, Holzgrefe HH *et al*. Myocardial thallium-201 kinetics in normal and ischaemic myocardium. *Circulation* 1981; **64**: 610–8

7 Leppo JA. Cardiac transport of single photon myocardial perfusion tracers. In: Zaret BL, Beller GA. (eds) *Nuclear Cardiology, State of the Art and Future Direction*, 2nd edn. St Louis: Mosby, 1993: 35–44

8 Li QS, Solot G, Frank TL, Wagner HNJ, Becker LC. Myocardial redistribution of technetium-99m-methoxyisobutyl isonitrile (SESTAMIBI). *J Nucl Med* 1990; **31**: 1069–76

9 Jain D, Wackers FJ, Mattera J, McMahon M, Sinusas AJ, Zaret BL. Biokinetics of technetium-99m-tetrofosmin: myocardial perfusion imaging agent: implications for a one-day imaging protocol. *J Nucl Med* 1993; **34**: 1254–9

10 Madahi J. Myocardial perfusion imaging for the detection and evaluation of coronary artery disease. In: Skorton DJ, Schelbert HR, Wolf GL, Brundage BH. (eds) *Cardiac Imaging. A Companion to Braunwald's Heart Disease*, 2nd edn. New York: WB Saunders, 1996; 971–94

11 Gianrossi R, Detrano R, Mulvihill D *et al*. Exercise induced ST depression in the diagnosis of coronary artery disease: a meta-analysis. *Circulation* 1989; **80**: 87–98

12 Underwood SR, Godman B, Salyani S, Ogle JR, Ell PJ. Economics of myocardial perfusion imaging in Europe: the EMPIRE study. *Eur Heart J* 1999; **20**: 157–66

13 de Bono D. Investigation and management of stable angina: revised guidelines 1998. *Heart* 1999; **81**: 546–55

14 Kontos MC, Jesse RL, Schmidt KL, Ornato JP, Tatum JL. Value of acute rest sestamibi perfusion imaging for evaluation of patients admitted to the emergency department with chest pain. *J Am Coll Cardiol* 1997; **30**: 976–82

15 Brown KA, Boucher CA, Okada RD *et al*. Prognostic value of exercise thallium-201 imaging in patients presenting for evaluation of chest pain. *J Am Coll Cardiol* 1983; **1**: 994–1001

16 Ladenheim ML, Kotler TS, Pollock BH, Berman DS, Diamond DA. Incremental prognostic power of clinical history, exercise electrocardiography and myocardial perfusion scintigraphy in suspected coronary artery disease. *Am J Cardiol* 1987; **59**: 270–7

17 Marie PY, Danchin N, Durand JF *et al*. Long-term prediction of major ischemic events by exercise thallium-201 single-photon emission computed tomography. Incremental prognostic value

compared with clinical, exercise testing, catheterization and radionuclide angiographic data. *J Am Coll Cardiol* 1995; **26**: 879–86

18  Gibson RS, Watson DD, Craddock GB *et al.* Prediction of cardiac events after uncomplicated myocardial infarction: a prospective study comparing predischarge exercise thallium-201 scintigraphy and coronary angiography. *Circulation* 1983; **68**: 321–36

19  Brown KA, Heller GV, Landin RS *et al.* tomographic imaging 2 to 4 days after acute myocardial infarction predicts in-hospital and postdischarge cardiac events: comparison with submaximal exercise imaging. *Circulation* 1999; **100**: 2060–6

20  American College of Physicians. Guidelines for assessing and managing the perioperative risk from coronary artery disease associated with major noncardiac surgery. *Ann Intern Med* 1997; **127**: 309–12

21  Hecht HS, Shaw RE, Bruce TR, Ryan C, Stertzer SH, Myler RK. Usefulness of tomographic thallium-201 imaging for detection of restenosis after percutaneous transluminal coronary angioplasty. *Am J Cardiol* 1990; **66**: 1314–8

22  Vom Dahl J, Altehoefer C, Sheehan FH *et al.* Effect of myocardial viability assessed by technetium-99m sestamibi SPECT and fluorine-18-FDG PET on clinical outcome in coronary artery disease. *J Nucl Med* 1997; **38**: 742–8

23  Tillisch JH, Brunken R, Marshall R *et al.* Reversibility of cardiac wall motion abnormalities predicted by positron tomography. *N Engl J Med* 1986; **314**: 884–8

24  Ragosta M, Beller GA, Watson DD, Kaul S, Gimple LW. Quantitative planar rest-redistribution Tl-201 imaging in detection of myocardial viability and prediction of improvement in left ventricular function after coronary bypass surgery in patients with severely depressed left ventricular function. *Circulation* 1993; **87**: 1630–41

25  Ohtani H, Tamaki N, Yonekura Y *et al.* Value of thallium-201 reinjection after delayed SPECT imaging for predicting reversible ischemia after coronary artery bypass grafting. *Am J Cardiol* 1990; **66**: 394–9

26  Kayden DS, Sigal S, Sonfer R *et al.* Thallium-201 for assessment of myocardial viability: quantitative comparison of 24 hour redistribution imaging with reinjection at rest. *J Am Coll Cardiol* 1991; **18**: 1480–6

27  Tamaki N, Ohtani H, Yamashita K *et al.* Metabolic activity in the areas of new fill-in after thallium-201 reinjection: comparison with positron emission tomography using fluorine-18-deoxyglucose. *J Nucl Med* 1991; **32**: 673–8

28  Udelson JE, Coleman PS, Metherall J *et al.* Predicting recovery of severe regional ventricular dysfunction. Comparison of resting scintigraphy with $^{201}$Tl and $^{99m}$Tc-sestamibi. *Circulation* 1994; **89**: 2552–61

29  Kauffman GJ, Boyne TS, Watson DD, Smith WH, Beller GA. Comparison of rest thallium-201 imaging and rest technetium-99m sestamibi imaging for assessment of myocardial viability in patients with coronary artery disease and severe left ventricular dysfunction. *J Am Coll Cardiol* 1996; **27**: 1592–7

30  Matsunari I, Fujino S, Taki J *et al.* Quantitative rest technetium-99m tetrofosmin imaging in predicting functional recovery after revascularization: comparison with rest-redistribution thallium-201. *J Am Coll Cardiol* 1997; **29**: 1226–33

31  Mintz GS, Nissen SE, Anderson WD *et al.* American College of Cardiology Clinical Expert Consensus document on Standards for Acquisition, Measurement and Reporting of Intravascular Ultrasound Studies (IVUS). A report of the American College of Cardiology Task Force on Clinical Expert Consensus Documents. *J Am Coll Cardiol* 2001; **37**: 1478–92

32  Rasmussen S, Corya BC, Feigenbaum H, Knoebel SB. Detection of myocardial scar tissue by M-mode echocardiography. *Circulation* 1978; **57**: 230–7

33  Henein MY, Anagnostopoulos C, Das SK, O'Sullivan C, Underwood SR, Gibson DG. Left ventricular long axis disturbances as predictors for thallium perfusion defects in patients with known peripheral vascular disease. *Heart* 1998; **79**: 295–300

34  Henein MY, Priestley K, Davarashvili T *et al.* Early changes in left ventricular subendocardial function after successful coronary angioplasty. *Br Heart J* 1993; **69**: 501–6

35  Alam M, Wardell J, Andersson E, Samad BA, Nordlander R. Characteristics of mitral and tricuspid annular velocities determined by pulsed wave Doppler tissue imaging in healthy subjects. *J Am Soc Echocardiogr* 1999; **12**: 618–28

36 Henein MY, Gibson DG. Abnormal subendocardial function in restrictive left ventricular disease. *Br Heart J* 1994; **72**: 237–42

37 Ryan T, Vasey CG, Presti CF *et al*. Exercise echocardiography: detection of coronary artery disease in patients with normal left ventricular wall motion at rest. *J Am Coll Cardiol* 1988; **11**: 993–9

38 Zoghbi W, Cherif J, Kleiman NS *et al*. Diagnosis of ischemic heart disease with adenosine echocardiography. *J Am Coll Cardiol*. 1991; **18**: 1271–9

39 Poli A, Previtali M, Lanzarini L *et al*. Comparison of dobutamine stress echocardiography with dipyridamole stress echocardiography for detection of viable myocardium after myocardial infarction treated with thrombolysis. *Heart* 1996; **75**: 240–6

40 Perrone-Filardi P, Pace L, Prastaro M *et al*. Dobutamine echocardiography predicts improvement of hypoperfused dysfunctional myocardium after revascularisation in patients with coronary artery disease. *Circulation* 1995; **91**: 2556–65

41 Previtali M, Lanzarini L, Fetiveau R *et al*. Comparison of dobutamine stress echocardiography, dipyridamole stress echocardiography and exercise testing for diagnosis of coronary artery disease. *Am J Cardiol* 1993; **72**: 865–70

42 Elhendy A, van Domburg RT, Bax JJ *et al*. Optimal criteria for the diagnosis of coronary artery disease by dobutamine stress echocardiography. *Am J Cardiol* 1998; **82**: 1339–44

43 Krivokapich J, Child JS, Walter DO, Garfinkel A. Prognostic value of dobutamine stress echocardiography in predicting cardiac events in patients with known coronary artery disease. *J Am Coll Cardiol* 1999; **33**: 708–16

44 Senior R, Glenville B, Basu S *et al*. Dobutamine echocardiography and thallium 201 imaging predict functional improvement after revascularisation in severe ischaemic left ventricular dysfunction. *Br Heart J* 1995; **74**: 358–64

45 Bax JJ, Wijns W, Cornel JH *et al*. Accuracy of currently available techniques for prediction of functional recovery after revascularisation in patients with left ventricular dysfunction due to chronic coronary artery disease – a comparison of pooled data. *J Am Coll Cardiol* 1997; **30**: 1451–60

46 Senior R, Soman R, Khattar RS, Lahiri A. Improved endocardial visualisation using second harmonic imaging compared to fundamental two-dimensional echocardiographic imaging. *Am Heart J* 1999; **138**: 163–8

47 Senior R. Role of contrast echocardiography in the evaluation of LV function. *Echocardiography* 1999; **167**: 747–52

48 LaCanna G, Rahimtoola SH, Visioli O *et al*. Sensitivity, specificity, and predictive accuracies of non-invasive tests, single and in combination, for diagnosis of hibernating myocardium. *Eur Heart J* 2000; **21**: 1358–67

49 Arnese M, Cornel JH, Salustri A *et al*. Prediction of improvement of regional left ventricular function after surgical revascularisation: a comparison of low dose dobutamine echocardiography with 201 Tl single photon emission computed tomography. *Circulation* 1995; **91**: 2748–52

50 Alfridi I, Grayburn PA, Panza JA *et al*. Myocardial viability during dobutamine echocardiography predicts survival in patients with coronary artery disease and severe left ventricular dysfunction. *J Am Coll Cardiol* 1998; **32**: 921–6

51 Meluzin J, Ciggaroa CG, Brickner ME *et al*. Dobutamine echocardiography in predicting improvement in global left ventricular systolic function after coronary bypass or angioplasty in patients with healed myocardial infarcts. *Am J Cardiol* 1995; **76**: 877–80

52 O'Sullivan CA, Henein MY, Sutton R, Coats AJ, Sutton GC, Gibson DG. Abnormal ventricular activation and repolarisation during dobutamine stress echocardiography in coronary artery disease. *Heart* 1998: **79**: 468–73

53 Duncan AM, O'Sullivan CA, Gibson DG, Henein MY. Electromechanical interrelations during dobutamine stress in normal subjects and patients with coronary artery disease: comparison of changes in activation and inotropic state. *Heart* 2001; **85**: 411–6

54 Xiao HB, Gibson DG. The effect of intermittent left bundle branch block on left ventricular diastolic function – a case report. *Heart* 2001; **85**: 411–6

55 Cooke FJ, Clague J, Henein MY. Stress long-axis function in coronary artery spasm. *Clin Cardiol* 1999; **22**: 757–8

# Invasive investigations and revascularisation

**S Chaubey, SW Davies** and **N Moat**

*Department of Invasive Cardiology, Royal Brompton Hospital, London, UK*

Invasive investigation of coronary artery disease is relatively expensive, and carries risks including a mortality of approximately 1 in 2000. It would not be practical or appropriate to perform invasive investigation in all patients with a clinical diagnosis of coronary artery disease, still less in the large numbers with chest pain and possible angina. Clinicians will refer for invasive investigation those: (i) with a high level of angina, needing revascularisation on symptomatic grounds; and (ii) who are likely to have a poor prognosis with medical treatment, and thus likely to benefit from revascularisation. Not all of these patients will have a high level of symptoms.

In the late 1950s and early 1960s, there were major advances in the treatment of coronary artery disease – the techniques of external cardiac massage, electrical cardioversion, and the introduction of lignocaine transformed the approach to acute myocardial infarction and arrhythmias, and led to coronary care units. At the same time, Sones and Judkins introduced methods of selective coronary arteriography, a prerequisite for coronary artery surgery. In the mid- and late-1960s, early forms of exercise ECG testing (Masters step test) and of isotope myocardial perfusion imaging (with caesium) were developed to identify those with severe coronary disease likely to benefit from coronary arteriography and revascularisation.

In the 1960s and 1970s, large registries charted the natural history of patients after their coronary artery disease had been defined by arteriography, and showed poor prognosis of those with triple vessel disease or left main stem disease. Randomised clinical trials of coronary artery surgery in the late 1970s and early 1980s showed that, for these groups of patients, surgery conferred prognostic benefit as well as symptomatic relief of angina. This established the value of coronary arteriography in deciding the correct treatment.

Invasive investigation is now taken to mean 'left heart catheterisation', comprising selective coronary arteriography with multiple views to show all major coronary vessels clearly without overlap or foreshortening, and contrast left ventriculography to show left ventricular function and any regional wall motion abnormality. It is used to assess the prognosis and hence need for revascularisation, as well as the anatomical (technical) suitability of the vessels for grafting or for angioplasty. In special circumstances, it may be used simply to confirm or refute the diagnosis of coronary artery disease, for example in airline pilots.

Correspondence to:
Dr SW Davies,
Department of Invasive
Cardiology, Royal
Brompton Hospital,
Sydney Street,
London SW3 6NP, UK

# Prognostic assessment (risk stratification)

Once the diagnosis of coronary artery disease has been made, it is important to assess the outlook to decide upon future treatment and the possible need for invasive investigation and revascularisation, as well as for the patient's information. The main determinants of prognosis are:

1  Left ventricular function – this is statistically the most powerful predictor not only in coronary artery disease, but also in cardiomyopathies, valvular heart disease, and many other conditions

2  The anatomical extent and severity of coronary artery disease – as defined precisely by angiography, or as estimated by one of the non-invasive tests discussed in the preceding section

3  Recent unstable angina or acute myocardial infarction – there is increased risk of death and of future infarction for at least 6 months following an acute coronary syndrome

4  General health – co-morbidity such as diabetes, renal disease, pulmonary disease, and age

Information may also be gained from the basic tests, such as the finding of pathological Q waves on the resting ECG, or noting a large heart and pulmonary venous congestion on the chest X-ray. Simple clinical risk scores have been devised, but they are not widely used in practice. Prediction is greatly strengthened by adding the results of a non-invasive test, for example the Duke exercise test treadmill score[1]. At present, these too are little used in practice, but the spread of information technology in medicine may change this – scores can easily be calculated from data already entered into an electronic patient record, and presented to the clinician on the desktop for 'decision support'.

Non-invasive testing has been discussed elsewhere in this issue, but we should make some general points. All the non-invasive tests are inaccurate to some degree. If we use coronary angiography as the gold standard to define the presence a stenosis of 50% or greater in a major epicardial vessel, then typically the sensitivity is 70–90% and specificity 70–90% for the above methodologies. Moreover, each method has specific weaknesses; for example, the treadmill exercise ECG is poor at reflecting disease in the circumflex territory. Interpretation of the exercise ECG is difficult if there is resting bundle branch block or other abnormality. CT coronary calcification scoring is only useful over the age range 40–70 years, as at younger ages there may be significant coronary plaques with little calcium. At ages over 70 years, there is often widespread coronary calcification irrespective of luminal narrowings. Stress echocardiography is perhaps the most operator-dependent technique and results will vary considerably according to the skill and experience of the echocardiographer obtaining and then interpreting the images, particularly at the high heart rates and respiratory movement associated with exercise or pharmacological stress. Myocardial perfusion scanning may have the highest predictive value, but involves a significant radiation dose to the patient. It is probably the investigation of choice if the patient is unable to exercise on a treadmill or cycle ergometer because of lower limb orthopaedic or vascular problems, or if there are resting ECG abnormalities.

If more than one non-invasive test is performed in a given patient, one test may give a result indicating normality and the other indicate coronary disease. When there are discrepant data, the clinician has to make a decision on the overall situation as to whether there is likely to be coronary artery disease or not. Performing additional tests is also of limited usefulness because of 'predictive redundancy' – the incremental information from performing a second non-invasive test is less than would be expected if they were independently predictive[2]. Patients who have an equivocal test with one modality are more likely to have an equivocal test with another modality, and those who are false positives with one are also more likely to be false positive with another – the reasons for this are unclear, but it is of practical importance. If the most appropriate non-invasive test has been correctly selected for the individual patient, then if the result is borderline or does not fit with the clinical picture, performing another different non-invasive test may not be helpful. However, all of the non-invasive tests have considerable prognostic value, aside from their ability to detect structural coronary artery disease – this is discussed in the chapter by Underwood.

## Invasive investigation

Selection of patients for left heart catheterisation for assessment of coronary artery disease can be summarised by the flow chart presented in Figure 1. This is greatly simplified, and in practice the correct decision for an individual patient will depend on many other factors, including patient preference, and co-morbidity. Across the world, local resources and availability of cardiac catheterisation will also affect referral for invasive investigation.

## Percutaneous coronary intervention

Balloon angioplasty of the coronary arteries was introduced by Gruntzig in 1977[3], and the results were greatly improved by the introduction of coronary stenting by Sigwart and by Puel in 1986. The term 'percutaneous coronary intervention' is now taken to include balloon angioplasty, stenting, and occasional other technologies such as atherectomy and laser methods.

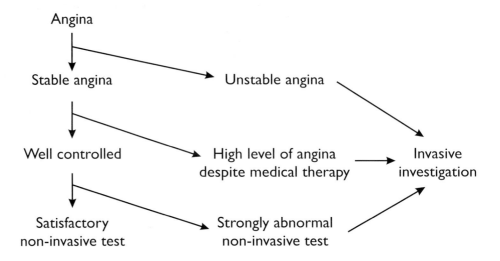

**Fig. 1** A simplified algorithm to select patients for invasive investigation of coronary artery disease. A 'satisfactory' non-invasive test is one that is normal, or has abnormalities which are minor and/or only appear at a high level of exercise or pharmacological stress. An example of a 'strongly abnormal' test is an exercise ECG with marked ST-segment depression at a low workload, or a thallium scan with widespread ischaemia.

The indications for percutaneous coronary intervention (PCI) have evolved over the years, as the quality of the evidence has improved. The initial experience was based on 'common sense' – when balloon angioplasty was first introduced, it seemed sensible to treat simple lesions in patients with single vessel disease, or in patients who were unsuitable for coronary artery surgery because of co-morbidity. When coronary stenting was first introduced, it was only used for 'bail-out' to restore flow in lesions that had dissected or occluded during conventional balloon angioplasty.

In the 1980s, large registries began to provide firm (non-randomised) data on the short-term success rates, complications, and long-term outcomes[4]. These data informed clinicians and patients when choosing between medical therapy, coronary surgery, and PCI.

In the 1990s, randomised controlled trials started to appear comparing PCI with medical therapy, and PCI with surgical revascularisation. Trials such as BENESTENT and STRESS compared elective stenting with conventional balloon angioplasty. Other trials have addressed technical aspects of PCI such the use of intravascular ultrasound to guide stent deployment, and the use of atherectomy devices, intravascular radiation to prevent re-stenosis, and adjuvant drug treatment with glycoprotein IIb/IIIa blockers and other drugs. As a result, there is now a large published literature on which recommendations and guidelines can be based.

A thorough digest of the evidence and of current recommendations has been published by the American College of Cardiology and the

**Table 1** Indications for percutaneous coronary intervention (PCI) as proposed by the American College of Cardiology and the American Heart Association[5]

* Patients with mild angina or currently asymptomatic, if there are significant lesions in 1 or 2 coronary arteries subtending a large area of viable myocardium, who are not diabetic

* Patients with moderate or severe angina, if there are significant lesions in 1 or 2 coronary arteries subtending an area of viable myocardium

* Patients with moderate or severe angina and previous coronary bypass surgery, if there are significant lesions in vein grafts which are focal stenoses or multiple vein graft stenoses in patients who are poor candidates for repeat surgery

* Patients with acute myocardial infarction who have a contra-indication to thrombolytic therapy, and/or who develop cardiogenic shock within 36 h of the onset of infarction

* Patients with acute myocardial infarction who present early (within 12 h) may be considered for PCI as an alternative to thrombolysis, if local PCI is readily available

* Patients with acute myocardial infarction who have continuing pain and ST elevation despite thrombolysis

American Heart Association in a joint document[5]. These are summarised in Table 1.

Less certain indication include patients with symptoms of angina and/or evidence of myocardial ischaemia, and more extensive coronary artery disease, who have relative contra-indications to coronary surgery. In these cases, it is important to discuss the options with the patient with regard to the features of their individual case and in the light of local experience and results.

## Surgical revascularisation – indications and trials

Coronary artery bypass grafting (CABG) is one of the most common operations performed today despite its recent beginnings. Cardiac revascularisation is undertaken either to minimise symptoms or to prevent premature death. CABG constitutes one of the three main categories of angina management, the other two being medical management or PCI.

A number of trials have now been conducted over the last three decades comparing these three management options resulting in the development of indications for surgery, PTCA or medical management for patients with chronic stable angina.

Three randomised controlled trials conducted in the 1970s[6–8] demonstrated that CABG had a survival benefit when compared to medical management for patients with significant (> 50%) left main stem stenosis, triple vessel disease or two vessel disease with left ventricular dysfunction.

No study has shown any survival benefits for CABG over medical management for patients with single or two vessel disease. Revascularisation in this group of patients is usually undertaken for symptom control when maximum medical management has been unsuccessful in improving their symptoms. PTCA or CABG are the two means of revascularisation available to this group of patients. Trials comparing CABG and PTCA for these patients show similar quality of life indices, stress test performance and clinical improvement. However, patients on whom PTCA was undertaken more often needed further revascularisation in the future due to re-stenosis[9]. Growing interest in stents has led to their use for sub-optimal PTCA, chronically occluded arteries and re-stenosis after PTCA along with other indications[10].

It is important that secondary preventive measures are also used. Aspirin should be used to lower the rate of graft occlusion following CABG (21% *versus* 30%). Lipid lowering drugs should also be commenced.

CABG may not be advisable on the elderly population or on high-risk patients due to their co-morbidity. There are scoring systems such as the Parsonnet or Euroscore which give an estimate of the risk of in-hospital death after CABG. These risks of intervention compared with non-intervention should be explained to the patient, especially when obtaining consent.

## Transmyocardial revascularisation

Patients unsuitable for revascularisation on whom medical management has been inadequate to control their symptoms can undergo transmyocardial revascularisation (TMR). TMR is a surgical procedure performed *via* a lateral thoracotomy. The surgeon places the laser on the epicardial surface of the left ventricle and discharges sufficient energy to create transmural channels in the myocardium. Percutaneous myocardial revascularisation (PMR) is performed *via* a cardiac catheter. Laser energy is applied to the endocardial surface of the heart to create partial thickness channels.

The precise mechanism of action of TMR is yet to be characterised. Randomised controlled trials of TMR *versus* medical management report improvements in the patient's symptoms[11–14]. These are sustained at 3 years in some reports making placebo as an explanation less likely.

PMR offers similar clinical benefits but with a better safety profile. It avoids a general anaesthetic and thoracotomy. The endocardial laser allows access to a greater surface area of the myocardium than TMR, which is largely limited to the anterior and lateral walls. Results from on-going trials are awaited.

## Surgical conduit

Saphenous vein has been the mainstay for CABG. However, there is now a shift to arterial revascularisation owing to the longer patency rates seen with arterial conduits. The saphenous vein is usually in plentiful supply and easy to harvest and is, therefore, very much still in use. However, due to thrombosis, fibro-intimal hyperplasia or continued atherosclerosis, only 50% of these grafts remain patent at 10 years. Interestingly, of the grafts that have not occluded at 5 years, 80% remain patent at 10 years[15].

The left internal thoracic artery (LITA) has superior patency rate when compared to the saphenous vein graft of 83–93% at 10 years. Remarkably, this artery is very often spared of any atherosclerotic changes allowing it to be used routinely as the first conduit of choice. It is usually used to graft the left anterior descending artery (LAD) which supplies a large territory of the heart. These facts have now made the LITA to the LAD one of the most commonly performed procedures. However the following conditions may preclude its use: brachiocephalic and subclavian disease, very poor left ventricular function, previous irradiation, or in an emergency where the saphenous vein is better as faster restoration of blood flow is required.

The right internal thoracic artery (RITA) can be used to graft the right coronary artery or the posterior descending artery. It is generally better not to cross the RITA to the left system as this can make subsequent sternotomy treacherous. The use of bilateral ITA is associated with less angina, fewer myocardial infarctions and a reduced need for re-operation. However, it shows no further survival benefits and is also associated with a greater incidence of sternal wound infection. Therefore, its use is generally avoided in patients prone to infection such as diabetics and the obese[16].

The radial artery is now being used more commonly as the second arterial conduit of choice. After initial disappointing results, its patency rate has improved (93% at 1 year) with the use of prophylactic calcium channel blockade to prevent spasm.

The gastro-epiploic artery constitutes the third arterial conduit for an initial operation. The vessel is harvested from the greater curvature of the stomach from where it runs either in front of or behind the pylorus and the left lobe of the liver and through the diaphragm. Alternatively, it can be taken as a free graft. The pedicled graft has a patency of 92% at 5 years as compared to 88% seen with the free graft. The artery can reach all the three main vessels of the heart but is usually used to graft the inferior and lateral portions of the heart.

The inferior epigastric artery, short saphenous vein and cephalic vein have all also been used as conduits. There is, however, no large follow-up to study long-term results. Artificial conduits have as yet proved unsuccessful, achieving rates of less than 40% at 1 year.

# Future developments in surgical revascularisation

Recently, there has been increasing interest in off-pump procedures. In such operations, a sternotomy is required but the operation is performed on the beating heart. Thus cardiopulmonary bypass is avoided along with all its associated inflammatory reaction[17]. The concern, however, about the quality of the anastomosis achieved as it is performed on the beating heart. Nevertheless, there are reports of results comparable to conventional CABG as assessed by follow-up angiography[18]. Improvement in stabiliser technology has resulted in some reports of people achieving total revascularisation off-pump. However, for more diffuse disease requiring multiple grafts, off-pump surgery is usually unsuitable.

Off-pump operations can be provided *via* a small anterior thoracotomy, thus avoiding a sternotomy. This minimally invasive, direct coronary artery bypass (MIDCAB) is also being developed with endoscopic and computer assisted techniques. Limited case series have been reported[19,20]. These show good graft patency, smaller wound size and reduced hospital stay.

How future studies develop indications for such procedures is awaited with interest. One will need to see how these procedures either replace the current conventional means of revascularisation or establish their own niche.

## Key points for clinical practice

- Left heart catheterisation (selective coronary arteriography and left ventriculography) helps to define prognosis, and the patient's technical suitability for revascularisation

- Referral for left heart catheterisation is a key step to identify patients needing revascularisation

- Coronary artery surgery effectively relieves angina in all categories of patient, and improves prognosis in those with extensive coronary disease

- Percutaneous coronary intervention (angioplasty) is used in patients with angina who have less extensive disease or who are unsuitable for coronary surgery because of pulmonary, renal, or cerebrovascular disease

- Developments in stenting and in adjuvant drug treatment have improved the results of PCI, and have extended the indications.

## References

1 Morise AP, Detrano R, Bobbio M, Diamond GA. Development and validation of a logistic regression-derived algorithm for estimating the incremental probability of coronary artery disease before and after exercise testing. *J Am Coll Cardiol* 1992; 20: 1187–96

2 Weissler AM. Assessment and use of cardiovascular tests in clinical prediction. In: Giuliani ER, Holmes DR, Hayes DL, *et al.* (eds) *Mayo Clinic Practice of Cardiology*, 3rd edn. St Louis, MO: Mosby-Yearbook, 1996; 400

3 Gruntzig AR, Senning A, Siegenthaler WE. Nonoperative dilatation of coronary artery stenosis:

percutaneous transluminal coronary angioplasty. *N Engl J Med* 1979; **301**: 61–8

4   Detre KM, Holubkov R, Kelsey S *et al*. Percutaneous coronary angioplasty in 1985–1986 and 1977–1981: the National Heart, Lung, and Blood Institute. *N Engl J Med* 1988; **318**: 265–70

5   Smith SS, Dove JT, Kern MJ, and members of the ACC/AHA Task Force on Practice Guidelines. ACC/AHA guidelines for percutaneous coronary intervention (revision of the 1993 PTCA guidelines). *J Am Coll Cardiol* 2001; **37**: 2239I–2239lxvi. Document downloadable from www.acc.org

6.  Veterans Administration. Coronary Artery Bypass Study: eleven year survival in the Veterans Administration Randomised Trial of coronary bypass surgery for stable angina. *N Engl J Med* 1984; **311**: 1333

7   CASS Principal Investigators and their Associates. Coronary Artery Surgery Study: a randomised trial of coronary artery bypass surgery; survival data. *Circulation* 1983; **68**: 939

8   Varnauskas E, European Coronary Surgery Study Group. Twelve year follow-up of survival in the randomised European Coronary Surgery Study. *N Engl J Med* 1988; **319**: 332

9   RITA Trial Participants. Coronary angioplasty *versus* coronary artery bypass surgery: The Randomised Intervention Treatment of Angina (RITA) Trial. *Lancet* 1993; **341**: 573

10  Macayac, Serruys PW, Ruygrak P, Supryapranata *et al*. Continued benefit of coronary stenting versus balloon angioplasty. BENESTENT Study Group. *J Am Coll Cardiol* 1996; **27**: 255–61

11  Allen KB, Dowling RD, Fudge T *et al*. Comparison of transmyocardial revascularisation with medical therapy in patients with refractory angina. *N Engl J Med* 1999; **341**: 1029–36

12  Burkhoff D, Schmidt S, Schulman SP *et al*. Transmyocardial laser revascularisation compared with continued medical therapy for treatment of refractory angina pectoris: a prospective randomised trial. *Lancet* 1999; **354**: 885–90

13  Schofield PM, Sharples LD, Caine N *et al*. Transmyocardial laser revascularisation in patients with refractory angina: a randomised controlled trial. *Lancet* 1999; **353**: 519–24

14  Frazier OH, March RJ, Horvath KA. Transmyocardial revascularisation with a carbon dioxide laser in patients with end stage coronary artery disease. *N Engl J Med* 1999; **341**: 1021–8

15  Campeau L, Enjalbert M, Lesperance J *et al*. Atherosclerosis and late closure of aortocoronary saphenous vein grafts: sequential angiographic studies at 2 weeks, 1 year, 5 and 7 year and 10–12 years after surgery. *Circulation* 1983; **68** (**Suppl II**): 1–7

16  Morris JJ, Smith LR, Glower DD *et al*. Clinical evaluation of single *versus* multiple internal mammary grafts. *Circulation* 1990; **82** (**Suppl IV**): 214–23

17  Cartier R, Brann S, Dagenois F, Martineau R, Couturier A. Systematic off-pump coronary artery revascularisation in multivessel disease: experience of 300 cases. *J Thorac Cardiovasc Surg* 2000; **119**: 221–9

18  Gill IS, Higginson LA, Maharajh GS, Keon WJ. Early follow-up angiography with minimally invasive coronary bypass without mechanical stabilisation. *Ann Thorac Surg* 2000; **69**: 56–60

19  Loulmet D, Carpentier A, Atelis N *et al*. Endoscopic coronary artery bypass grafting with the aid of robotic assisted instruments. *J Thorac Cardiovasc Surg* 1999; **118**: 4–10

20  Reichnespurner H, Damiano RJ, Mack M *et al*. Use of the voice controlled and computer assisted surgical system Zeas for endoscopic coronary artery bypass grafting. *J Thorac Cardiovasc Surg* 1999; **118**: 11–6

# Inflammatory mechanisms

**Afshin Farzaneh-Far, James Rudd** and **Peter L Weissberg**

*Division of Cardiovascular Medicine, University of Cambridge, Cambridge, UK*

Traditional concepts of the pathogenesis of acute coronary syndromes have changed over the last few years. In particular it has been demonstrated that high-risk lesions are not necessarily angiographically severe. Rather, unstable high risk lesions are the ones composed of large lipid cores and thin fibrous caps. It is now widely accepted that plaque instability is related to the development of inflammation within the intima. A consequence of this is that stabilization of lesions provides a new therapeutic target. Furthermore, there is growing evidence that statins may stabilize lesions by altering the inflammatory response. A brief overview of these developments and their impact on clinical practice is presented.

The process of atherosclerosis was considered for many years to merely represent a relentless, accumulation of lipids within the artery wall. However, over the last two decades, major developments in the field of vascular biology have made it clear that atherosclerotic lesions are in fact a series of highly specific, dynamic, cellular and molecular responses that are essentially inflammatory in nature. Indeed, the earliest lesion of atherosclerosis, the fatty streak, is a pure inflammatory lesion, consisting only of T lymphocytes and monocyte-derived macrophages[1]. A brief overview of these developments and their impact on clinical practice is presented below.

## Endothelial cell dysfunction

The original response-to-injury hypothesis put forward by Russell Ross and his colleagues postulated that endothelial denudation and injury were the first steps in the atherosclerotic process[2]. This was based on observations in which removal of endothelium by mechanical means dramatically enhanced the ability of a high lipid diet to induce atherosclerosis in animal models[3]. However, subsequent observations in humans and animal models in the late 1970s seemed to indicate that the endothelium overlying atherosclerotic lesions was anatomically intact. These apparently inconsistent observations were rationalized by Gimbrone who proposed the concept of 'endothelial dysfunction'. This acknowledged the importance of an intact, normally functioning endothelium in protecting against atherosclerosis but emphasized **functional** abnormalities of the endothelium in the setting of

Correspondence to:
Dr A Farzaneh-Far,
Division of Cardiovascular
Medicine, University
of Cambridge,
Addenbrooke's Hospital
(ACCI level 6), Hills Road,
Cambridge CB2 2QQ, UK

atherosclerosis. Ludmer and colleagues provided the first clinical evidence of endothelial dysfunction as an important component of coronary atherosclerosis[4]. They demonstrated that the muscarinic cholinergic agonist acetylcholine, was able to vasodilate angiographically normal coronary arteries but produced paradoxical vasoconstriction in segments with either minimal angiographic disease or severe stenosis. These abnormalities of vasomotor tone were assumed to reflect underlying endothelial dysfunction because of Furchgott's classical observations on endothelium-dependent vasorelaxation[5]. He had elegantly demonstrated an *in vitro* organ bath system in which preconstricted arterial rings would relax in response to muscarinic cholinergic agonists only if endothelial cells were present. Removal of the endothelium by any means abolished the vasorelaxation which was mediated by an undefined endothelium derived relaxing factor (EDRF). EDRF was subsequently shown to be, in large part, nitric oxide (NO)[6,7]. NO diffuses to the underlying vascular smooth muscle cells and stimulates the second messenger cGMP to cause relaxation. Ludmer's observations of abnormal vasomotor control in atherosclerotic vessels were, therefore, assumed to indicate abnormalities of NO production by the overlying endothelium.

It is now thought that the earliest detectable physiological manifestation of atherosclerosis is reduced production or bioavailability of NO in response to pharmacological or haemodynamic stimuli. This phenomenon is even observed in children with hypercholesterolaemia[8]. Other causes of this endothelial dysfunction include free radicals caused by cigarette smoking, hypertension, diabetes mellitus, elevated plasma homocysteine levels and infectious micro-organisms such as *Chlamydia pneumoniae*. Indeed, virtually every atherosclerotic risk factor is associated with endothelial dysfunction[1].

The above data are consistent with the idea that the primary event in atherogenesis is endothelial dysfunction. The endothelium can be damaged by a variety of means, leading to dysfunction and subendothelial lipid accumulation (due to increased permeability of the endothelium to plasma lipoproteins). In this situation, the normal homeostatic features of the endothelium break down. It becomes more adhesive to inflammatory cells and platelets, and it loses its anticoagulant properties. This is associated with reduced bioavailability of NO. Importantly, drugs that have been shown to improve the outcome of vascular disease – including statins and angiotensin converting enzyme inhibitors – have been shown to improve endothelial function.

## Oxidative stress

The initiating mechanisms leading to endothelial dysfunction have been the focus of a great deal of research activity. One of the major developments in vascular biology over the last 20 years has been the understanding of the importance of oxidation mechanisms in mediating pathophysiological responses in the arterial wall and endothelial dysfunction. In particular, the role of oxidised low density lipoprotein (LDL) has been intensively investigated. LDL appears to be a major cause of injury to the endothelium[9]. Moreover, increased permeability of the endothelium to plasma lipoproteins are amongst the earliest detectable changes of the atherosclerotic process. LDL particles trapped in the arterial wall can undergo progressive oxidation leading to internalization by macrophages by means of the scavenger receptors on the surface of these cells. The original observation which stimulated much of this work was that mononuclear cells in culture were unable to take up freshly isolated LDL to form lipid-rich foam cells, but that exposure of the LDL to cultured endothelial cells modified the lipoprotein so that it was taken up by monocyte/macrophages to form foam cells[10]. The modification of LDL that allowed recognition and uptake was oxidation, and oxidised LDL was found to have multiple biological and pro-inflammatory properties[11]. From observations such as these, it has become apparent that an extracellular oxidation mechanism is fundamentally important in the pathogenesis of atherosclerosis and endothelial dysfunction[12].

The importance of oxidative stress has been emphasized by a number of studies, which have provided compelling evidence that atherosclerosis is associated with enhanced production of oxygen free radicals at a time when NO production is continuing but endothelium dependent relaxation is impaired[12]. From these observations, it has been concluded that NO is being degraded and inactivated in the setting of atherosclerosis by reactive oxygen species. NO is itself an effective antioxidant and is produced from arginine by the enzyme NO synthase (NOS). NOS is a highly regulated enzyme whose activity is probably reduced in advanced atherosclerosis. Endothelial NOS is up-regulated by HMG-CoA inhibitors and this effect may be responsible for some of their clinical efficacy through enhancement of the antioxidant status of the arterial wall. Paradoxically, NO can, under certain circumstances, become highly pro-oxidant. High levels of NO – which can be produced by a different NOS isoform in macrophages/foam cells as well as by endothelial NOS – can combine with high concentrations of oxygen free radicals to form peroxynitrite. Peroxynitrite is a highly reactive pro-oxidant capable of changing protein functions and contributing to the vascular dysfunction in atherosclerosis.

## Inflammatory cells and the atherosclerotic plaque

As early as the 1950s, investigators were aware of the presence of inflammatory cells within atherosclerotic lesions, but this was not really appreciated until many decades later. Postmortem studies of infarct related lesions in coronary arteries demonstrated a localized inflammatory response manifested by accumulation of mononuclear cells[13].The mechanism by which these inflammatory cells are attracted into the arterial wall became an important focus of investigation. Important clues are provided by *in vitro* experiments that demonstrate the expression of leukocyte adhesion molecules on the surface of endothelial cells after cytokine stimulation[14]. Similar observations have been made in the arteries of rabbits after several days of cholesterol feeding. Monocyte adhesion has been observed at arterial branch points and regions of low flow or disturbed flow that are known to be sites of predilection for the development of atherosclerotic lesions. In some areas, the mononuclear cells were seen to have entered into the arterial wall and were located just beneath the overlying endothelial cells. On the endothelial cell surface there was evidence of expression of a new protein that was found to be the rabbit equivalent of human vascular cell adhesion molecule-1 (VCAM-1), which by interaction with its ligand VLA-4 causes adhesion of monocytes and T cells to endothelial cells. Therefore, VCAM-1 is the prototype of a set of molecules that are up-regulated during the very earliest stages of atherosclerosis and are involved in recruiting inflammatory cells into atherosclerotic lesions. Indeed, mice deficient in similar molecules such as intercellular adhesion molecule 1 (ICAM 1) and P selectin develop smaller lesions with less lipid and fewer inflammatory cells than control mice fed a high lipid diet. Interestingly, Marui *et al* have demonstrated that oxygen-derived radicals are involved in the intracellular signalling events controlling VCAM-1 gene expression[15]. They have shown that the VCAM-1 gene is regulated by a reduction/oxidation-dependent activation of the transcription factor NF-κB. Moreover, a number of intracellularly active antioxidants inhibit VCAM-1 expression *in vitro* in cultured endothelial cells and in hypercholesterolaemic animals. In these animals, fatty streak and foam cell formation has been inhibited by antioxidants, even in the presence of very high plasma cholesterol levels, suggesting that antioxidants may inhibit atherosclerosis by mechanisms other than the inhibition of LDL oxidation.

As previously mentioned, small accumulations of subendothelial lipid (particularly oxidised LDL) appear in the arterial wall at the very earliest stages of atherosclerosis. It is unclear to what extent this is a result of endothelial dysfunction and to what extent it causes it. Regardless of which process occurred first, oxidised LDL is a highly inflammatory substance leading to increased expression of selectins and adhesion molecules and also expression of chemokines, in particular monocyte chemo-attractant protein-1 (MCP-1)[16]. Chemokines are pro-inflammatory cytokines that lead to leukocyte chemo-attraction and activation. The importance of chemokines is highlighted by the observation that mice lacking MCP-1 develop much smaller atherosclerotic lesions than those expressing MCP-1. Inflammatory cells which have been 'attracted' in this way from the circulation migrate into the subendothelial space where, under the influence of local chemokines, they become activated. The monocytes develop into macrophages expressing the scavenger receptor necessary to ingest oxidised LDL to form foam cells. Removal of modified LDL is a critical part of the initial protective role of macrophages in the inflammatory response and minimizes the effects of modified LDL on endothelial and vascular smooth muscle cells. Unfortunately, the inflammatory response itself can lead to significant effects on lipoprotein movement into the arterial wall. Specifically, mediators of inflammation such as tumour necrosis factor-$\alpha$ (TNF-$\alpha$), interleukin-1 and macrophage colony stimulating factor increase binding of LDL to endothelium and vascular smooth muscle cells and increase transcription of the LDL receptor. Thus a vicious cycle is set up by the presence of modified lipids in the arterial wall that leads to inflammation which itself causes further modification of lipoproteins that in turn leads to further inflammation and so on.

## Vascular smooth muscle cells and the atherosclerotic plaque

As described above, inflammatory reactions in the subendothelial space result in the production of a large number of cytokines and inflammatory mediators. Many of these are chemo-attractant for the underlying medial VSMCs resulting in their migration into the intima where they form a fibrous cap over the lipid and inflammatory core. In the original response to injury hypothesis, this migration of VSMCs into the intima was seen as the initiating event in the development of a plaque and was thought of as being harmful by causing plaque growth and narrowing of the lumen. However, recent developments in the understanding of the cellular biology of VSMCs have led to a fundamental reversal of views on their effects in the atherosclerotic plaque. Medial VSMCs contain a substantial amount of contractile proteins, which allows them to maintain vascular tone. This contractile phenotype is partly maintained by extracellular signals in the VSMC environment. When VSMCs are taken out of this environment and placed in culture, they undergo a phenotypic change characterized by reduced production of contractile proteins and increased production of synthetic organelles. Interestingly, recent studies have shown a remarkable similarity between the gene expression pattern of intimal VSMCs in atherosclerosis and those in early developing blood vessels[17]. This has led to the hypothesis that intimal VSMCs may be acting in a reparative role. This reparative/synthetic phenotype is associated with the expression of proteinases which break down the underlying basement membrane to allow migration into the site of injury. They produce growth factors that facilitate their proliferation at the site of injury and they produce a range of matrix proteins such as collagens and elastin that may be used to repair injured tissues. It now seems that the expression of these genes is fundamental to the formation of the fibrous cap over the lipid core of atherosclerotic plaques[18]. This role of the VSMC is a critical defence mechanism against the progression of atherosclerosis because it separates the highly thrombogenic lipid core from circulating platelets and the proteins of the coagulation cascade. In addition, it confers structural stability to the plaque. The VSMC is in fact the only cell capable of synthesizing the cap and is, therefore, pivotal in maintaining plaque stability[18].

## Plaque stability

Atherosclerotic lesions can manifest themselves clinically by steady growth leading to a gradual restriction in blood flow such that nutrient supply cannot meet demand as in chronic angina pectoris. The growth of the plaque is gradual and is related to apoptotic death of macrophage foam cells and their incorporation into an enlarging necrotic lipid-laden core as well as the migration of medial VSMCs in response to inflammatory stimuli within the plaque. Alternatively, if the lesion either ruptures or erodes, there is exposure of the thrombogenic lipid core. This results in rapid platelet accumulation, fibrin deposition and thrombosis, leading to the acute coronary syndromes.

Over recent years, it has become apparent that some plaques are inherently more prone to rupture and complications than others of equal size. Careful *post mortem* pathological studies have described several characteristics that seem to be predictive of the risk of rupture in individual lesions[19]. Vulnerable plaques tend to have thin fibrous caps, a high ratio of inflammatory cells to VSMCs in the fibrous cap, a lipid core that occupies more than 50% of the volume of the plaque and a high tissue factor content. The most important of these is the cellular composition of the fibrous cap. Plaques with a heavy inflammatory cell infiltrate and relatively few VSMCs are at highest risk of rupturing. It is thought that the balance of power between the repairing effects of VSMCs and the destructive effects of the inflammatory cells determines fibrous cap integrity and, therefore, plaque stability.

Inflammatory cells can weaken and destroy the fibrous cap through a number of mechanisms. Firstly, activated T-lymphocytes can produce pro-inflammatory cytokines such as interferon-γ (INF-γ), that directly inhibit VSMC proliferation and almost completely shut down collagen synthesis. The result of this is that VSMCs in the vicinity of activated T-lymphocytes are unable to lay down or repair extracellular matrix effectively. Secondly, macrophage derived inflammatory cytokines such as interleukin-1β, TNF-α as well as INF-γ from T lymphocytes are cytotoxic to VSMCs in a synergistic fashion, leading to a reduction in cell numbers through apoptosis. Thirdly, work from our laboratory has shown that activated macrophages can induce VSMC apoptosis by direct cell–cell contact. Fourthly, and perhaps most importantly, macrophages produce a number of matrix metalloproteinases (MMPs) that are capable of degrading matrix components of the fibrous cap by proteolytic cleavage. MMP production appears to be up-regulated by inflammatory mediators such as TNF-α. Furthermore, for reasons that are not entirely clear, VSMCs from mature atherosclerotic plaques appear to have a reduced proliferative ability and an enhanced susceptibility to apoptosis. Thus, the inflammatory process which is central to atherosclerosis can lead to the destruction of intimal VSMCs and the structural framework of the plaque, leading to plaque instability and rupture. It is extremely important to realize that these features are often present in small, angiographically and haemodynamically insignificant atherosclerotic plaques that are clinically silent. In other words, plaque composition is much more important that plaque size in determining the propensity to rupture[20].

Atherosclerotic plaques can cause acute coronary syndromes either through rupture or endothelial cell erosion. Following plaque rupture, there is immediate exposure of the highly thrombogenic extracellular matrix of the cap as well as the tissue factor-rich lipid core to platelets and proteins of the coagulation cascade. This leads to platelet aggregation, activation and clot formation. Less commonly, erosion of the endothelial cells overlying the fibrous cap may occur which can also lead to the build-up of platelet-rich thrombi. Endothelial erosion seems to account for about 30% of acute coronary syndromes, but seems to be more common in women. Both forms of plaque destruction lead to platelet binding, aggregation and activation. This in turn leads to fibrin deposition and activation of the clotting cascade resulting in thrombus formation. However, thrombus extension and vessel occlusion are not inevitable consequences of this process. In a recent clinical study, up to 70% of plaques causing high grade stenosis were found to contain histological evidence of previous plaque rupture and subsequent repair in the absence of vessel occlusion or clinical events[21]. This is particularly likely to occur if high flow through the vessel prevents accumulation of occlusive thrombus. Platelet-rich thrombi contain many chemokines and mitogens, in particular platelet derived growth factor, thrombin and transforming factor β, which can induce migration and proliferation of VSMCs from the underlying media. This, therefore, helps drive formation of a new fibrous cap, thereby increasing the size of the lesion.

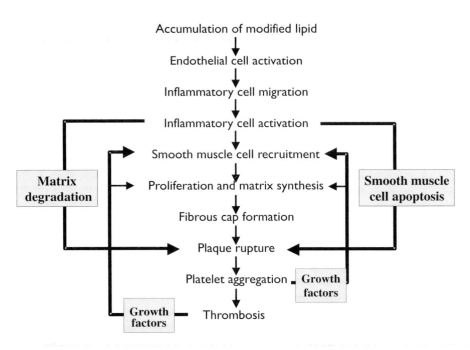

**Fig. 1** Plaque growth and stability.

Since this process occurs rapidly, there is presumably little opportunity for adaptive remodelling of the artery and the healed lesion may now impede flow sufficiently to cause ischaemic symptoms. A major clinical implication of this is that, potentially, pharmacological inhibition of these repeated episodes of plaque rupture would be expected to reduce progression of atherosclerotic lesions. This also explains and re-iterates the importance of antiplatelet drugs in the treatment of atherosclerosis. Thus atheromatous plaques may enlarge either gradually or in a sudden stepwise fashion. Gradual growth is through continued lipid deposition, macrophage apoptosis, and VSMC migration from the media. In contrast, the stepwise growth is due to repeated, often silent episodes of plaque rupture or erosion with secondary VSMC driven migration and repair (Fig. 1).

# Infection

One of the most interesting developments in recent years has been the hypothesis that infectious agents may play a role in atherosclerosis, either through a direct pro-inflammatory effect in the vessel wall or through a less specific, long distance pro-inflammatory effect[22]. *C. pneumoniae* probably remains the most plausible candidate pathogen. It is found within plaques, reaches high concentrations within macrophages and is rarely found in normal arteries. Furthermore, a high titre

(>1:1024) of *C. pneumoniae* is twice as frequent among cases than controls; and a high titre positive serology is associated with an odds ratio of 4 for cardiovascular events within 2 years. However, several prospective studies have failed to confirm these results. Therefore, although evidence for a link between viral and bacterial infections and atherosclerosis grows, a direct causal link remains tantalizingly out of reach. Studies have produced inconsistent results regarding the precise identity of the pathogens involved. It is not certain which organisms are culprits and which are innocent bystanders. Considerable interest was raised by the publication of a small British pilot study showing that short courses of azithromycin reduced coronary events[23]. However, in the subsequent ACADEMIC trial no reduction in cardiovascular events was seen in 2 years after a more reasonable 3 months of antibiotic treatment[24]. The results of two, large, on-going randomized, controlled trials of anti-chlamydia antibiotics (WIZARD and ACES) may give a more definitive answer. Although, the known anti-inflammatory effects of macrolide antibiotics, independent of their antibacterial effects, might cloud the issue.

# Clinical implications of recent scientific advances

*Risk factor evaluation*

The realization that atherosclerosis is essentially an inflammatory condition has prompted a great deal of research into identification of measurable biochemical markers of plaque inflammation. The presumption being that perhaps some of the multitudes of inflammatory mediators discussed above may be measurable in blood and reflect the degree of plaque inflammatory activity and, therefore, in some way relate to plaque instability. Some of these markers probably reflect the degree of plaque macrophage activation. Circulating levels of serum amyloid A (SAA), C-reactive protein (CRP) and TNF-α all correlate with risk of coronary events, but they are non-specific and may simply reflect inflammation or infection elsewhere in the body. The development of a highly sensitive assay to measure CRP (hs-CRP) has allowed the measurement of CRP levels below those of the routine assay. This was used in the Physicians' Health Study which revealed a strong correlation between CRP and the risk of myocardial infarction and stroke[25]. Furthermore, the subjects with the highest CRP levels (but still within the conventional normal range) derived most benefit from prophylactic aspirin. The recently reported Women's Health Study showed that women in the highest quartile of hs-CRP had a cardiovascular risk 4.4 times women in the lowest quartile. The recent CARE study, which was designed to look at the effects of pravastatin in post-myocardial infarction patients with a moderately raised cholesterol, confirmed the association between vascular risk and CRP levels[26]. Moreover, it also showed that even though the CRP level rose over 5 years in the placebo group, it fell in association with vascular event risk in the treatment group. Interestingly, this reduction was not correlated with the magnitude of the decrease in serum lipids in the treatment group.

Proteolysis of cell surface molecules such as ICAM-1, VCAM-1, E-selectin and P-selectin (which are up-regulated during atherosclerotic inflammation) may provide more specific markers of vascular risk than the general markers described above. In one study, Ridker and colleagues showed that soluble ICAM-1 levels were independently predictive of the risk of cardiovascular events in apparently healthy men, with levels in the highest quartile conferring an increased risk of 80% compared with those in the lowest quartile[27]. Although soluble ICAM-1 levels were strongly correlated with CRP levels, adjustment for CRP levels did not substantially decrease the relative risk associated with an elevated level of ICAM-1. This finding suggests that levels of soluble adhesion molecules may provide predictive information that is additive to the information provided by levels of general inflammatory markers.

What are the implications of the finding of multiple serum-based inflammatory markers that are predictive of the risk of cardiovascular events? It is now generally agreed that although evaluation of traditional factors produces reasonably accurate estimates of population risk, it fails to predict 40–50% of the variation in the absolute risk of an event in individual patients. Therefore, the addition of other factors that would increase the predictive ability would also probably improve the accuracy of decisions regarding the use of proven therapies for prevention. When Ridker made a comparison of the usefulness of various serum based markers, he found that the effects of inflammatory markers and those of lipids were obviously additive with respect to the ability to predict cardiovascular risk. Therefore, the argument has been made that the measurement of highly validated inflammatory markers such as CRP in selected patients may increase the clinical accuracy of assessments of cardiovascular risk. However, at the time of writing, more work is required before the levels of soluble, vascular specific, adhesion molecules such as ICAM-1 may be used for clinical risk assessment.

## Imaging

The realization that plaque composition is far more important than plaque size has important implications for the practice of clinical cardiology. The mainstay of much of clinical practice is the angiogram. However, angiography can only detect lesions which impinge significantly on the lumen. It provides little or no information on plaque composition. Since it is plaque composition which determines the risk of rupture, it follows that angiography is a poor predictor of clinical events[20]. Therefore, two lesions of equivalent size, one of which is stable and the other unstable, may look identical angiographically. Furthermore, as far back as the 1980s[28], it was known that arteries can accommodate large atherosclerotic plaques, without reducing lumen size, by 'remodelling'. This is a process in which the artery expands as the plaque increases in size. Therefore, large atherosclerotic plaques can be clinically silent and sometimes angiographically invisible. Falk and colleagues have convincingly demonstrated that most lesions which lead to myocardial infarction are due to rupture of plaques which cause less than 50% stenosis on angiography[20]. These observations emphasize the importance of developing newer and more useful diagnostic tools than angiography for the identification of unstable atherosclerotic plaques. One such approach has been the detection of coronary artery calcification using electron beam computed tomography (EBCT) since calcium apatite crystals are an intimate component of the plaque as early as the fatty streak stage[29]. A positive correlation has been shown between coronary calcium score, as measured by EBCT, and subsequent clinical events in patients with known coronary artery disease. However, the extent to which this predicts coronary events independently of traditional risk factors – particularly in asymptomatic patients – needs further study. The National Institutes of Health funded multi-ethnic study of atherosclerosis (MESA) will provide some of these data over the next decade.

Over the next few years, developments in magnetic resonance imaging (MRI) and radionucleotide-based techniques, especially positron emission tomography (PET), may allow non-invasive imaging of plaque composition. Presently, MRI can differentiate some plaque components in animal models and human vessels. However, image resolution and movement artefact remain obstacles to the use of MRI in coronary vessels. Furthermore, although MRI might provide fine anatomical detail, it seems unlikely that it will be able to provide information on plaque inflammatory activity. In contrast, PET provides very little anatomical detail but offers the potential of measuring and monitoring plaque inflammatory cell activity. Fuster and colleagues have demonstrated positive PET images of atherosclerotic plaques in cholesterol-fed rabbits using fluorinated deoxyglucose (a glucose substrate which is taken up by cells through the glucose transporter in proportion to their metabolic activity)[30]. This has been presumed to reflect inflammatory cell activity. Preliminary work in our laboratory has suggested that this technique may be applicable in human arteries.

*Statins*

Angiographic studies have shown that statins reduce the incidence of new lesion formation and produce significant, but haemodynamically negligible improvements in lumen diameter[31]. In contrast to these somewhat disappointing angiographic results, several large outcome studies, both in primary and secondary prevention of vascular events, have shown an impressive and consistent reduction (30–40%) in clinical events among patients receiving statins[32,33]. The only plausible explanation seems to be that statins are reducing new lesion formation and preventing rupture of pre-existing plaques. In other words, statins stabilize plaques. It is likely that most of this effect is directly due to lipid lowering because all lipid lowering studies have shown a reduction in cardiovascular events. However, statins do have a number of other biological properties that may influence plaque stability and inflammation. For example, statins have been shown to exert direct effects on endothelial cell function, inflammatory cell activity, VSMC proliferation, platelet aggregation and thrombus formation. The best evidence for the beneficial effects of statins independent of lipid lowering comes from the laboratory of Libby[34]. In this important study, monkeys were fed an atherogenic diet for 2 years so that they all developed atherosclerosis. The monkeys were then put on lipid lowering diets for a further 2 years and subdivided into two groups, one of which received pravastatin. The diet was adjusted so that each group had similar cholesterol levels. At the end of the study both groups had similar sized lesions but, compared with the untreated group, the pravastatin treated group had better endothelial function, and their atherosclerotic lesions contained fewer macrophages, less calcification and fewer new vessels, implying greater stability. More recent studies by Aikawa[35] and Crisby[36] strongly support the notion that statins act by reducing plaque inflammation.

## Conclusions

Atherosclerosis is a dynamic process in which the risk of plaque rupture and therefore outcome is determined by the balance between destructive inflammatory cell activity and the reparative effects of VSMCs. This balance can be modified beneficially by medical therapy, particularly with statins. Understanding the cellular events involved offers exciting therapeutic and diagnostic opportunities for the future. Possible therapeutic targets include adhesion molecules, MMPs, infectious pathogens, inflammatory cytokines and their receptors. Given the potential importance of oxidative stress in the pathogenesis of atherosclerosis, there are many theoretical reasons for believing that antioxidants might be beneficial. Unfortunately, results from recent clinical trials have been inconsistent and further work is required to resolve this issue. Stimulation of VSMC repair is also a potential therapeutic aim. This is currently achieved – rather crudely – with balloon angioplasty, which stimulates a vigorous VSMC response to create a matrix-rich neointima. Although this may lead to restenosis, the resulting lesion rarely, if ever, precipitates an acute coronary syndrome, even when the original target lesion was unstable. In the future, utilization of modulators of VSMC proliferation and matrix production may lead to new therapies aimed at strengthening the protective fibrous cap.

# Key points for clinical practice

- High-risk lesions are not necessarily angiographically severe

- Unstable, high risk lesions, are the ones composed of large lipid cores and thin fibrous caps

- Plaque instability is related to the development of inflammation

- Statins may stabilize lesions by altering the inflammatory response

## References

1   Ross R. Atherosclerosis – an inflammatory disease. *N Engl J Med* 1999; **340**: 115–26
2   Ross R, Glomset JA. The pathogenesis of atherosclerosis (first of two parts). *N Engl J Med* 1976; **295**: 369–77
3   Ross R, Glomset J, Harker L. Response to injury and atherogenesis. *Am J Pathol* 1977; **86**: 675–84
4   Ludmer PL, Selwyn AP, Shook TL *et al*. Paradoxical vasoconstriction induced by acetylcholine in atherosclerotic coronary arteries. *N Engl J Med* 1986; **315**: 1046–51
5   Furchgott RF, Zawadzki JV. The obligatory role of endothelial cells in the relaxation of arterial smooth muscle by acetylcholine. *Nature* 1980; **288**: 373–6
6   Forstermann U, Pollock JS, Schmidt HH, Heller M, Murad F. Calmodulin-dependent endothelium-derived relaxing factor/nitric oxide synthase activity is present in the particulate and cytosolic fractions of bovine aortic endothelial cells. *Proc Natl Acad Sci USA* 1991; **88**: 1788–92
7   Moncada S. The 1991 Ulf von Euler Lecture. The L-arginine: nitric oxide pathway. *Acta Physiol Scand* 1992; **145**: 201–27
8   Sorensen KE, Celermajer DS, Georgakopoulos D, Hatcher G, Betteridge DJ, Deanfield JE. Impairment of endothelium-dependent dilation is an early event in children with familial hypercholesterolemia and is related to the lipoprotein(a) level. *J Clin Invest* 1994; **93**: 50–5
9   Berliner JA, Navab M, Fogelman AM *et al*. Atherosclerosis: basic mechanisms. Oxidation, inflammation, and genetics. *Circulation* 1995; **91**: 2488–96
10  Steinbrecher UP, Parthasarathy S, Leake DS, Witztum JL, Steinberg D. Modification of low density lipoprotein by endothelial cells involves lipid peroxidation and degradation of low density lipoprotein phospholipids. *Proc Natl Acad Sci USA* 1984; **81**: 3883–7
11  Steinberg D, Parthasarathy S, Carew TE, Khoo JC, Witztum JL. Beyond cholesterol. Modifications of low-density lipoprotein that increase its atherogenicity. *N Engl J Med* 1989; **320**: 915–24
12  Harrison DG. Cellular and molecular mechanisms of endothelial cell dysfunction. *J Clin Invest* 1997; **100**: 2153–7
13  van der Wal AC, Becker AE, van der Loos CM, Das PK. Site of intimal rupture or erosion of thrombosed coronary atherosclerotic plaques is characterized by an inflammatory process irrespective of the dominant plaque morphology. *Circulation* 1994; **89**: 36–44
14  Cybulsky MI, Gimbrone MA. Endothelial expression of a mononuclear leukocyte adhesion molecule during atherogenesis. *Science* 1991; **251**: 788–91
15  Marui N, Offermann MK, Swerlick R *et al*. Vascular cell adhesion molecule-1 (VCAM-1) gene transcription and expression are regulated through an antioxidant-sensitive mechanism in human

vascular endothelial cells. *J Clin Invest* 1993; **92**: 1866–74

16  Berliner JA, Schwartz DS, Territo MC *et al*. Induction of chemotactic cytokines by minimally oxidized LDL. *Adv Exp Med Biol* 1993; **351**: 13–8

17  Shanahan CM, Weissberg PL. Smooth muscle cell phenotypes in atherosclerotic lesions. *Curr Opin Lipidol* 1999; **10**: 507–13

18  Libby P. Molecular bases of the acute coronary syndromes. *Circulation* 1995; **91**: 2844–50

19  Davies MJ. Stability and instability: two faces of coronary atherosclerosis. The Paul Dudley White Lecture 1995. *Circulation* 1996; **94**: 2013–20

20  Falk E, Shah PK, Fuster V. Coronary plaque disruption. *Circulation* 1995; **92**: 657–71

21  Davies MJ. Acute coronary thrombosis – the role of plaque disruption and its initiation and prevention. *Eur Heart J* 1995; **16 (Suppl L)**: 3–7

22  Shah PK. Link between infection and atherosclerosis: who are the culprits: viruses, bacteria, both, or neither? *Circulation* 2001; **103**: 5–6

23  Gupta S, Leatham EW, Carrington D, Mendall MA, Kaski JC, Camm AJ. Elevated *Chlamydia pneumoniae* antibodies, cardiovascular events, and azithromycin in male survivors of myocardial infarction. *Circulation* 1997; **96**: 404–7

24  Muhlestein JB, Anderson JL, Carlquist JF *et al*. Randomized secondary prevention trial of azithromycin in patients with coronary artery disease: primary clinical results of the ACADEMIC study. *Circulation* 2000; **102**: 1755–60

25  Ridker PM, Cushman M, Stampfer MJ, Tracy RP, Hennekens CH. Inflammation, aspirin, and the risk of cardiovascular disease in apparently healthy men. *N Engl J Med* 1997; **336**: 973–9

26  Ridker PM, Rifai N, Pfeffer MA *et al*. Inflammation, pravastatin, and the risk of coronary events after myocardial infarction in patients with average cholesterol levels. Cholesterol and Recurrent Events (CARE) Investigators. *Circulation* 1998; **98**: 839–44

27  Ridker PM, Hennekens CH, Roitman-Johnson B, Stampfer MJ, Allen J. Plasma concentration of soluble intercellular adhesion molecule 1 and risks of future myocardial infarction in apparently healthy men. *Lancet* 1998; **351**: 88–92

28  Glagov S, Weisenberg E, Zarins CK, Stankunavicius R, Kolettis GJ. Compensatory enlargement of human atherosclerotic coronary arteries. *N Engl J Med* 1987; **316**: 1371–5

29  Farzaneh-Far A, Proudfoot D, Shanahan C, Weissberg PL. Vascular and valvar calcification: recent advances. *Heart* 2001; **85**: 13–7

30  Vallabhajosula S. Radioisotopic imaging of atheroma. In: Fuster V. (ed) *The Vulnerable Atherosclerotic Plaque: Understanding, Identification, and Modification*. New York: Futura, 1999; 213–29

31  Anon. Effect of simvastatin on coronary atheroma: the Multicentre Anti-Atheroma Study (MAAS). *Lancet* 1994; **344**: 633–8

32  Anon. Prevention of cardiovascular events and death with pravastatin in patients with coronary heart disease and a broad range of initial cholesterol levels. The Long-Term Intervention with Pravastatin in Ischaemic Disease (LIPID) Study Group. *N Engl J Med* 1998; **339**: 1349–57

33  Anon. Randomised trial of cholesterol lowering in 4444 patients with coronary heart disease: the Scandinavian Simvastatin Survival Study (4S). *Lancet* 1994; **344**: 1383–9

34  Williams JK, Sukhova GK, Herrington DM, Libby P. Pravastatin has cholesterol-lowering independent effects on the artery wall of atherosclerotic monkeys. *J Am Coll Cardiol* 1998; **31**: 684–91

35  Aikawa M, Rabkin E, Sugiyama S *et al*. An HMG-CoA reductase inhibitor, cerivastatin, suppresses growth of macrophages expressing matrix metalloproteinases and tissue factor *in vivo* and *in vitro*. *Circulation* 2001; **103**: 276–83

36  Crisby M, Nordin-Fredriksson G, Shah PK, Yano J, Zhu J, Nilsson J. Pravastatin treatment increases collagen content and decreases lipid content, inflammation, metalloproteinases, and cell death in human carotid plaques: implications for plaque stabilization. *Circulation* 2001; **103**: 926–33

# Unstable angina: the first 48 hours and later in-hospital management

**David E Newby** and **Keith A A Fox**

*Department of Cardiology, Edinburgh Royal Infirmary, Edinburgh, UK*

Unstable angina is a common cardiovascular condition associated with major adverse clinical events. Over the last 15 years, therapeutic advances have dramatically reduced the complication and mortality rates of this serious condition. The standard of therapy in patients with unstable angina now incorporates the combined use of potent antithrombotic (aspirin, clopidogrel, heparin and glycoprotein IIb/IIIa receptor antagonists) and anti-anginal (β-blockade and intravenous nitrates) regimens complemented by the selective and judicious application of coronary revascularisation strategies. Increasingly, these invasive and non-invasive therapeutic interventions are being guided not only by the clinical risk profile but also by the determination of serum cardiac and inflammatory markers. Moreover, rapid and intensive management of associated risk factors, such as hypercholesterolaemia, would appear to have potentially substantial benefits even within the acute in-hospital phase of unstable angina.

Unstable angina can be ascribed to a range of patients with different clinical presentations and characteristics. Moreover, it should be recognised that much of the trial evidence, upon which this article is based, includes patients with non-Q-wave or non-ST elevation myocardial infarction. This reflects the common pattern of clinical presentation and the inevitable delay in obtaining cardiac enzyme estimations that ultimately determine the diagnostic category of the acute coronary syndrome.

Each year, unstable angina accounts for over 115,000 acute hospital admissions in the UK (~200 per 100,000 population) with a significant male preponderance. Throughout Europe, hospital admission rates for unstable angina exceed those of ST elevation myocardial infarction[1]. Ten years ago, before the advent of modern therapeutic interventions, 15% of patients with unstable angina progressed to sustain an acute myocardial infarction and the overall in-hospital mortality was up to 5%. The PRAIS-UK study[2] recently estimated the contemporary impact of unstable angina in the UK by collecting data on 20 consecutive admissions to 56 representative hospital centres. This observational

*Correspondence to:*
*Dr David E Newby,*
*Department of Cardiology,*
*The Royal Infirmary,*
*Lauriston Place,*
*Edinburgh EH3 9YW, UK*

**Table 1** Classification of unstable angina[3]

| | CLINICAL PRESENTATION |
|---|---|
| Class I | New onset, severe, or accelerated angina. |
| | Patients with angina of less than 2 months' duration, severe or occurring three or more times per day, or angina that is distinctly more frequent and precipitated by distinctly less exertion. No rest pain in the last 2 months. |
| Class II | Angina at rest – subacute. |
| | Patients with one or more episodes of angina at rest during the preceding month but not within the preceding 48 h. |
| Class III | Angina at rest – acute. |
| | Patients with one or more episodes of angina at rest during the preceding 48 h. |
| | CLINICAL CONTEXT |
| Class A | Secondary unstable angina. |
| | A clearly defined condition extrinsic to the coronary vascular bed that has intensified myocardial ischaemia, *e.g.* anaemia, infection, fever, hypotension, tachyarrhythmia, thyrotoxicosis, hypoxaemia. |
| Class B | Primary unstable angina. |
| Class C | Post-infarction unstable angina. |
| | Within 2 weeks of documented myocardial infarction. |
| | THERAPEUTIC INTERVENTION |
| 1 | Absence of, or minimal treatment. |
| 2 | Occurring in the presence of standard therapy for chronic stable angina. |
| 3 | Occurring despite maximally tolerated doses of all three categories of oral therapy, including intravenous nitrates. |

Class IIIB has been further sub-divided into IIIB-T$_{pos}$ and IIIB-T$_{neg}$ to reflect the marked differences in prognostic risk conferred by the presence or absence of an elevation in troponin I or T concentrations.[3]

study reported that the in-hospital event rates for unstable angina included a 2% mortality rate, 4% progression to myocardial infarction and 3% recurrence of refractory ischaemia. By 6 months this had risen to 7% mortality, 7% myocardial infarction and 17% recurrent myocardial ischaemia. One year after the index episode of unstable angina, the cardiovascular event rate had returned to that of patients with stable angina and a similar risk factor profile.

# Clinical presentation

Patients with unstable angina present with prolonged anginal chest pain that may occur at rest or be precipitated by progressively less exertion. This may present on a background of chronic stable angina or as a *de novo* phenomenon. Although this is a heterogeneous group of patients, the Braunwald classification attempts to provide an objective description of the clinical presentation and context as well as the response to therapy (Table 1).

Physical examination is directed towards the identification of potential precipitants such as anaemia, confounding cardiac conditions such as critical aortic stenosis and complications of cardiac ischaemia such as hypotension or heart failure. This may also reveal the extent of co-existent vascular disease such as the presence of vascular bruits or absence of peripheral pulses.

# Preliminary investigations

## Electrocardiogram

The electrocardiogram will often, but not always, show evidence of ischaemia that classically takes the form of ST segment depression, T wave inversion and new bundle branch block. Frequent repeated recordings should be made, particularly in the early acute phase and/or in the presence of ongoing chest pain. Ischaemic electrocardiographic changes provide important markers of an adverse prognosis[2] with the presence, and degree, of ST segment depression being independent predictors of mortality[4,5]. They also identify those patients with the most to gain from therapeutic interventions such as percutaneous coronary intervention[6].

## Cardiac and inflammatory markers

The measurement of cardiac enzymes in the first 24 h provides not only diagnostic but also prognostic information in patients with unstable angina[5,7]. As with the electrocardiogram, an elevation in the cardiac troponin identifies those patients who benefit most from interventions such as glycoprotein IIb/IIIa receptor antagonism[8,9] and percutaneous coronary intervention[6].

C-reactive protein, a marker of inflammation, provides further prognostic information in patients presenting with unstable angina[10] that is independent of the presence of myocardial damage. Recent evidence has also suggested that the combined measure of C-reactive protein and troponin provides additive information and that together they are powerful predictors of long-term outcome in patients with unstable angina[5].

## Secondary causes of unstable angina

Occasionally, unstable angina may be precipitated, or exacerbated, by an intercurrent illness (Braunwald class A). Therefore, guided investigation of potential precipitants should be undertaken, but as a

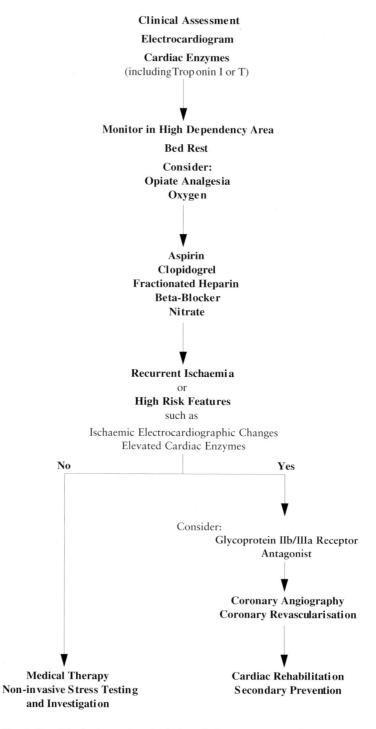

**Fig. 1** Simplified scheme for the in-hospital management of patients with unstable angina.

minimum haemoglobin concentration, oxygen saturation, and thyroid function should be assessed. In patients presenting within 24 h of pain onset, serum total cholesterol concentration may be determined although the full serum lipid profile will need to be re-assessed following complete recovery.

# Immediate management – the first 48 h

Patients should be transferred to a high dependency area with the provision of haemodynamic and cardiac monitoring, and ready access to resuscitation facilities. The patient should be restricted to bed rest, and opiate analgesia and oxygen therapy given as appropriate. Complications of severe myocardial ischaemia, such as haemodynamic compromise or arrhythmias, should be treated as appropriate (see elsewhere in this volume).

Initial specific therapeutic interventions are targeted at the prevention of thrombotic vessel occlusion, the reduction in myocardial oxygen demand and the enhancement of coronary blood flow (Fig. 1).

## Antithrombotic therapy

### Antiplatelet therapy

#### Aspirin

Aspirin has a relatively short plasma half-life of 1–2 h, but is able to inhibit long-term platelet activity by irreversible acetylation of the platelet cyclooxygenase enzyme, thereby preventing thromboxane $A_2$ formation. Although a weak inhibitor of platelet aggregation, aspirin is associated with major clinical benefits[11] that may, in part, relate to its additional anti-inflammatory action[12].

The efficacy of aspirin therapy in patients with unstable angina was first described nearly 20 years ago. The Veterans Administration Cooperative Study[13] of 1266 men with unstable angina demonstrated a 50% reduction in the risk of death or myocardial infarction. The more recent meta-analysis by the Antiplatelet Trialists Collaboration incontrovertibly confirmed the benefits of aspirin therapy in patients with unstable angina[11]. Because of this marked reduction in the risk of cardiovascular death, MI and stroke, all patients with unstable angina pectoris should be commenced on aspirin therapy.

Aspirin has been used at various dosages (80–325 mg) but a reasonable dosage regimen is an initial 300 mg stat followed by a maintenance dose of 75 mg daily. The initial 300 mg dose is sufficient to achieve maximal anti-platelet effects and maintenance inhibition is achieved by 75 mg daily. This attempts to achieve maximum efficacy whilst minimising the dose related gastrointestinal side effects of aspirin.

*Thienopyridines*

Thienopyridines inhibit platelet aggregation through blockade of the platelet adenosine diphosphate receptor. Ticlopidine was the first licensed thienopyridine to achieve widespread clinical use. In the STAI trial, administration of ticlopidine (250 mg bd) was associated with a halving of event rates in patients with unstable angina[14]. However, this trial was conducted in the absence of aspirin therapy and it is unclear whether combination therapy would achieve additional benefits.

Ticlopidine has been largely superceded by a closely related analogue, clopidogrel, since the latter is better tolerated and, unlike ticlopidine, does not cause significant bone marrow toxicity. In the CAPRIE trial[15], long-term clopidogrel treatment (75 mg daily) was at least as efficacious as aspirin in preventing ischaemic stroke, myocardial infarction or cardiovascular death in patients with atherosclerotic vascular disease. Although the overall secondary preventative benefits of clopidogrel statistically exceeded that of aspirin, the relative benefits were modest (relative risk reduction, 8.7%; $P = 0.04$). Recently, the preliminary results from the CURE study have been reported[16]. This trial was a comparison of aspirin with the combination of aspirin and clopidogrel in 12,562 patients with unstable angina. At a mean follow-up of 9 months, there was a 20% relative risk reduction in the composite primary end point of cardiovascular death, myocardial infarction or stroke (odds ratio of 0.80, 95% confidence intervals of 0.72–0.89; $P < 0.001$). The benefits of therapy were apparent within the first 24 h and were predominantly seen within the first 90 days. As expected, there was a modest increase in the risk of bleeding, but this was predominantly confined to minor bleeding events.

*Glycoprotein IIb/IIIa receptor antagonists*

The evidence for the use of glycoprotein IIb/IIIa receptor antagonists in the treatment of patients with unstable angina is confusing and, at times, contradictory. This, in part, results from the diversity of compounds (peptidic, non-peptidic and oral agents), receptor binding avidity (short and long receptor dissociation half lives) and pharmacokinetic profiles. Although glycoprotein IIb/IIIa receptor antagonists effectively prevent platelet aggregation, they do not inhibit platelet activation, secretion or adhesion. Indeed, this class of compounds may paradoxically cause platelet activation.

Clinical trials have demonstrated that certain agents appear to be most appropriate under specific circumstances. In patients with unstable angina, intravenous tirofiban or eptifibatide administration is associated with a significant reduction in the composite end-point of death, myocardial infarction or refractory ischaemia out to 6 months of follow-up[17,18]. This benefit was independent of percutaneous coronary intervention. In contrast, intravenous abciximab has been shown to be of benefit in the context of percutaneous coronary intervention[19,20] and has superior efficacy in comparison to tirofiban in this setting[21]. However, abciximab administration does not appear to be beneficial in patients with unstable angina outwith the context of percutaneous coronary intervention[23].

A meta-analysis of 16 randomized controlled trials incorporating 32,135 patients confirmed glycoprotein IIb/IIIa receptor antagonists have modest beneficial effects (relative risk reduction of 14%) in patients during percutaneous coronary intervention or acute coronary syndromes[24].

### Summary of antiplatelet therapy

All patients with unstable angina should be given oral aspirin and clopidogrel therapy (300 mg stat and 75 mg maintenance for both). The use of intravenous glycoprotein IIb/IIIa receptor antagonists should be reserved for patients with severe refractory ischaemia or, in particular, those undergoing urgent percutaneous coronary intervention.

## Anti-coagulant therapy

### Unfractionated heparin

Heparin is composed of a range of different sized glycosaminoglycans that bind to antithrombin III and accentuate the inhibition of thrombin and factor Xa. The benefits of heparin therapy in patients with unstable angina are well established and widely accepted. A meta-analysis of six randomised controlled trials demonstrated that, in addition to aspirin, intravenous heparin conferred a relative risk reduction of 33% in the risk of death or myocardial infarction[25].

The use of unfractionated heparin is hindered by its unpredictable efficacy that necessitates monitoring of its anticoagulant effects and dose adjustments. Moreover, idiosyncratic reactions, such as heparin-induced thrombocytopaenia, do occur and can cause serious clinical problems.

### Fractionated heparin

Fractionated or low molecular weight heparins have several advantages over unfractionated heparin. They have a greater selectivity for factor Xa inhibition, have less non-specific protein binding properties and produce more potent inhibition of thrombin generation. In particular, their ease of administration, the reduced incidence of idiosyncratic reactions, and the more predictable pharmacokinetics and pharmacodynamics makes their clinical use especially attractive.

There have been four major randomised controlled trials that have compared fractionated and unfractionated heparin in patients with unstable angina – the FRIC[26], ESSENCE[27], TIMI-11B[28] and FRAXIS[29] trials. Fractionated heparins appear to have equivalent benefits to unfractionated heparin[30] and, particularly in the case of enoxaparin, may have superior efficacy in the prevention of death, myocardial infarction or recurrent angina: relative risk reduction of 15–18%[27,28]. These potential additional benefits are modest, but are predominantly seen in high-risk patients during the early acute phase and are sustained at 1-year follow-up[31]. There is little evidence to suggest that the continuation of fractionated heparin therapy beyond 7 days confers any additional benefit[30,55].

### Antithrombin therapy

Hirudin is a peptidic and direct thrombin inhibitor that, in comparison to heparin, may possess additional and more complete anticoagulant actions. However, in the GUSTO IIb trial[32] of patients with unstable angina, hirudin (desirudin) had only modest benefits in comparison to unfractionated heparin. These benefits principally consisted of an early reduction in the rate of myocardial infarction at 24 h, but this was not sustained at 30 days (relative risk reduction 11%, $P = 0.06$). The subsequent OASIS-1[33] and OASIS-2[34] trials of hirudin (lepirudin) again showed a small benefit above unfractionated heparin at 30 days (relative risk reduction 14%, $P = 0.04$)[35]. Other direct thrombin inhibitors, such as inogatran and hirulog, are also under clinical evaluation and development, but again have yet to demonstrate clinically meaningful superior efficacy in comparison to heparin. Given the potential additional benefits of fractionated heparin, the routine use of direct antithrombins has not been widely accepted or implemented.

### Summary of anticoagulant therapy

The major clinical benefits of anticoagulant therapy in patients with unstable angina are clear. In a recent meta-analysis, the use of fractionated or unfractionated heparin is associated with a relative risk reduction of 47% ($P < 0.001$) in comparison to placebo or control[30]. Although the superiority of a specific anticoagulant therapeutic approach has yet to be definitively established, the use of fractionated heparin has the advantage of ease of administration without the requirement for therapeutic monitoring. Moreover, enoxaparin may confer a sustained small reduction in clinical events with evidence to suggest a reduction in health care costs[36].

## Reduction in myocardial oxygen demand and enhancement of coronary blood flow

### Beta-blockers

β-Blockers inhibit the $\beta_1$-adrenergic receptors of the myocardium to produce negative chronotropism and negative inotropism of the heart. The attenuation of the heart rate response to exercise and stress reduces the myocardial oxygen demand and severity of ischaemia. The impact is also to prolong diastole, a major determinant of myocardial perfusion time. Randomised controlled trials in chronic stable angina have demonstrated that β-blocker therapy is efficacious in reducing symptoms of angina, episodes of ischaemia and improving exercise capacity[37,38]. Moreover, a meta-analysis of post-myocardial infarction trials has demonstrated a 23% relative risk reduction in mortality in patients maintained on long-term β-blocker therapy[39].

The direct evidence for unstable angina is limited but, in a meta-analysis of trials incorporating nearly 5000 patients with unstable angina, β-blocker therapy reduced the risk of myocardial infarction by 13% (1–23 %; $P$ <0.04)[40]. Because of the inferred benefit from post-myocardial infarction trials, β-blocker therapy has become established as the first line medication in unstable angina. Intravenous preparations should be considered particularly in the presence of on-going pain or tachycardia, and titrated to reduce the resting heart rate below 70 beats per minute. Caution should be exercised in patients with acute pulmonary oedema, bradycardia and bronchospasm.

### Nitrates

Nitrates were the first form of anti-anginal drug therapy to be discovered and utilized. Their mechanism of action is exerted through the direct or indirect release of nitric oxide causing vaso- and venodilatation. This results in a reduction in cardiac preload and afterload as well as causing epicardial vasodilatation to increase coronary blood flow.

Nitrates are an effective method of alleviating acute anginal chest pain and, in order to produce rapid control of symptoms, should be administered intravenously to all patients with unstable angina, particularly where it is complicated by pulmonary oedema[41]. Randomised controlled trials in patients with chronic stable angina have demonstrated that nitrates are also effective in reducing the long-term frequency of anginal symptoms and improving exercise capacity[42,43]. However, there is no trial evidence to show that acute or chronic nitrate use has any prognostic or long-term benefits in patients with unstable or stable angina.

One of the main limitations of nitrate use is the development of tolerance that can occur from 24 h after the initiation of continuous parenteral administration. The development of nitrate tolerance appears, at least in part, to be due to the depletion of sulphydryl groups and can be rectified by the provision of a nitrate-free period.

### Calcium channel blockers

Dihydropyridine calcium channel blockers, such as nifedipine and amlodipine, cause coronary and systemic vasodilatation thereby improving coronary blood flow and reducing cardiac afterload. Reflex tachycardia may, however, limit their use in the absence of rate limiting medication, such as β-blockers. Non-dihydropyridine calcium channel blockers, such as verapamil and diltiazem, have additional negative chronotropic and more pronounced negative inotropic actions that also serve to reduce myocardial oxygen demand.

Although there is a suggestion that dihydropyridines, especially nifedipine, are associated with an adverse outcome in patients with unstable angina[44], overall calcium antagonists appear to have a neutral effect on outcome[40]. Moreover, post-myocardial infarction trials suggest that rate limiting non-dihydropyridine calcium channel antagonist, such as verapamil[45] and diltiazem[46], may have modest prognostic benefits in the absence of heart failure. Therefore, rate-limiting non-dihydropyridine calcium antagonists should be reserved as second line agents in patients with contra-indications to β-blocker therapy or those with resistant anginal symptoms.

### Potassium channel openers

This is a novel class of anti-anginal therapy that has vasodilator and potential cardioprotective actions. Potassium channel openers act on the ion channels of the vascular smooth muscle cell and cardiac myocyte. Consequently, they may have a role in enhancing ischaemic precon-ditioning and improving the myocardial response to an ischaemic insult.

Currently, nicorandil is the only preparation of this class in clinical use. It is effective in the treatment of angina and has both nitrate and potassium channel opening properties. In the first small randomised controlled trial of patients with unstable angina[47], nicorandil use was associated with a reduction in myocardial ischaemia and arrhythmias. However, whether this translates into reductions in major clinical events has yet to be established.

### Intra-aortic balloon pump

Intra-aortic balloon counterpulsation has two main beneficial haemo-dynamic effects in the setting of unstable angina: the augmentation of diastolic aortic and coronary perfusion pressure as well as the reduction in cardiac afterload and myocardial oxygen demand. Reflecting the invasive nature and the associated potential vascular complications of this approach, the insertion of an intra-aortic balloon pump is usually reserved for patients with haemodynamic instability or severe refractory angina, especially as a bridge to coronary angiography and definitive coronary revascularisation. Although there have been no randomised controlled trials in patients with unstable angina, its use is associated with marked clinical improvements in refractory unstable cases.

# Later in-hospital management

## Risk assessment

The identification of patients at risk of future events will help guide the further investigation and management of patients with unstable angina. Those at particular high risk, have most to gain from further intensive and invasive treatment[6,22].

There are several useful clinical markers of risk that have been identified from trial data (Table 2)[48,49]. These factors are associated with failure of medical therapy and can be used to help guide the identification of patients who should be considered for cardiac catheterisation and potential coronary revascularisation.

### Non-invasive stress testing

Pre-discharge non-invasive stress testing is often employed in low-risk patients who have been free of ischaemia for 12–24 h, or intermediate risk for 2 or more days. This is performed in the absence of direct evidence since the prognostic information it provides is based on patients with stable ischaemic heart disease. It should be appreciated that non-invasive testing may be falsely re-assuring since in many cases unstable angina is precipitated by thrombus formation on a small non-stenotic plaque. Moreover, an initially positive stress test may become negative following a period of convalescence due to plaque remodelling.

There are three main modalities of stress testing: electrocardiography, radionuclide myocardial perfusion scintigraphy and echocardiography. There are significant advantages and disadvantages with each modality, but exercise electrocardiography remains the most widely used non-invasive test since it is easily performed and has been extensively validated. However, the sensitivity and specificity of exercise electrocardiography is

**Table 2** Variables associated with an adverse prognosis in patients with unstable angina[48,49]

- Age 65 years or older
- Three or more risk factors for coronary artery disease*, particular family history of coronary disease
- Prior coronary stenosis of more than 50% or previous history of angina
- ST segment deviation on the electrocardiogram at presentation
- ST segment deviation despite medical therapy
- Two or more anginal episodes within previous 24 h
- Aspirin use prior to admission
- Elevated cardiac markers (creatinine kinase and troponin)

•*Family history of coronary artery disease, hypertension, diabetes mellitus, smoking habit, hypercholesterolaemia.

**Table 3** Non-invasive stress testing in patients with ischaemic heart disease: features that are particularly associated with a poor prognosis and indicative of severe disease

EXERCISE ELECTROCARDIOGRAM

- Poor maximal exercise capacity (< stage 3 of the Bruce Protocol)
- ≥ 1 mm ST depression during stage 2 or less (Bruce Protocol)
- ≥ 2 mm ST depression at any time
- Limited blood pressure response, *i.e.* fall or no rise from baseline

MYOCARDIAL PERFUSION SCINTIGRAPHY

- Reversible radionuclide perfusion defect in more than one territory
- Reduced radionuclide ejection fraction with exercise
- Increased lung uptake of radionuclide

STRESS ECHOCARDIOGRAPHY

- Wall motion abnormality involving more than two segments developing at low stress
- (dobutamine dose of ≤ 10 mg/mg/min) or heart rate
- Evidence of extensive ischaemia

reduced by intraventricular conduction defects, repolarization abnormalities, poor exercise tolerance and concomitant cardiac medications such as digitalis. Myocardial perfusion scintigraphy, during pharmacological or exertional stress, provides a method of visualizing myocardial perfusion more directly and can circumvent some of the electrocardiographic artefactual problems associated with, for example, digitalis therapy or repolarization abnormalities. The indicators of high risk during non-invasive stress testing are shown in Table 3.

## Coronary angiography

The American Heart Association and American College of Cardiology guidelines[50] recommend cardiac catheterisation in patients with unstable angina in the following circumstances:

- recurrent angina/ischaemia at rest or low-level exercise despite therapy
- recurrent angina/ischaemia with symptoms or signs of acute heart failure
- high-risk findings on non-invasive stress testing
- reduced left ventricular function (ejection fraction <40%)
- haemodynamic instability or angina at rest accompanied by hypotension
- sustained ventricular tachycardia
- percutaneous coronary intervention (PCI) within the previous 6 months
- prior CABG

In the light of the evidence from the FRISC II and TACTICS trials[6,22] (see below), patients with raised cardiac troponins or electrocardiographic abnormalities should also be considered for cardiac catheterisation with a view to coronary revascularisation.

There are a number of patients who continue to have chest pain but either cannot perform an exercise tolerance test or have satisfactory non-invasive investigations. These patients may have frequent admissions to hospital with chest pain and take empirical anti-anginal medication with little objective evidence of its benefit to them. In this context, a normal coronary angiogram can be very helpful in excluding obstructive coronary artery disease, removing uncertainty about the diagnosis, reassuring the patient, and thereby reducing their use of health care resources.

## Coronary revascularisation

Initial randomised studies looking at early invasive interventions suggested that there was either a neutral or harmful effect of such approaches in patients with acute coronary syndromes[51,52]. However, these studies have been heavily criticised for the high cross over rates with a half of the patients in the conservative management group undergoing cardiac catheterisation. Moreover, the coronary revascularisation rates were very similar at 44% and 33% for the invasive and non-invasive groups, respectively. It is likely, therefore, that high-risk patients had an intervention irrespective of their randomised treatment and the lower risk patients only received revascularisation if they were in the invasive treatment group. From the ACME and RITA-2 trials, we already know that there is an excess of events in lower risk patients treated with percutaneous coronary intervention[53].

Observational data from the OASIS registry have indicated that an early invasive strategy is likely to be particularly beneficial in patients with refractory symptoms and may reduce the rate of re-admission with unstable angina[54]. Recently, two randomised controlled trials have been reported that demonstrate an early invasive strategy is appropriate, especially in the presence of electrocardiographic changes or elevations in cardiac enzymes[6,22]. From the 1-year follow-up of the FRISC II trial, an early strategy of coronary revascularisation is associated with major reductions in the risk of death (RR 0.57, CI 0.36–0.90; $P < 0.02$), myocardial infarction (RR 0.74, CI 0.59–0.94; $P < 0.02$) or re-hospitalisation (RR 0.67, CI 0.62–0.72; $P < 0.001$)[55]. These findings have been supported by the subsequent TACTICS trial of 2220 patients that demonstrated a 22% risk reduction ($P = 0.03$) in the primary end-point of death, myocardial infarction or re-hospitalisation for an acute coronary syndrome at 6 months' follow-up. Both these trials had significant differences in the rate of early intervention between the invasive and non-invasive strategy groups: for example, 71% *versus* 9%, respectively, in the FRISC II trial[55]. However, the benefits of interventional strategies are not yet clear as they may first appear. Both trials employed a more sensitive threshold for the diagnosis of myocardial infarction for non-procedure related myocardial infarction, thereby favouring the diagnosis of myocardial infarction in the conservative group. This is particularly pertinent given that the majority of the absolute clinical benefit was seen in the incidence of myocardial infarction.

### Coronary artery bypass surgery or percutaneous coronary intervention

Selection of the type of revascularisation procedure will be heavily influenced by technical aspects of the coronary anatomy as well as factors such as co-morbidity and patient preference. For example, in many patients, a policy of initial percutaneous coronary intervention may simply delay the subsequent need for revascularization with coronary artery bypass surgery, especially in younger patients.

Meta-analysis[56] of the three major randomised controlled trials comparing coronary artery bypass surgery with medical therapy in patients with chronic stable angina has suggested that this is the most appropriate in patients with a significant left main stem stenosis of 50% or more, triple vessel disease or two vessel disease including a significant proximal LAD stenosis. These benefits are most marked if the left ventricular function is impaired or the stress test is strongly positive. Patients with single or two-vessel coronary artery disease may be appropriately revascularised by either coronary artery bypass surgery or percutaneous coronary intervention.

## Early in-hospital initiation of secondary prevention

Cardiac rehabilitation, risk factor management and the use of secondary prevention therapy in patients recovering from an episode of unstable angina are discussed elsewhere in this volume.

Where appropriate, all patients should be maintained on aspirin, clopidogrel and β-blocker therapy at the time of hospital discharge. However, in the LIPID trial incorporating patients with unstable angina, the initiation of lipid lowering therapy was between 3–24 months from the index event. Recently, the MIRACL trial assessed the effect of early in-hospital initiation (within 24–96 h of admission) of atorvastatin 80 mg daily in 3086 patients with unstable angina and non-Q wave myocardial infarction[57]. Within 16 weeks of therapy, the composite end-point of death, myocardial infarction or re-hospitalisation for myocardial ischaemia was reduced by 16% ($P = 0.048$), predominantly due to a reduction in re-hospitalisation for myocardial ischaemia (26%, $P = 0.02$). These data require confirmation but it would, therefore, appear that aggressive lipid lowering therapy can be safely initiated in-hospital[57].

## Conclusions

There is now a substantial evidence base to guide therapeutic interventions in the treatment of patients presenting with unstable angina (Fig. 2). The combined use of potent anti-platelet and anti-coagulant therapies has markedly reduced the rate of thrombotic coronary artery occlusion. Moreover, targeted invasive intervention and revascularisation in high-risk patients is associated with major clinical benefits with a reduction in the rate of progression to myocardial infarction and associated cardiovascular death. Finally, intensive secondary preventative strategies in the early acute phase appear to be associated with substantial benefits.

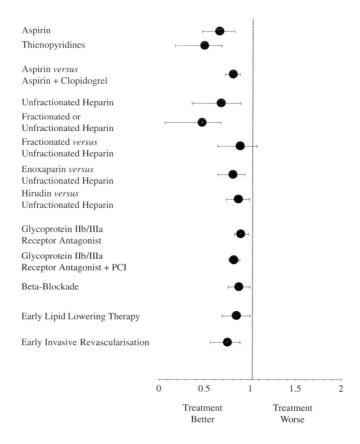

**Fig. 2** Evidence base for the in-hospital treatment of patients with unstable angina.

## References

1   Fox KAA, Cokkinos DV, Deckers J, Keil U, Maggioni A, Steg G. The ENACT study: a pan-European survey of acute coronary syndromes. European Network for Acute Coronary Treatment. *Eur Heart J* 2000; **21**: 1440–9

2   Collinson J, Flather MD, Fox KA *et al.* Clinical outcomes, risk stratification and practice patterns of unstable angina and myocardial infarction without ST elevation: Prospective Registry of Acute Ischaemic Syndromes in the UK (PRAIS-UK). *Eur Heart J* 2000; **21**: 1450–7

3   Hamm CW, Braunwald E. A classification of unstable angina revisited. *Circulation* 2000; **102**: 118–22

4   Holmvang L, Clemmensen P, Wagner G, Grande P. Admission standard electrocardiogram for early risk stratification in patients with unstable coronary artery disease not eligible for acute revascularization therapy: a TRIM substudy. ThRombin Inhibition in Myocardial Infarction. *Am Heart J* 1999; **137**: 24–33

5   Lindahl B, Toss H, Siegbahn A, Venge P, Wallentin L. Markers of myocardial damage and inflammation in relation to long-term mortality in unstable coronary artery disease. FRISC Study Group. Fragmin during instability in coronary artery disease. *N Engl J Med* 2000; **343**: 1139–47

6   The Fragmin and Fast Revascularisation during InStability in Coronary artery disease (FRISC II) investigators. Invasive compared with non-invasive treatment in unstable coronary-artery disease: FRISC II prospective randomised multicentre study. *Lancet* 1999; **354**: 708–15

7   Antman EM, Tanasijevic MJ, Thompson B *et al.* Cardiac-specific troponin I levels to predict the risk of mortality in patients with acute coronary syndromes. *N Engl J Med* 1996; **335**: 1342–9

8   Hamm CW, Heeschen C, Goldmann B *et al.* Benefit of abciximab in patients with refractory unstable angina in relation to serum troponin T levels. c7E3 Fab Antiplatelet Therapy in Unstable Refractory Angina (CAPTURE) Study Investigators. *N Engl J Med* 1999; **340**: 1623–9

9   Heeschen C, Hamm CW, Goldmann B, Deu A, Langenbrink L, White HD. Troponin concentrations for stratification of patients with acute coronary syndromes in relation to therapeutic efficacy of tirofiban. PRISM Study Investigators. Platelet Receptor Inhibition in Ischemic Syndrome Management. *Lancet* 1999; **354**: 1757–62

10  Haverkate F, Thompson SG, Pyke SD, Gallimore JR, Pepys MB. Production of C-reactive protein and risk of coronary events in stable and unstable angina. European Concerted Action on Thrombosis and Disabilities Angina Pectoris Study Group. *Lancet* 1997; **349**: 462–6

11  The Antiplatelet Trialists' Collaboration. Collaborative overview of randomised trials of antiplatelet therapy – I: prevention of death, myocardial infarction, and stroke by prolonged antiplatelet therapy in various categories of patients. *BMJ* 1994; **308**: 81–106

12  Ridker PM, Cushman M, Stampfer MJ, Tracy RP, Hennekens CH. Inflammation, aspirin, and the risk of cardiovascular disease in apparently healthy men. *N Engl J Med* 1997; **336**: 973–9

13  Lewis HD, Davis JW, Archibald DG *et al.* Protective effects of aspirin against acute myocardial infarction and death in men with unstable angina. Results of a Veterans Administration Cooperative Study. *N Engl J Med* 1983; **309**: 396–403

14  Balsano F, Rizzon P, Violi F *et al.* Antiplatelet treatment with ticlopidine in unstable angina. A controlled multicenter clinical trial. The Studio della Ticlopidina nell'Angina Instabile Group. *Circulation* 1990; **82**: 17–26

15  The CAPRIE Steering Committee. A randomised, blinded, trial of clopidogrel versus aspirin in patients at risk of ischaemic events. *Lancet* 1996; **348**: 1329–39

16  The CURE investigators. Effects of clopidogrel in addition to aspirin in patients with acute coronary syndromes without ST-segment elevation. N Engl J Med 2001; 345: 494–502

17  The Platelet Receptor inhibition in Ischemic Syndrome Management in Patients Limited by Unstable Signs and symptoms (PRISM-PLUS) study investigators. Inhibition of the platelet glycoprotein IIb/IIIa receptor with tirofiban in unstable angina and non-Q wave myocardial infarction. *N Engl J Med* 1998; **338**: 1488–97

18  The Platelet glycoprotein IIb/IIIa in Unstable angina: Receptor Suppression Using Integrilin Therapy (PURSUIT) trial investigators. Inhibition of platelet glycoprotein IIb/IIIa with

eptifibatide in patients with acute coronary syndromes. *N Engl J Med* 1998; **339**: 436–43

19 The EPIC investigators. Use of a monoclonal antibody directed against the platelet glycoprotein IIb/IIIa receptor in high-risk coronary angioplasty. *N Engl J Med* 1994; **330**: 956–61

20 The CAPTURE study investigators. Randomised placebo-controlled trial of abciximab before and during coronary intervention in refractory unstable angina: the CAPTURE Study. *Lancet* 1997; **349**: 1429–35

21 The TARGET Investigators. *Do Tirofiban and ReoPro give Similar Efficacy Trial*. New Orleans, LA: The American Heart Association, 2000

22 The TACTICS investigators. *Treat angina with Aggrastat and determine the Cost of Therapy with Invasive or Conservative Strategies*. New Orleans, LA: The American Heart Association, 2000

23 The Global Use of Strategies To Open occluded coronary arteries (GUSTO) IV investigators. *GUSTO-IV: Abciximab in Unstable Angina*. Amsterdam: The European Society of Cardiology, 2000

24 Kong DF, Califf RM, Miller DP *et al*. Clinical outcomes of therapeutic agents that block the glycoprotein IIb/IIIa integrin in ischemic heart disease. *Circulation* 1998; **98**: 2829–35

25 Oler A, Whooley MA, Oler J, Grady D. Adding heparin to aspirin reduces the incidence of myocardial infarction and death in patients with unstable angina. A meta-analysis. *JAMA* 1996; **276**: 811–5

26 Klein W, BuchWald A, Hillis SE *et al* for the FRagmin In unstable Coronary artery disease (FRIC) study investigators. Comparison of low-molecular-weight heparin with unfractionated heparin acutely and with placebo for 6 weeks in the management of unstable coronary artery disease. *Circulation* 1997; **96**: 61–8

27 Cohen M, Demers C, Gurfinkel EP *et al* for the Efficacy and Safety of Subcutaneous Enoxaparin in Non-Q-wave Coronary Events (ESSENCE) study group. A comparison of low-molecular-weight heparin with unfractionated heparin for unstable coronary artery disease. *N Engl J Med* 1997; **337**: 447–52

28 Antman EM, McCabe CH, Gurfinkel EP *et al*. Enoxaparin prevents death and cardiac ischemic events in unstable angina/non-Q-wave myocardial infarction. Results of the thrombolysis in myocardial infarction (TIMI) 11B trial. *Circulation* 1999; **100**: 1593–601

29 The FRAXIS Study Group. Comparison of two treatment durations (6 days and 14 days) of a low molecular weight heparin with a 6-day treatment of unfractionated heparin in the initial management of unstable angina or non-Q-wave myocardial infarction: FRAXIS (FRAXiparine in Ischaemic Syndrome). *Eur Heart J* 1999; **20**: 1553–62

30 Eikelboom JW, Anand SS, Malmberg K, Weitz JI, Ginsberg JS, Yusuf S. Unfractionated heparin and low-molecular-weight heparin in acute coronary syndrome without ST elevation: a meta-analysis. *Lancet* 2000; **355**: 1936–42

31 Goodman SG, Cohen M, Bigonzi F *et al*. Randomized trial of low molecular weight heparin (enoxaparin) versus unfractionated heparin for unstable coronary artery disease: one-year results of the ESSENCE Study. Efficacy and Safety of Subcutaneous Enoxaparin in Non-Q Wave Coronary Events. *J Am Coll Cardiol* 2000; **36**: 693–8

32 The Global Use of Strategies To Open occluded coronary arteries (GUSTO) IIb investigators. A comparison of recombinant hirudin with heparin for the treatment of acute coronary syndromes. *N Engl J Med* 1996; **335**: 775–82

33 The Organisation to Assess Strategies for Ischemic Syndromes (OASIS-1) investigators. Comparison of the effects of two doses of recombinant hirudin compared with heparin in patients with acute myocardial ischemia without ST elevation: a pilot study. *Circulation* 1997; **96**: 769–77

34 The Organisation to Assess Strategies for Ischemic Syndromes (OASIS-2) investigators. Effects of recombinant hirudin (lepirudin) compared with heparin on death, myocardial infarction, refractory angina, and revascularisation procedures in patients with acute myocardial ischaemia without ST elevation: a randomised trial. *Lancet* 1999; **353**: 429–38

35 Greinacher A, Lubenow N. Recombinant hirudin in clinical practice : focus on lepirudin. *Circulation* 2001; **103**: 1479–84

36 Mark DB, Cowper PA, Berkowitz SD *et al*. Economic assessment of low-molecular-weight heparin (enoxaparin) versus unfractionated heparin in acute coronary syndrome patients:

results from the ESSENCE randomized trial. Efficacy and Safety of Subcutaneous Enoxaparin in Non-Q wave Coronary Events. *Circulation* 1998; **97**: 1702–7

37 Stone PH, Gibson RS, Glasser SP *et al*. Comparison of propranolol, diltiazem and nifedipine in the treatment of ambulatory ischemia in patients with stable angina. *Circulation* 1990; **82**: 1962–72

38 Dargie HJ, Ford I, Fox KM. Total Ischaemic Burden European Trial (TIBET). Effects of ischaemia and treatment with atenolol, nifedipine SR and their combination on outcome in patients with chronic stable angina. *Eur Heart J* 1996; **17**: 104–12

39 Freemantle N, Cleland J, Young P, Mason J, Harrison J. β-blockade after myocardial infarction: systematic review and meta regression analysis. *BMJ* 1999; **318**: 1730–7

40 Yusuf S, Wittes J, Friedman L. Overview of results of randomized clinical trials in heart disease. II. Unstable angina, heart failure, primary prevention with aspirin, and risk factor modification. *JAMA* 1988; **260**: 2259–63

41 Cotter G, Metzkor E, Kaluski E *et al*. Randomised trial of high-dose isosorbide dinitrate plus low-dose furosemide versus high-dose furosemide plus low-dose isosorbide dinitrate in severe pulmonary oedema. *Lancet* 1998; **351**: 389–93

42 Friedensohn A, Meshulam R, Schlesinger Z. Randomised double-blind comparison of the effects of isosorbide dinitrate retard, verapamil sustained-release, and their combination on myocardial ischaemic episodes. *Cardiology* 1991; **79** (**Suppl 2**): 31–40

43 Chrysant SG, Glasser SP, Bittar N *et al*. Efficacy and safety of extended release isosorbide mononitrate for stable effort angina pectoris. *Am J Cardiol* 1993; **72**: 1249–56

44 Lubsen J, Tijssen JG. Efficacy of nifedipine and metoprolol in the early treatment of unstable angina in the coronary care unit: findings from the Holland Interuniversity Nifedipine/metoprolol Trial (HINT). *Am J Cardiol* 1987; **60**: 18A–25A

45 The Danish Study Group on Verapamil in Myocardial Infarction. Effect of verapamil on mortality and major events after acute myocardial infarction (The Danish Verapamil Infarction Trial – DAVIT II). *Am J Cardiol* 1990; **66**: 779–85

46 The Multicenter Diltiazem Post Infarction Trial (MDPIT) research group. The effect of diltiazem on mortality and reinfarction after myocardial infarction. *N Engl J Med* 1988; **319**: 385–92

47 Patel DJ, Purcell HJ, Fox KM. Cardioprotection by opening of the K(ATP) channel in unstable angina. Is this a clinical manifestation of myocardial preconditioning? Results of a randomized study with nicorandil. CESAR 2 investigation. Clinical European studies in angina and revascularization. *Eur Heart J* 1999; **20**: 51–7

48 Stone PH, Thompson B, Zaret BL *et al*. Factors associated with failure of medical therapy in patients with unstable angina and non-Q wave myocardial infarction. A TIMI-IIIB database study. *Eur Heart J* 1999; **20**: 1084–93

49 Antman EM, Cohen M, Bernink PJ *et al*. The TIMI risk score for unstable angina/non-ST elevation MI: a method for prognostication and therapeutic decision making. *JAMA* 2000; **284**: 835–42

50 Braunwald E, Antman EM, Beasley JW *et al*. ACC/AHA guidelines for the management of patients with unstable angina and non-ST-segment elevation myocardial infarction. A report of the American College of Cardiology/American Heart Association Task Force on Practice Guidelines (Committee on the Management of Patients With Unstable Angina). *J Am Coll Cardiol* 2000; **36**: 970–1062

51 Anderson HV, Cannon CP, Stone PH *et al*. One year results of the Thrombolysis In Myocardial Infarction (TIMI) IIIB clinical trial: a randomized comparison of tissue-type plasminogen activator versus placebo and early invasive versus early conservative strategies in unstable angina and non-Q wave myocardial infarction. *J Am Coll Cardiol* 1995; **26**: 1643–50

53 The RITA-2 Trial Participants. Coronary angioplasty versus medical therapy for angina: the second Randomised Intervention Treatment of Angina (RITA-2) trial. *Lancet* 1997; **350**: 461–8

52 Boden WE, O'Rourke RA, Crawford MH *et al*. Outcomes in patients with acute non-Q wave myocardial infarction randomly assigned to an invasive as compared with a conservative management strategy: Veterans Affairs Non-Q-Wave Infarction Strategies in Hospital (VANQWISH) trial investigators. *N Engl J Med* 1998; **338**: 1785–92

54 Yusuf S, Flather M, Pogue J *et al* for the OASIS registry investigators. Variations between countries in invasive cardiac procedures and outcomes in patients with suspected unstable angina or myocardial infarction without initial ST elevation. *Lancet* 1998; **352**: 507–14

55 Wallentin L, Lagerqvist B, Husted S, Kontny F, Ståhle, Swahn E for the FRISC II investigators. Outcome at 1 year after invasive compared with a non-invasive strategy in unstable coronary-artery disease: the FRISC II invasive randomised trial. *Lancet* 2000; **356**: 9–16

56 Yusuf S, Zucker D, Peduzzi P *et al*. Effect of coronary artery bypass graft surgery on survival: overview of 10-year results from randomised trials by the Coronary Artery Bypass Graft Surgery Trialists Collaboration. *Lancet* 1994; **344**: 563–70

57 Schwartz GG, Olsson AG, Egekowitz MD *et al*. Effects of atonastatin on early recurrent ischemic events in acute coronary syndromes. JAMA 2001; 285:1711–18

# The acute management of myocardial infarction

## A H Gershlick

*Academic Department of Cardiology, University Hospitals Leicester, Leicester, UK*

Acute myocardial infarction (AMI) is a common and potentially fatal condition. Primary prevention by reducing the risk of developing coronary atheroma disease has had an important effect on the incidence of the disease. However, for many, the first clinical presentation of their coronary atheroma is the development of acute coronary occlusion[1]. The acute nature of such presentation is the result of the dynamic nature of the plaque event. Thus while measures such as increasing public education in areas of primary prevention are always important it needs to be recognised that real differences in outcome need to and can be made even once the event has occurred. Individuals developing chest pain need to be encouraged to present early, especially if they have a history of ischaemic heart disease. Once they have arrived at point of medical contact, rapid triage, early diagnosis and the institution of therapies designed to reduce the extent of myocardial damage are paramount.

While evidence-based use of established treatments is important, the urgency with which they are instituted may also be critical. Much of what is practised has become standard management for a number of years so it is easy to presume that the current management of acute myocardial infarction is optimal. This is not the case and many contentious issues remain. This article will address some of these.

## The natural history of AMI

Correspondence to:
Mr A H Gershlick,
Academic Department of
Cardiology, Clinical
Sciences Building,
Glenfield Hospital,
University Hospitals
Leicester,
Leicester LE3 9QP, UK

In the UK, acute myocardial infarction accounts for up to 250,000 deaths each year with 150,000 admissions to hospital. Many deaths thus occur before help arrives, with up to 30% occurring within the first 2 h. Many of these deaths are due to malignant arrhythymias. To date, out-of-hospital mortality has changed little. However, the establishment of coronary care units in the 1960s showed that having access to defibrillators had a significant impact on outcome once the patient had reached hospital, with an overall reduction in mortality from about 30% to about 20%. The importance of having defibrillators available has thus been recognised and more than 20 airline companies now have such equipment (and trained staff) available. Some have suggested that defibrillators should be made available wherever the public are (shopping malls, football stadia). It will be interesting to see if prehospital mortality changes. It has been estimated that the lives of 29/1000 patients can be saved by out of hospital resuscitation and that 86% of these patients are discharged from hospital when the arrest is witnessed compared to 34% when it is not[2]. However, to date, the most important therapeutic impact has been with the introduction of thrombolytic in-hospital therapy in the 1980s and this reduced mortality further, currently estimated to be 10–20%[3]. This is still a worryingly high figure and the reasons for it being so high need to be examined.

## Understanding the pathology of AMI: impact on early strategies

Important studies by Davies[4], Conti[5] and others helped explain clinical progression or regression in patients with coronary disease and identified targets for therapy. In essence, these authors described the coronary arteries from patients who had died following acute coronary syndromes. It became clear that the primary event was plaque disruption, the consequences of which depended on the patient's response to it[6]. Thus, following a plaque event, unstable angina (through the continuing presence of

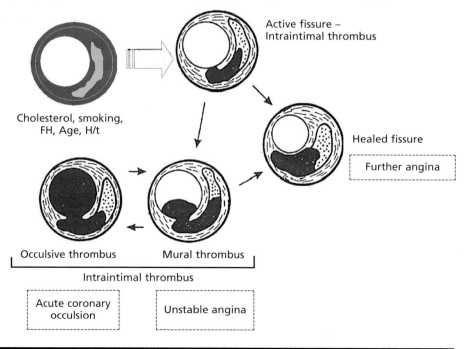

**Fig. 1** The pathological and clinical consequences of plaque rupture (adapted with permission from Davies et al[4]).

thrombus), stable angina (incorporation of the thrombus) or acute vessel closure could all result (Fig. 1). While factors such as initial severity of luminal narrowing clearly influence outcome, the dynamic theory of coronary syndrome pathology meant that having a plaque that significantly reduced the arterial lumen was not essential. The patient can suffer a very prothrombogenic response to the plaque event, especially for example, if they are smokers or have high lipid levels, both of which increase platelet aggregation.

The development of these concepts, by placing the thrombus central to the clinical problem was important for a number of reasons. First, it confirmed various clinical observations. As early as 1980, de Wood had undertaken sequential angiography on patients with acute myocardial infarction (AMI). He reported a 90% thrombotic occlusion (suggesting that thrombus was not formed after infarction), but more importantly showed spontaneous recanalisation by demonstrating a 54% occlusion rate only, in those studied 12–24 h after onset. More importantly, it became clear that the first presentation of AMI was not necessarily preceded by symptoms of angina. The cornerstone of treatment thus became dissolution of the thrombus which had formed after a plaque event, so-called thrombo- or fibrinolysis. However, the acute management of AMI involves other important therapeutic measures as well.

# Managing the patient with acute coronary occlusion

The aims of managing patients with acute infarction are quite simple. They can be divided into those aimed at treating the patient's symptoms and those that will influence prognosis. Thus relieving pain and anxiety are critical. At the same time, limiting myocardial cell death and so preventing myocardial damage in order to reduce the impact on prognosis should be the absolute end-point of therapeutic strategies. Thus once a patient has sought medical help, the goals are early diagnosis, rapid symptom relief and imperative reperfusion. There remain a number of issues that need to be discussed before these absolute goals can be achieved in all patients.

## Prehospital thrombolysis

Since the availability of defibrillators and thrombolysis have been shown to influence outcome, the first priority when managing someone with a suspected infarct is to ensure rapid access to these. Public education strategies aimed at ensuring that those with chest pain summon help quickly are vitally important, especially if the patient is at higher risk as, for example are those with previous angina. Since loss of muscle cells starts to become irreversible following 45 min of ischaemia[7], and death is common within the first 2 h, speed is critical. While provision of immediate care will need to reflect local conditions (such as whether the area is urban or rural), evidence suggests that patients' needs may be best served by them calling for an ambulance or for the general practitioner (GP) to call an ambulance, rather than the GP going to the patient and assessing them first. Local arrangements should be discussed and agreed between the GPs, the ambulance service and representatives from the hospital medical staff. Local guidelines should be drawn up, adhered to, and audited. A number of rural areas now have early triage systems in place. In some areas of the UK providers of care are looking at delivering thrombolysis by appropriately trained paramedics. Setting up of such a system requires a number of prerequisites. First, it requires enthusiasm from ambulance crews and the emergency services administrators. Second, there needs to be the ability to diagnose accurately the presence of an AMI, which may involve electronic transmission of ECGs to the hospital or full paramedic training in ECG diagnosis, or both. Finally, there needs to be demonstration through the audit process not only of an increase in rapidity of thrombolytic delivery but also of better outcomes with no increase in incidence of adverse side effects.

## Acute management following arrival in hospital

The aim of all treatments is to reduce the impact of coronary artery occlusion on the myocardium. Speed is of the essence. A system that allows immediate triage of patients with chest pain is vital. The first contact should be with someone experienced in directing the patient towards the immediate management of their infarct. In some hospitals, this is an accident and emergency nurse, in some there is an admission ward evaluation, and in others the patient is seen on the coronary care unit. Whichever system is used, it should be structured and audited such that standard guideline directives (*e.g.* door-to-needle time) are met. Once the diagnosis has been made on history and ECG, then the patient needs to be in an area where monitoring and treatment can be undertaken, expeditiously and safely.

If the patient has not yet received pain relief, then this is a mandatory first step. Pain often exacerbates anxiety, which in turn increases catecholamine release and peripheral increase in systemic resistance. Pain should be relieved using intravenous opiate. Morphine, in the form of diamorphine (2.5–5 mg, repeated if necessary) should be given. Since opiate analgesia can induce vomiting, metoclopramide (10 mg i.v.) or cyclazine (50 mg i.v.) should also be given. Oxygen administration and obtaining venous access are early important actions.

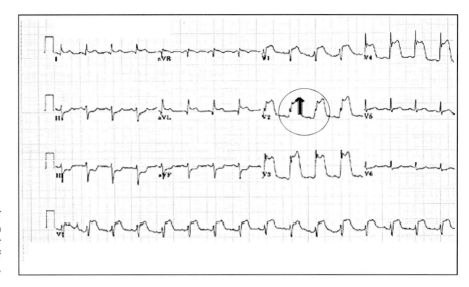

**Fig. 2** Anterior ST segment elevation indicating need for consideration of thrombolytics.

Establishing an early diagnosis is important in order to start appropriate treatment. Thus a history of severe chest pain lasting for greater than 15 min, unrelieved by GTN should raise a high index of suspicion but so should less obvious presentations such as pain predominantly in the jaw or teeth, or in one or both arms or occasionally unusual presentations such as syncope. Breathlessness may be the presenting complaint in the elderly.

An ECG may confirm the diagnosis and help determine whether thrombolysis is indicated. It should be remembered that an apparently normal early ECG does not exclude myocardial infarction. Repeated ECGs may help show changes. In the thrombolysis trials, patients with the ECG changes of left bundle branch block, anterior ST elevation (Fig. 2) and inferior ST elevation in association with a history of chest pain were all shown to benefit from thrombolytic therapy. ST depression, equivocal T wave changes and normal ECGs were not. Patients with other ECG changes may still have acute manifestations of ischaemic heart disease and, in the era of glycoprotein IIb/IIIa (GPIIb/IIIa) receptor blockers, the use of markers such as troponin tests may be essential. Thus, where there is a difficulty in making a diagnosis, early evaluation of standard cardiac enzymes or measurement of troponin, especially in those with stuttering syndromes may help. Measurement of troponin T or I (myocardial myofibrillar proteins) may be a specific and rapid aid to such diagnoses[8]. How troponin testing influences the appropriateness of thrombolytic therapy in those without standard ECG changes has not been established. Since standard enzyme measurement usually takes too long and since the thrombolytic trials indicated that those patients who clearly benefit are those with obvious ECG changes (rather than patients whose diagnosis continues to be equivocal), it becomes clear that it is **at the point of ECG diagnosis** that thrombolytic therapy is mandated, provided there are no contra-indications.

### Thrombolysis

The aim of all therapies should be the early, complete and maintained patency of the infarct related artery. Currently, in the UK and elsewhere, thrombolysis remains the cornerstone of treatment, but percutaneous coronary intervention has a role to play and may become increasingly used in the future.

If there is a suspicion that the patient is suffering an acute infarct, then an aspirin (150 mg) should be given[9] (chewing it is an effective method of absorption). Aspirin has been shown to have an independent influence on 30-day mortality. If the patient presents to a unit that does not have a policy of direct intervention, then once the diagnosis is confirmed on ECG, a thrombolytic should be administered without delay.

Natural thrombolysis occurs via the action of plasmin on fibrin thrombi. Plasmin is formed from plasminogen by cleavage of a single peptide bond. Plasmin is a non-specific protease and dissolves coagulation factors as well as fibrin based clots. Three thrombolytic agents are currently available. Streptokinase (SK) forms a non-covalent link with plasminogen. The resultant conformational change exposes the active site on plasminogen to induce the formation of plasmin. Tissue plasminogen activator (tPA) is a serine protease and binds directly to fibrin via a lysine site, activating fibrin-bound plasminogen. The theoretical advantages of tPA are its increased specificity and potency because of its direct affect on fibrin-bound plasminogen. It should have a greater effect than streptokinase on vessel patency which should translate into better clinical outcome. Being the product of recombinant DNA technology, there should be no allergic reaction. Unlike SK which because of neutralising antibody production can be used only once, tPA can be used repeatedly. Some of these theoretical advantages translate into definite clinical benefit with tPA but not all. Reteplase, a modified plasminogen activator, theoretically designed to overcome some of the limitations of tPA by having an increased resistance to breakdown, has now been introduced as an alternative to tPA as has TNK-PA.

There is true evidence of benefit from thrombolytic treatment. More than 100,000 patients have been randomised in large clinical trials testing thrombolytic agent against controls or against other thrombolytic agents; these trials have been summarised in the Fibrinolytic Therapy Trialists Collaborative Group[10]. The overall relative risk reduction in 35-day mortality with treatment was 18% ($P < 0.00001$). The mortality at this time point was reduced from about 13% in controls to about 8–9% with treatment. However, in real life where the population is older than in the trials, the true mortality may be higher in treated patients with figures up to 18–20% thought likely.

Despite this, the beneficial effect of thrombolytic therapy still holds for those presenting within 12 h of onset of symptoms. This holds true irrespective of age, sex, history of hypertension or diabetes, or previous MI. It is clear, however, that the earlier patients are treated, the better. Administration of a thrombolytic saves about 30 lives in a 1000 in those presenting within 6 h of symptom onset, but only 20 lives per 1000 when patients receive treatment 6–12 h after symptom onset. After 12 h, there appears to be only a small and statistically uncertain benefit. The LATE Trial, for example, clearly showed lack of benefit 12 h after onset of symptoms[11]. Judging the onset of symptoms can be difficult and may be influenced by collateral flow from another artery. If, for example, a patient presents with stuttering symptoms over 24 h or so, but has had severe pain over a few hours and then has an appropriately abnormal ECG, thrombolytic treatment should be seriously considered. Many patients do not have optimal outcome from treatment because too little notice is taken of the symptoms. The specific question 'from the history is it likely that this patient with this diagnostic ECG will benefit from thrombolytic therapy' is too infrequently asked.

Thrombolytic dissolution of extracardiac thrombus that was perhaps maintaining the cerebral vascular integrity can lead to strokes. The overall risk of stroke is about 1.2% in treated patients compared to 0.8% in controls, an overall excess risk of 4 per 1000 treated patients ($P < 0.00001$). There is some suggestion that patients who suffer cerebral haemorrhage may do so because of a general lytic ooze. Risk factors for ICH, such as hypertension and age have been well established. While the risk is clearly greater in the elderly, the overall benefit from lytic therapy exceeds the risk in these patients.

Prehospital thrombolysis has been shown to reduce the cardiac mortality compared to in-hospital thrombolysis by 17% ($P = 0.03$) almost certainly by reducing the mean time to treatment by about 1 h[12]. Despite this, prehospital thrombolysis has, in general, not been taken up for logistical reasons. Some of these are now being seriously addressed through the use of paramedics and strategies designed to provide treatment expeditiously and safely before reaching hospital.

# Initial management

## Agents that should be given

Care of the patient during their in-hospital stay involves continued monitoring for arrhythymias, careful daily clinical examination for new murmurs indicating the presence of mitral regurgitation or VSD, and examination to detect early signs of heart failure.

Apart from aspirin, the only adjunctive medication shown to improve outcome when administered **acutely** is intravenous β-blockade (ISIS-1) trial[13]. Given within 12 h of onset of the infarct intravenous β-blocker reduced a composite end-point of death, cardiac arrest and re-infarction ($P$ <0.002). The benefit was most evident in the first 2 days following administration (25% reduction), most likely due to a reduction in ventricular fibrillation and cardiac rupture. It should be given to patients with inappropriate tachycardia and hypertension. It is generally underused.

The benefits of continuing β-blockers in the longer term have been well established. It has been suggested that a β-blocker given only in the acute phase is in itself a strategy that has no longer term benefit. In an overview published in the *British Medical Journal* in 1999, Freemantle and colleagues reviewed 82 β-blocker trials. Overall, the longer term trials indicate the pooled OR as being 0.77 (95% CI, 0.69–0.85). Over 2 years, 42 patients would need to be treated with β-blockers to avoid one death, whereas 292 patients would need to be treated over the same period with antiplatelet agents to achieve the same benefit[14]. There appears to be no time cut-off after which β-blockers no longer benefit, so it would seem that these agents need to be continued indefinitely.

A number of studies[15,16] have demonstrated that early administration of an ACE inhibitor in unselected patients improves outcome. Even in the absence of any clinical signs of heart failure, early (day 1) treatment improves outcome (Table 1). Subgroup analysis of GISSI-3 and ISIS-4 indicate greater benefit in high-risk patients treated after day 1. Continued treatment improves longer term outcome. In a meta-analysis, Domanski[17] reviewed 15 trials (15,104 patients). ACE inhibitor administration significantly reduced the risk of death (OR, 0.83; 95% CI, 0.71–0.97), cardiovascular death (OR, 0.82; 95% CI, 0.69–0.97) and sudden cardiac death (OR, 0.80; 95% CI, 0.70–0.92). The recent HOPE study showed that treatment with ramipril ($n = 651$) resulted in a lower primary end-point (14%) compared to placebo (17.8%; RR, 0.78; 95% CI, 0.70–0.86; $P < 0.001$)[18], and has raised the profile of this particular ACE inhibitor.

## Agents tested and shown not to be of benefit

### Nitrates

Nitrates might be expected to have a beneficial effect in acute myocardial infarction by dilating arterial resistance vessels, venous capacitance vessels and coronary arteries and so opening up collaterals. Reducing afterload and preload, reduced wall tension and oxygen demand are also theoretical

**Table 1** Effect of starting ACE inhibitor early after MI on short-term mortality

| Randomised comparison | | | ACEI better | Control better |
|---|---|---|---|---|
| CONSENSUS-II | 6.9% | 7.2% | | |
| GISSI-3 | 6.3% | 7.1% | | |
| CCS-1 | 9.1% | 9.6% | | |
| ISIS-4 | 7.2% | 7.7% | | |
| All Trials | 7.27% | 7.73% | | |

0.5    0.75    1.0    1.25

6.5 % odds reduction

4.6 lives saved/1000 treated

Adapted from ISIS-1[13].

benefits. Nitrates are also known to affect platelet aggregation. However, in the ISIS-4 trial[15], the 35-day mortality was 7.34% in the group treated for 4 weeks with isosobide mononitrate *versus* 7.54% in controls. Benefit was also not shown in the GISSI-3 trial[46].

### Magnesium

Small studies and a larger trial based in Leicester (LIMIT-2) suggested a benefit from use of magnesium. However, in the larger ISIS-4 trial no benefit was seen. Controversy continues, however, since in the LIMIT-2 study not all patients received thrombolysis whereas all did in ISIS-4. The magnesium was also administered at different times. Thus a small advantage from magnesium may be being masked in the patients treated with thrombolysis. Advocates would argue that magnesium is beneficial only if present at appropriate blood levels at the time of reperfusion, *i.e.* it needs to be given early. Longer-term surveillance of the LIMIT–2 patients by the investigators suggests a continued benefit (K Woods, personal communication).

### Prophylactic anti-arrhythmic agents

A number of studies have shown a trend towards an increase in mortality in patients given class IB agents prophylactically. This does not mean that an individual patient with a ventricular arrhythmia should not be considered for a drug like lignocaine. That stated, there is also some data to suggest that those patients with frequent premature ventricular beats (10 h) or repetitive (>1 run ventricular tachycardia) do better at 2-year follow-up treated with amioderone in terms of resuscitated ventricular death or arrhythmic death (4.5% *versus* 6.9% placebo; RRR, 34.3%; 95% CI,

1.9–66.8; $P$ <0.03)[19]. Further, a meta-analysis of 13 trials (8 in patients with a history of AMI, 5 in patients with a history of congestive heart failure total; $n$ = 6500) indicated that amioderone provides a modest reduction in all-cause mortality, death from arrhythmia or sudden death[20].

# Opening the artery: the absolute goal

## Thrombolytics

In theory, tPA and reteplase should be more effective agents at opening coronary arteries than SK. This has been supported in a number of angiographic studies which showed a higher percentage of patients with patent arteries after tPA treatment than with SK (~70% *versus* ~35%). There followed a number of studies that set out to compare the clinical efficacy of the two agents. Neither the GISSI-2 study[21] nor the ISIS-3 study found any difference in 30-day mortality rate (8.5% SK *versus* 8.9% tPA) and (10.6% for SK and 10.3% for tPA, respectively). In the GUSTO trial, a more aggressive regimen was used, the so-called front loaded tPA. This produced a small, but significant, benefit favouring tPA (6.3% *versus* 7.3%; $P$ >0.04). There was, however, an excess of strokes with this accelerated or front loaded regimen (0.72% for tPA *versus* 0.54% for SK) which translates into 5 or 6 new haemorrhagic strokes per 1000 treated. Combining deaths and strokes, there was still a benefit favouring tPA (6.9 % *versus* 7.8%)[22].

In the UK, streptokinase remains the first line treatment for most AMIs. This is because the advantage for tPA is modest at most and tPA is expensive compared to SK, allowing more patients to be treated overall for the same amount of money. Since streptokinase neutralising antibodies are formed from about day 4 onwards, then tPA will need to be administered should the patient re-infarct after this time. This accounts for about 20% of the market. Based on the GUSTO trial there are also patients who should receive tPA first time out. They include the younger patient, those presenting early and in those with larger, and in particular anterior, infarcts.

The lack of any large difference in clinical outcome between tPA and SK despite the difference in angiographic patency needs to be explained. tPA being locally effective has little systemic thrombolytic effects (for example on circulating plasminogen). It is, however, very specific which is the likely cause for the excess in strokes. It has a short half-life compared to SK. It has been clearly shown in animal models of arterial thrombotic occlusion that opening of the vessel by administration of tPA may be followed by early reclosure, perhaps within minutes. The 90-min angiogram cannot reflect the consequent re-occlusion of the artery, which will happen less with SK which has a longer half-life. Thus, the increased early patency with tPA may not translate into a decrease in 30-day mortality. The short half-life of tPA means that heparin should be co-administered and continued for 24 h, although true benefit has never actually been proven. The addition of subcutaneous heparin to streptokinase produced no improvement in outcome in the GISSI-2 trial and was associated with an excess of bleeding. In the GUSTO trial, the addition of subcutaneous or i.v. heparin made no difference to outcome in the SK groups, but it is indirectly assumed that the addition of heparin to the tPA group in this study contributed to its benefit.

### What to give

In the absence of previous administration, the first line thrombolytic in the UK is streptokinase: 1.5 million units are given in 100 ml 5% dextrose or 0.9% saline over 30–60 min. Side-effects and complications with streptokinase include hypotension, but severe allergic reactions are rare. Routine hydrocortisone is not required and hypotension should be managed simply by lying the patient flat, raising their legs and administering atropine or volume expanders if necessary. The infusion should be temporarily halted.

If SK has been given >5 days previously, then tPA as a 15 mg bolus followed by 50 mg over 60 min and the residual 35 mg over a further 30 min or reteplase (10 IU bolus + a further 10 IU after 30 min) should be given. Choice between these two agents will be based on hospital or individual policy. Trials comparing efficacy show equivalence, which is interesting considering reteplase was 'designed' to have advantages over standard thrombolytics.

It should also be remembered that, during the early stages of thrombolysis, patients are at risk of bleeding and care about placing temporary pacing wires and arterial sampling for blood gases should be paramount. If the patient has a spontaneous bleed large enough to be life-threatening, then the infusion should be stopped, fresh frozen plasma given and, if necessary, i.v. aprotinin (4 mg/kg) administered, with or without tranexamic acid (25 mg/kg orally 6 hourly).

Thrombolysis should not be given if standard contra-indications are present (Table 2).

In the ISIS-2 trial, aspirin (~150 mg) was shown to have an effect additional to streptokinase and should be continued at this dose indefinitely.

## Problems with thrombolysis

The 'open artery' theory suggests that the short- and longer-term outcome after acute infarction is determined by the degree of patency

**Table 2** Contra-indications to thrombolysis

- Recent major surgery
- Risk of bleeding from a peptic ulcer
- Risk of bleeding from a subarachnoid haemorrhage
- Recent head injury (*e.g.* if patient collapsed and sustained head trauma during infarct
- Prolonged or vigorous cardiopulmonary resuscitation
- Avoid vascular puncture for up to 30 min after tPA and for up to 6 h after streptokinase
- If needed, pacing wires or Swann-Ganz catheters should be introduced via the brachial vein

obtained with treatment following initial vessel closure, and that when optimal patency is achieved it is also maintained. In other words, benefit is lost if the vessel re-occludes. Degree of patency is graded according to the TIMI classification, where TIMI flow 0 = total closure and TIMI flow 3 = flow equivalent to that in unaffected arteries. A number of studies have clearly shown that longer-term outcome correlates with the TIMI flow seen, especially at 90-min angiogram. For example, data from the angiographic study arm of the GUSTO trial[23] clearly demonstrate that patients with TIMI grade 0 flow (*i.e.* complete occlusion) at 90-min angiogram had a 30-day mortality of 8.4%, whereas in those with TIMI grade 3 this was only 4%.

Other non-randomised data are available to support the belief that the better the patency the better the long-term outcome. Thus a retrospective meta-analysis of 4607 patients showed that mortality was 3.7% for TIMI grade 3 flow, but 6.6% ($P <0.0003$) for TIMI grade 2 and 9.2% ($P <0.0001$) for TIMI 0/1 flow[24]. Five and ten year follow-up suggests a continued benefit in those patients with initial grade 3 flow[25].

There are two problems with thrombolytic therapy. Thrombolytic therapy alone is unable to produce 'adequate patency'. TIMI grade 3 flow is seen in only 54% of patients treated with front loaded tPA and in only 30% with SK. Thus thrombolysis with current agents appears to have a therapeutic plateau. This may be due to a number of factors: atheromatous bulk, degree of intimal disruption or lytic resistance being some.

The second problem with current thrombolytic regimens is vessel re-occlusion. A number of studies have compared early (usually the 90 min patency) with late patency to determine the re-occlusion rate. Re-occlusion is a time-related phenomenon, and reaches an astonishing, albeit plateaued, rate of 30% by 3 months[26]. Reasons for this include re-release of thrombin, residual prothrombogenic plaque and activation of coagulation factors V and VIII by plasmin. Patients who have re-occluded have a much lower 1-year event-free survival (83% *versus* 63%; $P < 0.001$) and the 3-year event rate is 73% in the re-occluded group *versus* 33% in the group whose arteries are patent at 3 months.

Current goals are aimed at dealing with these two problems: optimal TIMI flow and re-occlusion. Strategies include the development of new thrombolytics, altering adjunctive therapy or by treating the occluded artery mechanically with balloon angioplasty and stenting.

## Can adjunctive therapy help?

### New thrombolytics

Various investigators have studied tPA mutants or variants of tPA. These agents may possess altered resistance to inhibitors such as plasminogen activator inhibitor-1 (PAI-1) or require binding to fibrin to become active. Other approaches have involved altering thrombolytic molecules to reduce their plasma clearance, although such modifications may lessen their thrombolytic effectiveness. One mutant produced by an alteration at the kringle 2 region of the tPA molecule appears to have a prolonged half-life, which may prove to be of value[27]. Some early trials in patients using tPA mutants have shown promise. Whether these and other mutants, such as those with increased resistance to plasma inhibitors, are any better in clinical practice than current agents is as yet unclear and will need to be tested in large, randomised, clinical trials against tPA.

Reteplase or rPA, a non-glycosylated deletion mutant of wild-type tPA, was the first member of the third generation thrombolytics and is one successful variant of tPA. Unfortunately, patency rates have been shown to be no greater with reteplase than with tPA and choice between these agents is frequently a commercial one.

Naturally occurring thrombolytics such as the vampire bat plasminogen activator (bat-PA) have also attracted attention. This latter agent is similar to human tPA but does not have a plasmin-sensitive processing site. It thus appears resistant to PAI-1 (one inhibitor of tPA) and has greater fibrin selectivity than tPA. Experimental data have shown that bat-PA is efficacious without activating systemic plasminogen and thus may partly circumvent bleeding complications associated with thrombolytics. Clinical trials were planned and are still awaited.

Staphylokinase is a protein with known profibrinolytic properties and is produced by *Staphylococcus aureus*. A recombinant form (STAR) has been produced and observed in experimental studies to be less immunogenic, but more active, against platelet-rich arterial clots than streptokinase. This agent has now been evaluated in small published clinical trials. STAR (10–20 mg) given intravenously over 30 min to patients with acute myocardial infarction resulted in similar coronary recanalisation rates to accelerated tPA, but without any fibrinogen

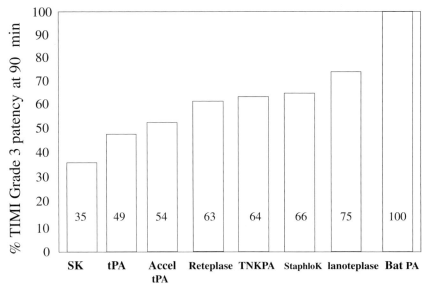

**Fig. 3** TIMI flow grade for the various thrombolytics from phase 2 and phase 3 trials.

breakdown (*i.e.* significantly more fibrin-specific than accelerated tPA)[28]. However, all patients developed STAR-neutralising antibodies from the second week after treatment, suggesting that, at least in man, this agent may not be as hypo-allergenic as originally hoped.

All these agents will need testing against current best therapy, tPA, in large trials. The TIMI patency of all the newer thrombolytics compared to those currently available is shown in Figure 3. Perhaps the most promising new agent is tenecteplase (single bolus) TNK-tPA which has been tested in the ASSENT-2 and ASSENT–3 trials[29,30]. It has slower plasma clearance, better fibrin specificity and high resistance to plasminogen-activator inhibitor 1. It seems easier to administer than tPA, and this may be its main advantage.

*In vitro* and *ex vivo* work is starting in our laboratory to assess whether there is increased efficacy of thrombolytic when it is targeted to the thrombus using monoclonal antibodies, with the aim of increasing local concentration and reducing side-effects. In theory, a systemic injection of targeted thrombolytic would be concentrated at site of the infarct.

### Adjunctive therapy

Heparin has limitations as an antithrombin: it needs a cofactor, has little action against bound thrombin and can be inactivated. Three large clinical trials designed to evaluate the value of hirudin (a powerful direct anti-thrombin originally extracted from the leech) in the setting of myocardial infarction have been undertaken and reported in 1994 (GUSTO-II, TIMI-9 and HIT-III)[31–33]. Given with tPA, the dose of hirudin used in these trials was as an intravenous bolus of 0.6 mg/kg, followed by a fixed dose infusion of 0.2 mg/kg/h for 96 h (GUSTO-II) or 72–120 h (TIMI-9). It became clear to the Event and Safety Committees during the trials, however, that bleeding, and in particular intracerebral haemorrhage, was occurring to excess in patients given hirudin. In the HIT-III trial, the incidence of haemorrhagic stroke was 3.4% in the hirudin group and 0% in the heparin group. These trials were stopped.

The TIMI-9 and GUSTO-II trials were then restarted using lower doses of hirudin (0.1 mg/kg bolus and 0.1 mg/kg/h infusion) and the lessons from the first trials on the need for APTT monitoring were incorporated (APTT value 2–3 times baseline). Unfortunately, early reports suggest that at this dose of hirudin no benefits may be seen. This suggests that the therapeutic window for these agents is very narrow. These studies taught us that increases in patency rates may come only at the cost of extra bleeding.

### GPIIb/IIIa antagonists

Regardless of the mechanism of activation, the final common pathway for platelet aggregation is the cross-linking of platelets through fibrinogen bound to GPIIb/IIIa. The importance of GPIIb/IIIa has been known for many years because of the evidence that Glanzmann's thrombasthenia (GT), an hereditary deficiency of GPIIb/IIIa, results in a moderately severe bleeding tendency. Early animal studies with monoclonal antibodies to GPIIb/IIIa demonstrated the potent antiplatelet effects accruing from blocking the binding of fibrinogen to activated GPIIb/IIIa. This has lead to a number of fibrinogen receptor antagonists currently in various stages of clinical application. Their value in interventional cardiology and in the management of acute coronary syndromes has been proven in various well-controlled trials. Since the overall aim is to attempt to reduce thrombotic occlusion and since thrombus in the arterial system is both platelet initiated and platelet propagated, then these agents have come under some scrutiny to see if there is any benefit in the setting of acute infarction. Thus phase I studies and early safety pilot studies have shown an increase in TIMI grade 3 patency at 60 and 90 min when half dose thrombolytic was given in combination with glycoprotein IIb/IIIa receptor blocker (Fig. 4)[34–36].

These studies have led to the initiation and recently reported GUSTO-V (previously GUSTO-IV) study[37], which tested the efficacy and safety of half-dose reteplase with full-dose GPIIb/IIIa (a chimeric monoclonal antibody abciximab aka ReoPro). Taking into account the ICH rate for the antithrombin trials and the implied narrow therapeutic window, these studies implied it was possible to predict that the complication rates would form an important part of the trial report. This the 'non-inferiority' trial study of 16,588 patients was published in *The Lancet* in June 2001[35]. It showed that the mortality rate for the full-dose reteplase was 5.9% (*n* = 488), and for the half-dose reteplase plus full-dose abciximab was

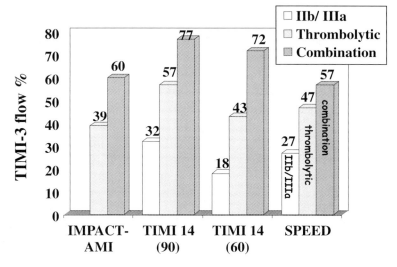

**Fig. 4** Effect of GP IIb/IIIa receptor blockers plus reduced dose thrombolytics on 60 or 90 min TIMI grade 3 flow.

5.6% (*n* = 468) – clearly no mortality benefit. There was, however, a significant benefit for the combined end point of 'death, re-infarction and need for coronary intervention' (20.6% for lytic alone group *versus* 16% for lytic plus abciximab; OR, 0.75; CI, 0.69–0.81; *P* <0.0001). Re-infarction was the significant factor driving this combined end point benefit (3.5% reteplase *versus* 2.3% half-dose reteplase plus abciximab; *P* <0.0001). However, not only was this an open label trial, but re-infarction was investigator determined. Additionally, there was a cost for the reduction in this softer end-point with an increase in bleeding for the combined therapy group, some of which were severe and spontaneous (combined therapy 1.1% *versus* reteplase alone 0.5%; *P* <0.0001); any bleeding occurred in 24.6% *versus* 11.4% reteplase alone; *P* <0.0001. What did this trial tell us? It confirmed that the therapeutic window for agents or combinations is narrow. However, there is some suggestion from this trial, albeit unpublished, that those patients who went onto angioplasty did better if they were on the combined treatment.

However, medication to produce maximal patency may have limited potential. It is likely that a trial comparing Clopidogrel (the so-called 'super-aspirin') with aspirin will be compared with aspirin alone after myocardial infarction. There will always be patients who fail thrombolytic therapy for mechanical reasons such as atheroma bulk or large spontaneous intimal disruption (Fig. 5). Perhaps mechanical strategies are better.

## Primary angioplasty

Grade 3 TIMI flow can only be achieved in 54% of patients with thrombolysis; perhaps it will be shown to be more with lytic therapy plus powerful antiplatelet agent. Currently, however, the only treatment shown to be better than thrombolysis is to open the artery at the time of

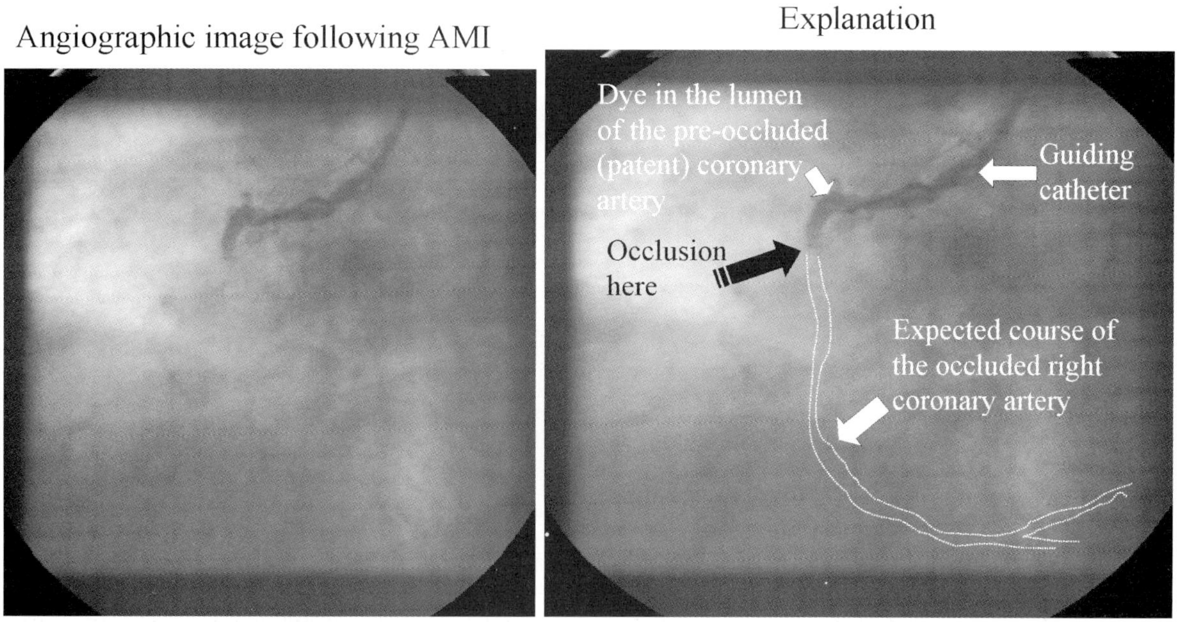

Angiographic image following AMI

Explanation

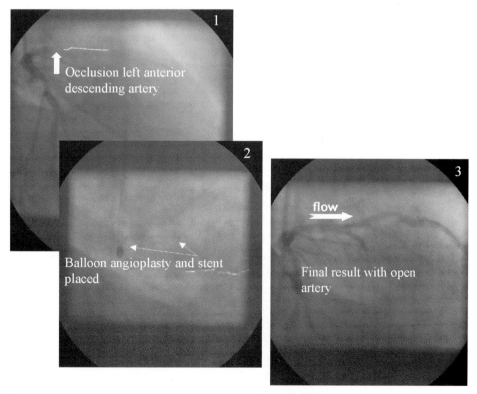

Dye in the lumen of the pre-occluded (patent) coronary artery

Guiding catheter

Occlusion here

Expected course of the occluded right coronary artery

**Fig. 5** Totally occluded right coronary artery with disrupted plaque: penetration of lesion by systemically administered lytic may be difficult

1

Occlusion left anterior descending artery

2

Balloon angioplasty and stent placed

3

flow

Final result with open artery

**Fig. 6** Angioplasty and stenting in acute myocardial infarction

presentation with balloon angioplasty (plus stent; Fig. 6). A number of studies, albeit with small numbers, have shown that if a patient can be taken to the catheter laboratory within 12 h and the artery successfully opened and dilated, TIMI grade 3 flow can be obtained in 80–97% of cases[38]. Short- and long-term survival and morbidity have been improved compared to thrombolysis. Re-occlusion of the vessel remains a real problem with thrombolytic therapy (reaching 30–40% by 3–6 months, and remaining at 25% at 1 year). The comparable 3–6 month vessel patency after primary angioplasty is much higher (87–91%)[39]. Pooled data from the various thrombolytic trials not surprisingly suggest a worse longer term outcome compared to direct angioplasty (death 6.4% *versus* 2.5%; re-infarction 7.9% *versus* 2.0%; stroke 2.5% *versus* 0.3%; death and/or re-infarction 13.1% *versus* 4.3%, respectively). Recurrent ischaemia in the three comparative trials (MAYO clinic, PAMI-I and Zwolle) varied between 27% and 36% for thrombolytic-treated patients and between 9% and 15% for direct angioplasty patients. The 2-year event-free survival (*i.e.* no myocardial infarction, cardiac death or need for re-intervention) for the PAMI-I trial patients was reported to be 85%, indicating that the early separation of the outcome curves for thrombolytic-treated and angioplasty-treated patients is maintained.

However, there are difficulties with these trials. The small numbers of centres and patients results in wide confidence intervals. The data, therefore, have been pooled and evaluated on the basis of 'high' and 'low' risk patients. It would appear that the high-risk patients (older age, larger infarcts and anterior infarcts) benefit both in terms of mortality and re-infarction from direct angioplasty, whereas the low-risk group benefit only in terms of re-infarction. The GUSTO-IIb study[40] failed to demonstrate longer term benefit. This was undoubtedly due, in part, to inadequate angioplasty. More recent trials in which stenting has been employed have shown significant improvement in immediate patency rates which may be the critical factor.

The same factors that influence benefit in thrombolytic treatment need also to be considered in primary angioplasty. Thus Cannon *et al*[41] found that in 27,080 patients treated with primary angioplasty, the door-to-balloon time was a significant factor in mortality outcome (adjusted odds of mortality OR, 1.41; 95% CI, 1.08–1.84; $P = 0.01$ for door-to-balloon time > 2 h: and OR, 1.61; 95% CI, 1.25–2.08; $P < 0.001$ for > 3 h). Others have asserted that even late after the event, primary PCI may beneficially influence left ventricular re-modelling[42]; this is not current practice in the absence of recurrent symptoms or ECG changes, however.

The most important factor determining an improved outcome in patients undergoing intervention for acute myocardial infarction appears to be the use of stents. In a small study, Maillard found the 6-month event-free survival rates were 81.2% in those stented *versus* 72.7%[43]. The major study, however, was published by the Beaumont Hospital group. They studied patients who only received PCI for the primary treatment of their infarct. The acute result was significantly better in the stented group. The 6-month event-free survival rate was also higher in the stented group (12.6% *n*= 452 *versus* PTCA 20.1% *n* = 448; *P* <0.01)[44].

There are now compelling data to suggest that the addition of glycoprotein IIb/IIIa inhibitor to the strategy (the ADMIRAL trial) improves outcome even further[45].

**What are the advantages of primary angioplasty?**
Although still a matter for debate, the case for direct angioplasty for acute MI appears compelling, particularly for selected high-risk cases presenting within 12 h to an hospital with a catheter laboratory. It appears as effective or more effective than thrombolysis with significantly lower risk of stroke and lower risk of the high mortality risk associated with cerebral bleeding (stroke – PTCA = 0.7% *versus* lytic = 2.0%; OR, 0.35; 95% CI, 0.14–0.77; *P* = 0.007: intracerebral – haemorrhage PTCA = 0.1% *versus* lytic = 1.1%; OR, 0.07; 95% CI, 0.0–0.42; *P* <0.001). These figures do not of course take account of current strategies that incorporate glycoprotein IIb/IIIa receptor blocker use. Importantly, intervention deals with the stenosis which lytic agents cannot do. There are data to support the concept that the greater the residual stenosis the more likely the artery will re-occlude[46]. Failure of reperfusion is more likely with lytic therapy when there is significant atheroma bulk or severe disruption of the plaque. Finally, knowing the state of the coronary arteries allows for better triage of patients post-infarct. Thus the normal 5–7 day in-patient stay may be reduced if the infarct-related artery is open and we know the rest of the arteries are normal[47].

**What are the problems with primary angioplasty?**
Primary and rescue angioplasty may be being undertaken in patients who are unwell and the best outcomes may require the most experienced operators. In a retrospective study, Magid *et al*[48] showed the benefits of primary angioplasty outweighed those of thrombolysis in high and intermediate volume centres, but not in low volume centres ( high volume – mortality 3.4% PTCA *versus* 5.4% thrombolysis; *P* < 0.001: low volume centres – 6.2% *versus* 5.9%; *P* = 0.58). Poor outcome for patients with cardiogenic shock remains high no matter what treatment is instigated. Cost-effectiveness data are less available for the current interventional strategy of using stents and glycoprotein IIb/IIIa receptor blocker, than for just balloon angioplasty.

While better early patency rates can be achieved with primary PTCA which translates into improved clinical outcome, both in the short and medium-term, this treatment is not available to all. The problem is that most patients are admitted to hospitals without interventional facilities. There is neither the personnel nor financial resources to place such facilities in all hospitals receiving AMI patients.

## Dealing with the thrombolysis versus angioplasty for AMI problem

There are a number of options. Some have advocated a policy of thrombolysis followed by angiography in **all** patients with angioplasty when indicated (occlusion or significant residual stenosis in the infarct-related artery). Thus Ross[49] found a tPA patency rate of 61% on arrival on the catheter table which was increased to 77% after intervention. Others believe that, in the current resource-limited climate, primary angioplasty for acute infarction cannot be delivered and that angiography and angioplasty where indicated should be reserved for those who demonstrate failure of lytic therapy. There are two UK trials on-going of such a policy. The first, the MERLIN trial[50], has reported preliminary data. In 179 patients undergoing emergency angiography for failed thrombolysis, 156 were deemed to need angioplasty. Providing at least TIMI grade 2 flow was attained (124/135 patients), they showed the mortality was low (5.9%). In the 11 patients in whom TIMI grade 2 flow was not successful, the mortality was very high at 48%. Interestingly, re-infarction or need for revascularisation was 37% in the 41 patients deemed not to need intervention following their angiogram. In the second ongoing trial, the UK-based British Heart Foundation funded on-going REACT trial, patients shown on 90 min ECG to have failed thrombolysis (failure of resolution ST to $\geq 50\%$) were randomised to conservative therapy, second thrombolytic or intervention.

Whether high risk patients will do better receiving thrombolysis at their admission hospital or primary angioplasty after transfer to another hospital is also currently being tested both in the UK and in Europe.

Yet others are developing strategies for early out-of-hospital triage. Thus, on arrival at a patient suffering chest pain, the paramedic would record an ECG and electronically transmit it to a dedicated co-ordinator in a dedicated catheter laboratory. The patient would then be received to this laboratory and undergo angiography and intervention if necessary. Such concepts will need serious resource examination

Understanding that there are significant benefits that can be attributed having an open artery is important[51]. While current measures of patency may be deemed crude in that the TIMI grade flow only measure epicardial flow rather than perfusion[52], this is currently the best indicator in that it has correlated well with short, medium and longer term outcome. There are data to support the benefit of an open artery on short-term commonly recognised complications such as electrical instability[53]. However, whatever the initial treatment prognosis for the infarct, be it lytic or primary PTCA, certain complications occur and need to be treated since these too may influence prognostic outcome.

The most important action, taking account of what has been stated about the importance of having an open artery is that if a patient either fails to settle after thrombolysis (on-going pain or recurrent ECG changes) intervention (with transfer if necessary, for so-called rescue angioplasty) remains an important option[54].

The future is likely to see the advent of facilitated PCI (percutaneous coronary intervention). In this scenario, a rapid onset-of-action lytic (tPA or TNK-PA) will be given as soon as possible (including in ambulances). The additive benefits of subcutaneous heparin and/or glycoprotein IIb/IIIa inhibitors (ASSENT-3)[30] will be utilised and the patient will either undergo coronary angiography and intervention on arrival at the hospital or careful assessment of success of medical treatment be undertaken prior to consideration for coronary angiography. Of course the practicality, bleeding and other side-effect risk and cost effectiveness of such strategies will need to be tested in appropriately conducted clinical trials. Trial data suggest mortality is about 5–6%. Real life mortality in 2001 according to registries such as the GRACE Registry and EuroASPIRE suggest it is closer to 10–12%. Even so, the numbers of patients required to prove benefit with such aggressive interventions will need to be very large.

## Summary and conclusions

Effective opening of the infarct-related artery is of paramount importance. It saves lives in the short, medium and long-term and reduces complications. Thrombolytic therapy with adjunctive aspirin has significantly improved the outcome following acute myocardial infarction. It is cheap and relatively safe. It must be given as early as possible. On-going efforts in public education about the need to recognise the implications of chest pain particularly in those with increased risk factors or who already have angina is imperative in order to reduce the delay in administration of thrombolytics. Beyond this there remains a need to optimise the vessel patency rate since this definitively correlates with both early and longer term survival. New thrombolytics are becoming available, which may improve patency. These agents, however, will need to be tested against current regimens in large clinical trials. Testing of the new antithrombins for reducing vessel re-occlusion in such a setting have indicated that these agents have a relatively narrow therapeutic window. We await the assessment of half-dose thrombolytics with full dose glycoprotein IIb/IIIa receptor blockers. Primary angioplasty may prove the definitive treatment for myocardial infarction in selected cases such as young or elderly patients with anterior infarction, provided the procedure can be undertaken early enough to be of benefit. Limited resources may be the inhibiting factor in wide-spread use of this treatment modality. However, ways to provide primary angioplasty to appropriate patients and importantly in a cost-effective manner should be the strategic aim over the next few years. Facilitated angioplasty may become a strategy to be tested. Early assessment of the thrombolysed patients or triage at the prehospital stage is the way forward.

## References

1  Thaulow E, Erikssen J, Sandvik L *et al.* Initial clinical presentation of cardiac disease in asymptomatic men with silent myocardial ischemia and angiographically documented coronary artery disease. *Am J Cardiol* 1993; **72**: 629–33

2  Norris RM. A new performance indicator for acute myocardial infarction. *Heart* 2001; **85**: 395–401

3  Stevenson R, Ranjadayalan K, Wilkinson P *et al.* Short and long term prognosis of acute myocardial infarction since the introduction of thrombolysis. *BMJ* 1993; **307**: 349–53

4  Davies MJ, Thomas AC. Plaque fissuring – the cause of acute myocardial infarction, sudden ischaemic death, and crescendo angina. *Br Hosp J* 1985; **53**: 363–73

5  Conti CR. Vascular events responsible for thrombotic occlusion of a blood vessel. *Clin Cardiol* 1993; **16**: 761–2

6  Gershlick AH, Syndercombe Court D, Mills P. Young infarct patients with single-vessel occlusion do not have an underlying prothrombotic state to explain their coronary occlusion. *Int J Cardiol* 1992; **36**: 49–56

7  Reimer KA, Lowe JE, Ramussen MM *et al.* The wavefront phenomenon of ischemic cell death. *Circulation* 1977; **56**: 786–94

8  Ohman EM, Armstrong P, Califf RM *et al.* Risk stratification in acute ischemic syndromes using serum troponin T. *J Am Coll Cardiol* 1995; **30**: 148A

9  ISIS-2 (Second International Study of Infarct Survival) Collaborative Group. Randomised trial of intravenous streptokinase, oral aspirin, both or neither among 17187 cases of suspected acute myocardial infarction. *Lancet* 1988; **ii**: 349–60

10  Fibrinolytic Therapy Trialists (FTT) Collaborative Group. Indications for fibrinolytic therapy in suspected acute myocardial infarction: collaborative overview of early mortality and major morbidity from all randomised trials of more than 1000 patients. *Lancet* 1994; **343**: 311–22

11  LATE Study Group. Late assessment of thrombolytic efficiency (LATE) study with alteplase 6–24 hours after onset of acute myocardial infarction. *Lancet* 1993; **342**: 759–66

12  The European Myocardial Infarction Project Group. Pre hospital thrombolytic therapy in patients with suspected acute myocardial infarction. *N Engl J Med* 1993; **329**: 383–9

13  Anonymous. Randomised trial of intravenous atenolol among 16 027 cases of suspected acute myocardial infarction: ISIS-1. First International Study of Infarct Survival Collaborative Group. *Lancet* 1986; **ii**: 57–66

14  Freemantle N, Cleland J, Mason P *et al.* Beta–blockade after myocardial infarction: systematic review and meta regression analysis. *BMJ* 1999; **31**: 1730–7

15  ISIS-4. A randomised trial comparing oral captopril versus placebo, oral mononitrate versus placebo, and intravenous magnesium sulphate versus control among 58,043 patients with suspected

acute myocardial infarction. *Lancet* 1995; **345**: 669–85

16  GISSI-3. Effects of lisinopril and transdermal glyceryl trinitrate singly and together on 6-week mortality and ventricular function after acute myocardial infarction. *Lancet* 1994; **343**: 1115–22

17  Domanski MJ, Exner DV, Borkowf CB *et al*. Effect of angiotensin converting enzyme inhibition on sudden cardiac death in patients following acute myocardial infarction. A meta-analysis of randomised clinical trials. *J Am Coll Cardiol* 1999; **33**: 598–604

18  Yusuf S, Sleight P, Pogue J *et al*. Effects of an angiotensin-converting enzyme inhibitor, ramipril on cardiovascular events in high-risk patients. *N Engl J Med* 2000; **342**: 145–53

19  Cairns JA, Connolly SJ, Roberts R *et al*. Randomised trial of outcome after myocardial infarction in patients with frequent or repetitive ventricular premature depolarisations: CAMIAT. *Lancet* 1997; **349**: 675–82

20  Connolly SJ, Amiodarone Trials Meta-Analysis Investigators. Effect of prophylactic amiodarone on mortality after acute myocardial infarction and in congestive heart failure: meta-analysis of individual data from 6500 patients in randomised trials. *Circulation* 1999; **100**: 2025–34

21  GISSI-2. A factorial randomised trial of alteplase versus streptokinase and heparin versus no heparin among 12,490 patients with acute myocardial infarction. *Lancet* 1990; **336**: 65–71

22  The GUSTO Investigators. An international randomized trial comparing four thrombolytic strategies for acute myocardial infarction. *N Engl J Med* 1993; **329**: 673–82

23  The GUSTO Angiographic Investigators. The effects of tissue plasminogen activator, streptokinase, or both on coronary patency, ventricular function, and survival after acute myocardial infarction. *N Engl J Med* 1993; **329**: 1615–22

24  Fath-Ordoubadi F, Huehns T, Al-Mohammad A *et al*. Significance of the thrombolysis in myocardial infarction scoring system in assessing infarct-related artery reperfusion and mortality rates after acute myocardial infarction. *Am Heart J* 1997; **134**: 62–8

25  French JK, Hyde TA, Patel H *et al*. Survival 12 years after randomisation to streptokinase: the influence of thrombolysis in myocardial infarction flow at three to four weeks. *J Am Coll Cardiol* 1999; **34**: 62–9

26  Meijer A, Verheugt FW, Werter CJ, Lie KI, van der Pol JM, van Eenige MJ. Aspirin versus coumadin in the prevention of reocclusion and recurrent ischemia after successful thrombolysis: a prospective placebo-controlled angiographic study. Results of the APRICOT Study . *Circulation* 1993; **87**: 1524–30

27  Suzuki S, Satio M, Suzuk N *et al*. Thrombolytic properties of novel modified human tissue type plasminogen activator (E6010): a bolus injection of E6010 has equivalent potency of lysing young and aged canine coronary thrombi. *J Cardiovasc Pharmacol* 1991; **17**: 738–46

28  Collen D, Van der Werf F. Coronary thrombolysis with recombinant staphylokinase patients with evolving myocardial infarction. *Circulation* 1993; **87**: 1850–3

29  Anonymous. Single-bolus tenecteplase compared with front-loaded alteplase in acute myocardial infarction: the ASSENT-2 double-blind randomised trial. Assessment of the Safety and Efficacy of a New Thrombolytic Investigators. *Lancet* 1999; **354**: 716–22

30  Anonymous. Efficacy and safety of tenecteplase in combination with enoxaparin, abciximab, or unfractionated heparin: the ASSENT-3 randomised trial in acute myocardial infarction. *Lancet* 2001; **358**: 605–13

31  Anonymous. Randomized trial of intravenous heparin versus recombinant hirudin for acute coronary syndromes. The Global Use of Strategies to Open Occluded Coronary Arteries (GUSTO) IIa Investigators. *Circulation* 1994; **90**: 1631–7

32  Antman EM. Hirudin in acute myocardial infarction. Safety report from the Thrombolysis and Thrombin Inhibition in Myocardial Infarction (TIMI) 9A Trial. *Circulation* 1994; **90**: 1624–30

33  Neuhaus KL, von Essen R, Tebbe U. Safety observations from the pilot phase of the randomized r-Hirudin for Improvement of Thrombolysis (HIT-III) study. A study of the Arbeitsgemeinschaft Leitender Kardiologischer Krankenhausarzte (ALKK). *Circulation* 1994; **90**: 1638–42

34  Ohman E, Magnus MD, Kleiman NS *et al*. Combined accelerated tissue-plasminogen activator and platelet glycoprotein IIb/IIIa integrin receptor blockade with integrilin in acute myocardial infarction: results of a randomized, placebo controlled, dose-ranging trial. *Am Heart J* 1997; **95**: 846–54

35  de Lemos JA, Antman EM, Gibson C *et al*. Abciximab improves both epicardial flow and myocardial reperfusion in ST elevation myocardial infarction: observations from the TIMI 14 trial. *Am Heart J* 2000; **101**: 239

36  Anonymous. Trial of abciximab with and without low-dose reteplase for acute myocardial infarction. Strategies for Patency Enhancement in the Emergency Department (SPEED) Group. *Circulation* 2000; **101**: 2788–94

37  Topol EJ, The GUSTO V Investigators. Reperfusion therapy for acute myocardial infarction with fibrinolytic therapy or combination reduced fibrinolytic therapy and platelet glycoprotein IIb/IIIa inhibition: the GUSTO V randomised trial. *Lancet* 2001; **357**: 1905–14

38  Grines CL, Browne KF, Marco J. A comparison of immediate angioplasty with thrombolytic therapy for acute myocardial infarction. The Primary Angioplasty in Myocardial Infarction Study Group. *N Engl J Med* 1993; **328**: 673–9

39  Mark DB, O'Neill WW, Brodie BR. Baseline and six-month costs of primary angioplasty therapy for acute myocardial infarction: results from the Primary Angioplasty Registry. *J Am Coll Cardiol* 1995; **26**: 688–95

40  Anonymous. A clinical trial comparing primary coronary angioplasty with tissue plasminogen activator for acute myocardial infarction. The Global use of Strategies to Open Occluded Coronary Arteries in Acute coronary Syndromes (GUSTO IIb). *N Engl J Med* 1997; **336**: 1621-8

41  Cannon CP, Gibson CM, Lambrew CT *et al*. Relationship of symptom-onset-to-balloon time and door-to-balloon time with mortality in patients undergoing angioplasty for acute myocardial infarction. *JAMA* 2000; **283**; 2941–7

42  Kanamasa K, Nakabayashi T, Hayashi T *et al*. Percutaneous transluminal coronary angioplasty performed 24–48 hours after the onset of acute myocardial infarction improves chronic-phase left ventricular regional wall motion. *Angiology* 2000 **51**: 281–8

43  Maillard L, Hamon M, Khalife K *et al*. A comparison of systematic stenting and conventional balloon angioplasty during primary percutaneous transluminal coronary angioplasty for acute myocardial infarction. STENTIM-2 Investigators. *J Am Coll Cardiol* 2000; **35**: 1729–36

44  Grines CL, Cox DA, Stone GW *et al*. Coronary angioplasty with or without stent implantation for acute myocardial infarction. Stent Primary Angioplasty in Myocardial Infarction Study Group. *N Engl J Med* 1999; **341**: 1949–56

45  Montalescot G, Barragan P, Wittenberg O *et al*. Platelet glycoprotein IIb/IIIa inhibition with coronary stenting for acute myocardial infarction. *N Engl J Med* 2001; **344**: 1895–903

46  Lenderink T, Simoons ML, Van Es GA *et al*. Benefit of thrombolytic therapy is sustained throughout five years and is related to TIMI perfusion grade 3 but not grade 2 flow at discharge. The European Cooperative Study Group. *Circulation* 1995; **92**: 1110–6

47  Grines CL, Marsalese DL, Brodie B *et al*. Safety and cost-effectiveness of early discharge after primary angioplasty in low risk patients with acute myocardial infarction. PAMI-II Investigators. Primary Angioplasty in Myocardial Infarction. *J Am Coll Cardiol* 1998; **31**: 967–72

48  Magid DJ, Calonge BN, Rumsfeld JS *et al*. Relation between hospital primary angioplasty volume and mortality for patients with acute MI treated with primary angioplasty vs thrombolytic therapy. *JAMA* 2000; **284**: 3131–8

49  Ross AM, Coyne KS, Reiner JS *et al*. A randomized trial comparing primary angioplasty with a strategy of short-acting thrombolysis and immediate planned rescue angioplasty in acute myocardial infarction: the PACT trial. PACT Investigators. Plasminogen-activator Angioplasty Compatibility Trial. *J Am Coll Cardiol* 1999; **34**: 1954–62

50  Sutton AG, Campbell PG, Grech ED *et al*. Failure of thrombolysis: experience with a policy of early angiography and rescue angioplasty for electrocardiographic evidence of failed thrombolysis. *Heart* 2000; **84**: 197–204

51  Sadanandan S, Hochman JS. Early reperfusion, late reperfusion, and the open artery hypothesis: an overview. *Prog Cardiovasc Dis* 2000; **42**: 397–404

52  Roe MT, Ohman EM, Maas AC *et al*. Shifting the open-artery hypothesis downstream: the quest for optimal reperfusion. *J Am Coll Cardiol* 2001; **37**: 9–18

53  Carnendran L, Steinberg JS. Does an open infarct-related artery after myocardial infarction improve electrical stability? *Prog Cardiovasc Dis* 2000; **42**: 439–54

54  Kovac JD, Gershlick AH. How should we detect and manage failed thrombolysis? *Eur Heart J* 2001; **22**: 450–8

# Later management of documented ischaemic heart disease: secondary prevention and rehabilitation

## A A McLeod

*Department of Cardiology, Poole Hospital NHS Trust, Poole, UK*

Patients may present with a variety of syndromes related to ischaemic heart disease. These include unstable or stable angina pectoris, acute myocardial infarction, and occasionally cardiac failure without prior anginal pain or infarction. For the purposes of this review, it will generally be assumed that the condition has been stabilised, though one important aspect of the rehabilitation process is the recognition of continuing or recurrent problems such as angina pectoris and cardiac decompensation. This should then be followed by appropriate intervention. The key components of post-hospital management of such patients are: (i) support; (ii) education; (iii) assessment; (iv) intervention (if necessary); (v) therapy; and (vi) lifestyle modification.

A comprehensive programme of cardiac rehabilitation will contain all of these components, and will place varying emphasis on each one in a manner which is tailored to the individual patient. In the computer age, this could be called the 'menu driven' approach, in which the doctor or therapist chooses the most appropriate course of action for the ischaemic heart disease patient from a selection of options. Although many reviews and texts of cardiac rehabilitation exist, a brief summary of the process is appropriate.

## Cardiac rehabilitation

The definition of this process has altered subtly over recent years. The most commonly quoted definition is:

*The rehabilitation of cardiac patients is the sum of activities required to influence favourably the underlying cause of the disease, as well as the best possible physical, mental and social conditions, so that they may, by their own efforts preserve or resume when lost, as normal a place as possible in the community. Rehabilitation cannot be regarded as an isolated form of therapy, but must be integrated with the whole treatment of which it forms only one facet[1].*

Correspondence to:
Dr A A McLeod,
Department of
Cardiology, Poole
Hospital NHS Trust,
Longfleet Road, Poole,
Dorset BH15 2JB, UK

The US Agency for Health Care Policy and Research expands this concept thus:

*Cardiac rehabilitation services are an essential component of the contemporary management of patients with multiple presentations of CHD and with heart failure. Cardiac rehabilitation is a multifactorial process that includes exercise training, education, counselling regarding risk reduction and lifestyle changes, and use of behavioural interventions; these services should be integrated into the comprehensive care of cardiac patients. The objective of cardiac rehabilitation services is to improve both the physiologic and psychosocial status of cardiac patients. The physiologic outcomes targeted include improvement in exercise capacity and exercise habits and optimization of risk-factor status, including improvement in blood lipid and lipoprotein profiles, body weight, and blood glucose and blood pressure levels, and the cessation of smoking. Enhancements of myocardial perfusion and performance, as well as reduction in progression of the underlying atherosclerotic process, are additional goals. The psychosocial functioning of patients should be improved when needed, including reduction of stress, anxiety, and depression. Functional independence of patients, particularly the elderly, is an essential goal of cardiac rehabilitation services. Return to appropriate and satisfactory work could benefit both patients and society[2].*

The WHO definition emphasizes a particular aspect of treatment for chronic diseases such as ischaemic heart disease, namely that improvements in health should be 'by their own efforts'. In modern medical practice, the patient becomes a partner in a concerted effort to improve their health status. An exclusively paternalistic approach, where the doctor dictates the treatment that is followed by the patient, means that treatment for a condition where the patient can also help himself or herself is necessarily incomplete.

## The phases of rehabilitation

These are commonly divided into four time periods.

### Phase I: the in-hospital treatment phase

A variety of interventions, endorsed by a substantial evidence base, are applied in acute myocardial infarction. These include therapy with fibrinolytic drugs, beta-blocking drugs, and Angiotensin Converting Enzyme (ACE) inhibitors. The goals of rehabilitation in this phase are to speed recovery and to minimise risk from deconditioning and immobility such as muscle wasting and deep venous thrombosis. Although an extremely vulnerable phase psychologically, this period provides a valuable opportunity to begin imparting lifestyle advice such as the cessation of cigarette smoking. Studies indicate that uptake of health-related information during this phase is limited, and needs to be re-inforced during subsequent phases.

### Phase II: the immediate post-hospital phase

A peak of anxiety is recorded at, or immediately after, hospital discharge. Poor resources or poor planning often mean that patients are not well supported during this period. Potentially life threatening problems such as early recurrent myocardial ischaemia, deterioration in or the emergence of heart failure symptoms, and occasionally the emergence of cardiac arrhythmias may jeopardise recovery at a time when the specialist cardiac services present in hospital are no longer available to provide support. This phase represents one where potentially the impact of a well organized cardiac support team can minimise anxiety and react to the development of the specific medical problems mentioned above.

### Phase III: the formal rehabilitation programme phase

Many programmes of rehabilitation focus on the provision of services during this phase. The specialized skills of physiotherapists, exercise physiologists, occupational therapists, pharmacists, dieticians, cardiac nurses, and clinical psychologists may be used in educational and lifestyle modification programmes. Many programmes focus on exercise as a means of promoting both physical fitness and healthy behaviour in general. Unfortunately, many programmes are delayed until 6–8 weeks after the index cardiac event. Patient education (the re-inforcement of information already given in hospital) and progressive exercise rehabilitation should ideally start as soon as the patient leaves phase I.

### Phase IV: the maintenance phase

After the formal intervention of phase III, this phase which is life-long focuses on the maintenance of a healthy lifestyle, and aims to avoid the loss of previously achieved goals such as improved physical fitness, the maintenance of weight loss, and continued abstinence from tobacco products. Many studies attest to the difficulties of long-term health maintenance.

## Post-hospital cardiac care

All rehabilitation phases after phase I can be thought of under the above heading. The original development of ischaemic heart disease can be thought of as the net result of the interplay of risk factors, and the impact of measures to reduce these after the acute phase of illness is known as secondary prevention. Before discussing pharmacological and non-pharmacological interventions, it is necessary to consider the optimum management of specific medical problems. Adjunctive therapy after myocardial infarction has been reviewed by multiple authorities[3].

## Myocardial ischaemia

An aggressive approach to the management of acute myocardial ischaemia is validated by the results of recent trials[4] and by the knowledge that optimum flow in a coronary artery which has occluded and caused myocardial infarction is associated with reduced mortality. The degree to which a patient has been treated with interventional therapies during acute myocardial ischaemia or infarction varies substantially world-wide. However, a consistent goal for cardiologists, prior to a patient's discharge, is the abolition of evident ischaemia by intervention, or by ischaemia-reducing drugs. The efficacy of in-hospital therapy is often assessed by formal exercise testing on a stationary bicycle ergometer, or by motor-driven treadmill.

Unfortunately, treadmill testing, despite its simplicity and obvious relevance to physical stress in everyday life, has substantial limitations in practice. The Italian GISSI-2 study concluded that even being able to perform a treadmill test was a predictor of a good outcome after a myocardial infarct. The mortality of patients who were not subjected to treadmill testing or in whom treadmill testing was thought to be contra-indicated was 4-fold greater than those who undertook a treadmill test[5,6].

Substantial limitation on a treadmill test is associated with a poor outcome. Two major factors underlie this. The first is left ventricular impairment. The second is marked ischaemic limitation. Evidence of ischaemia at a low workload on exercise testing may indicate unresolved coronary flow limitation, or multivessel coronary artery disease. Some centres will further investigate these patients with a view to angioplasty or coronary artery surgery. There will always be some patients, however, in whom these problems are either unresolved or unavoidable. In such patients, it is important to check that the role of drug therapy has been fully explored. Exercise and other forms of stress testing are however relatively poorly predictive of re-occlusion in an infarct-related artery, and close surveillance is advised to detect recurrent ischaemia[7].

## Cardiac failure therapy

ACE inhibitors are the most obviously beneficial agents in this condition. A wealth of evidence supports their use in asymptomatic left ventricular dysfunction (LVEF 0.40 or less) or in overt left ventricular failure, even if the failure has been transient. It seems likely that the angiotensin (AT) II inhibitors are as beneficial, though at present none are licensed for this indication[8].

β-Blocking drugs are also valuable in patients with cardiac impairment. A paradox exists, however, in this form of therapy. When ACE inhibitors are given, it can immediately be appreciated that their actions are likely to be beneficial. Sudden loss of left ventricular pump function results in a substantial stimulus to the renin-angiotensin axis. The deleterious effects of ACE and angiotensin activation such as salt and water retention, and increased left ventricular afterload are blocked by ACE inhibitors and ATII antagonists. In acute cardiac failure, however, there is substantial stimulation of adrenergic activity, primarily through sympathetic nerves (noradrenaline), but also through the adrenal medulla (adrenaline) if the stress is severe enough. Acute blockade of this response is dangerous. Nonetheless, in chronic stable cardiac impairment, considerable evidence for deleterious effects of chronic sympathetic stimulation exists. A large number of trials have been conducted with β-adrenoceptor antagonists following myocardial infarction, with a consistent indication of benefit to both reduction of re-infarction risk, and also to mortality. An interesting feature of these studies has been that the more severe or damaging the infarct, the greater the evidence of benefit. For example the Beta Blocker Heart Attack Trial (BHAT) showed that the mortality reduction with propranolol when compared with placebo was most substantial in the group of patients who had either suffered electrical complications (such as cardiac arrest) or cardiac failure during their index infarct[9]. In clinical practice, it is common to control overt cardiac failure with an ACE inhibitor and if necessary a diuretic, but to try and introduce a β-blocker before hospital discharge. The long-term benefit of β-blockade in chronic heart failure is also incontestable. Many studies, however, show that all too often drugs such as β-blockers are not given to patients who could benefit from them. There is a particular bias in this respect against the elderly, and a national bias is also evident. β-Blockers are less commonly prescribed in the UK than in Scandinavia, Italy and the US. Some physicians point to the real adverse effects of these drugs such as fatigue. This is not a reason for not trying the agents in the first instance, however, particularly when the mortality benefits are so striking. Although β-blockers experimentally show an antifibrillatory action, it is unclear if this is important in clinical practice. Some evidence exists, however, to show that there is less ventricular irritability when patients receive these drugs in the post-infarction period. There is little evidence for such a role for any other purely anti-arrhythmic drugs. Although some evidence of benefit for amiodarone has been found in several studies, no other anti-arrhythmic drugs have been shown to be beneficial and most have shown increased mortality. An interesting case in point is sotalol, a non-selective β-blocker with class III (action potential and refractoriness prolongation) anti-arrhythmic effect. Commercially available sotalol is a racemic mixture, but its β-blocking effect resides in the l-isomer. When d-sotalol (only class III action) was tested in the Survival With Oral d-sotalol (SWORD) trial, increased mortality in the active treatment group was found[10].

Anticoagulation with warfarin or other drugs has also been tested after myocardial infarction. There is considerable heterogeneity in the studies (some are in heart failure, some post-infarction) though overall a meta-analysis found a reduction in mortality when patients with coronary artery disease were treated with high-intensity warfarin therapy[11]. An excess of major bleeding events is to be expected with this treatment strategy. In addition, the possible complementary roles of anticoagulant drugs such as warfarin, and antiplatelet drugs such as aspirin, remains to be determined. Aspirin is routinely prescribed to most patients with chronic coronary artery disease. It does appear to interact with ACE inhibitors reducing the efficacy of the latter. There is interest, therefore, in the thienopyridines – antiplatelet drugs with apparently similar efficacy to aspirin. At present, their use is generally short-term following coronary intervention, or when aspirin is genuinely contra-indicated[12].

## Anti-ischaemic therapy

As discussed above, modern management of coronary artery disease attempts to eliminate ischaemia where possible, often using physical intervention techniques. Despite this, overt (symptomatic) ischaemia or silent ischaemia is often present and not amenable to angioplasty or coronary bypass techniques. Where treatment with β-blockade is not possible, there is reasonable evidence to support the use of heart rate lowering calcium antagonists (diltiazem and verapamil) post-myocardial infarction. Their use appears deleterious when heart failure is present. The routine use of dihydropyridine calcium antagonists or of nitrates does not appear to add benefit, though they synergise well with β-blockers in patients with symptomatic angina[3].

## Plasma lipid modification

Westernized populations have high circulating levels of plasma cholesterol when compared with countries whose food intake is closer to subsistence level. Although plasma cholesterol was considered a marker for increased coronary risk for many years, conclusive proof that manipulation of the circulating cholesterol level affected coronary heart disease risk was only obtained when the hydroxymethyl glutaryl coenzyme A reductase (HMGCoA) antagonists became available and were tested in large-scale clinical trials. These drugs act at an important rate-limiting step in cholesterol synthesis. Since the landmark 4S (Scandinavian Simvastatin Survival Study) was published in 1994, a wealth of evidence has confirmed the very substantial effect on coronary event rates and mortality that these compounds confer[13]. There is dispute (largely for economic reasons) over the use of these drugs in patients whose coronary risk is low, or in whom for reasons that are unclear, very low LDL cholesterol levels co-exist with coronary artery disease. The majority of patients with overt ischaemic heart disease, including unstable angina pectoris[14], can benefit from therapy however. More recently, gemfibrozil, which has little effect on LDL cholesterol, but which increases HDL cholesterol and reduces triglycerides, has also been shown to be beneficial[15]. During the rehabilitation process, the key issue with these drugs (as well as with drugs such as ACE inhibitors and β-blockers) is not whether they work, but how is it possible to ensure that patients receive them, and whether they should be titrated to produce optimal effect in the individual patient. Compliance with therapy is therefore a vital issue.

## Compliance and psychological issues in the rehabilitation process

Thus far we have focused on the classical 'disease model' of coronary artery disease, familiar to all doctors from their training in medical school. Firm evidence shows that implementation of specific therapies can make a major impact on the disease process. But there is another model of disease, the 'illness perspective'. In this model, familiar to clinical psychologists, the subjective responses of patients, and indeed those close to them determine how they make sense of and respond to the symptoms. It is vital for the patient to overcome the psychological hurdles that the disease has placed in his or her path. Both the patient and the family must adapt to the illness, and also react positively to the advice given. It is of little import how great the *P* value of a trial indicating benefit from β-blockade after myocardial infarction is if the patient does not comply with the therapy. If significant clinical depression, or poor understanding of the condition is present after infarction and is not addressed, then improvements in lifestyle behaviour such as smoking cessation, weight reduction, compliance with therapy, and modification of diet are unlikely. Skilled rehabilitation therapists can work with a patient to encourage positive change, and should be alert to the need to refer for appropriate clinical help where necessary. Other treatments such as better diabetic control and improved antihypertensive regimens may also be needed. The process of conveying information to the patient has recently been formally reviewed by Scott *et al*[16].

Observations within and without cardiac rehabilitation programmes indicate that important lifestyle interventions are not adhered to long-term[17]. Three specific areas can be identified. These are: (i) patient-related factors – these can be predicted by the patient's initial adherence, their self-efficacy, and social support; (ii) regimen-related factors – a more complex treatment regimen predicts non-adherence; and (iii) provider-related factors – these relate to the empathic and communication and motivational skills of the healthcare professional delivering therapy.

As well as exploring the patient's readiness to change behaviour[18], it is important to emphasise the concept of self-efficacy, where the power to change is seen to reside within the patient himself or herself. Other strategies include the involvement of partners, self-monitoring, re-inforcement, multiple contacts and goal setting. When lifestyle modification advice is delivered in a cardiac rehabilitation programme, extended-length participation predicts better control of body weight, physical fitness, and lipoprotein subfractions, and may be an argument for continuing centre-based programmes[19]. Lack of funding and other practical issues suggest, however, that strategies for enhancing adherence to home-exercise and dietary programmes will be needed.

# Lifestyle modification of coronary risk factors in the rehabilitation process

Although much emphasis is rightly placed on pharmacological therapy in ischaemic heart disease, many patients are reluctant to take drugs. Even when the patient accepts that appropriate medication is needed, many will also wish to try and avert further cardiac events, and will readily accept lifestyle change advice. The implementation of such advice is problematic. This section of the review now focuses on areas where patients can help themselves.

## Physical inactivity and exercise

Physical inactivity continues to increase in Westernised populations and is associated with increasing levels of obesity[20]. Physical inactivity is itself a risk factor for the development of coronary artery disease[21,22].

A number of studies link physical inactivity with increased risk of coronary artery disease. The largest single trial of exercise and its potential beneficial effects on coronary artery disease patients was the National

Exercise and Heart Disease Project, sponsored by the National Heart, Lung, and Blood Institute (NHLBI) in the US[23]. Premature withdrawal of funding compromised the conclusions of this study, which showed trends in favour of an intensive 1-year exercise programme compared with 'usual care'. This study, however, was incorporated into both of the two substantial overviews of exercise and cardiac rehabilitation published within a short time of each other[24,25]. These analyses independently reached broadly similar conclusions. After approximately 3 years, the reduction in risk of cardiovascular death following participation in a cardiac rehabilitation programme is of the order of 20–25%. But trials included were performed between 1972 and 1985, and the exercise intervention applied varied widely. Follow-up of more than 1 year was required for the O'Connor analysis and 2 years for the Oldridge analysis. Almost all trials recruited exclusively male patients under the age of 65 years. A more recent systematic review suggests that exercise trials *per se* have favourably influenced mortality[26]. Recent data from the British Regional Heart Study also suggest that exercise in subjects with coronary artery disease is associated with reduced cardiovascular disease mortality[27].

Physical exercise can aid symptom management after myocardial infarction. The 'training effect' whereby the patient can achieve an external workload with reduced heart rate and blood pressure compared with the levels before training is valuable in clinical practice. Both heart rate and systolic blood pressure are important determinants of myocardial oxygen consumption[28]. It follows that patients may achieve a level of external work after exercise training that they cannot achieve without experiencing angina pectoris prior to training. Myocardial function may also be improved after training in cardiac patients, particularly if prolonged and intensive[29]. Much of the training effect, however, is due to enhanced oxygen extraction by exercising in the trained muscle groups (increased arteriovenous oxygen difference), and is, therefore, largely obtained at a reduced overall cardiac output[30]. This training effect can be quite potent, comparable in clinical results with anti-anginal therapy[31,32].

Exercise is important life-long, but has particular and attractive benefits for the elderly. Longitudinal studies of the age-related decline in maximal aerobic performance, as assessed by maximal oxygen uptake ($VO_2$ max), indicate that between 60–90 years minimal aerobic requirement for survival is reached. Exercise conditioning attenuates this decline[33]. But exercise in older people brings other benefits too, some as apparently mundane as the prevention of disabilities caused by immobility – faecal impaction, incontinence, deep vein thrombosis[34]. Exercise also increases safety for older people[35,36]. Exercise and its contribution to lipid management is further reviewed below, but its continuation in a life-long pattern is important. Many exercise benefits are lost with discontinuation[37]. Exercise is not 'bankable'.

## Exercise in heart failure

Exercise in this group of patients has evolved from complete contra-indication: 'rest for the body; rest for the mind; rest for the heart'[38] to accepted practice[39]. Although there is general agreement on rest for acute heart failure, patients with chronic left ventricular dysfunction can undergo exercise training safely and show benefit. Improvements in peak oxygen consumption and exercise duration are associated with reduced catecholamine levels and other neuro-endocrine responses, and improved heart rate variability. These latter markers are known to be associated with poorer prognosis in heart failure, though the conceptual leap between the observation of more favourable neuro-endocrine profiles, and improved prognosis has not been demonstrated in adequately sized trials as yet.

The US Agency for Health Care Policy and Research consensus document endorses the opinions expressed above[2]. An independently constituted group has also endorsed the need for greater physical activity in the maintenance of cardiovascular health and prevention of recurrent disease[40].

Anxiety exists about the possible adverse effects of exercise. It is a common anecdotal experience that some people die suddenly during exercise, due to coronary artery disease, or sustain a heart attack shortly afterward. This phenomenon is sometimes called 'triggering'. Current knowledge of acute coronary syndromes and myocardial infarction suggests that frequently this is triggered by rupture of a 'vulnerable' coronary artery plaque, though instantaneous death is more commonly due to arrhythmia[41]. During violent isometric exercise, substantial increases in cardiac afterload occur, and direct mechanical stress is imposed on the whole of the central vasculature. The phenomenon of 'triggering' has been explored in both Augsburg, Germany, and in Boston, USA[42]. Although a substantial amount of debate was engendered by the papers discussed by Curfman[42] (see correspondence[43]), the essential message is 2-fold: (i) exercise can act as a trigger of myocardial infarction; and (ii) paradoxically, perhaps, exercise taken regularly is nonetheless protective. The worst thing to do is never to exercise, and then to have to do so! Pushing a broken-down car, or shovelling snow, are not only fixed in the layman's mind as associated with heart attack, they are also borne out by the evidence. All exercise programmes with physiological demonstrable benefits to patients utilize an aerobic, graded, exercise programme with repetitive, rythmic exercise of large muscle groupos to steadily increase whole body oxygen uptake and cardiac output. In heart failure patients who may initially be very deconditioned and sedentary, this level of exercise may be very low indeed. In young uncomplicated, previously fit, post-myocasrdial infarction patients the level of exercise may be much greater than this. A safe starting point for most subjects ia approximately 50% of an individual's maximal oxygen uptake.

## Smoking cessation

Cigarette smoking is the single largest avoidable environmental and behavioural cause of cardiovascular disease, and of course the cause of several forms of cancer[44]. Its highly addictive nature can be seen in studies carried out in drug addiction clinics, in that opiate addicts generally find it easier to give up heroin than to give up smoking. Interventions to promote smoking cessation have been costed at less than £1000 per life-year gained, in contrast with over 310 other medical interventions with a median cost of about £17,000 per life-year gained. Smoking is, therefore, a 'best buy' target for healthcare professionals. Intensive support and nicotine replacement therapy are important components of any serious attempts to help heavy smokers, though even brief but assertive medical advice is helpful. Kottke and colleagues reviewed the attributes of successful smoking cessation interventions in medical practice[45]. Programmes with multiple advisers in the team, multiple methods of approach, and sustained and regular contacts with clients were the most successful. Fiscal measures are also important[46]. Full details of guidelines can be found elsewhere[47].

## Dietary modification

Rigorous dieting can improve cholesterol levels, though generally only of the order of 0.3–0.6 mmol/l. It is noteworthy that in the Scandinavian 4S trial, although the placebo group was given advice on dietary modification, the run-in levels of cholesterol prior to initiation of randomized therapy showed no difference over several months, and continued without any real change on randomized placebo therapy for 5 years or more[13]. This, therefore, probably represents the 'real world' of treatment effect (or lack of it) with simple dietary advice alone. A systematic overview of dietary intervention trials indicated that diets equivalent to the American Heart Association Step 2 diet (*vide infra*) lowered blood total cholesterol by 6.1% and diets equivalent to the American Heart Association Step 1 schema lowered blood total cholesterol by 3.0% ($P$ <0.0001)[48]. Efficacy was limited by lack of compliance. Overviews of complex interventions, however, are fraught with statistical problems, and the paper by Tang and colleagues has been criticized for inappropriately excluding trials and for drawing conclusions when statistical testing reveals substantial heterogeneity between studies[49]. Although there is little doubt that such interventions do good, the modest effects on plasma cholesterol should be compared with the 30–40% reduction in cholesterol achievable by HMGCoA reductase inhibitors.

In a number of small-scale studies, however, relatively large effects on plasma lipids have been found, and in some cases these have been associated with favourable angiographic changes. In the Lifestyle Heart Trial, Ornish and colleagues sought to modify risk in a multifactorial manner, though with an approach which eschewed drug therapy in favour of major dietary changes, meditation and relaxation therapy, and moderate physical exercise[50]. Although the study populations were small, changes in LDL cholesterol were quite striking, and this was associated with improved coronary angiographic appearances. In the dietary component, however, only about 10% of total calories were made up of fat. This intake is very markedly below most dietary levels in the Western world. Current US fat intake is 33% of calories; the National Cholesterol Education Program recommends 30% (Step I) and 20% (Step II)[51]. Dramatic changes in fat intake as in the Lifestyle Heart Trial require very careful dietary planning. In this study there was one chef for every 8 patients enrolled! Another study incorporating diet in the management of coronary artery disease was the St Thomas' Atherosclerosis Regression Study (STARS)[52]. Although an examination of cholestyramine added to dietary treatment, the diet alone group in whom the primary aim was to reduce fat intake to 27% of dietary energy also showed significant falls in LDL cholesterol compared with a control group over 39 months. Triglyceride levels were also reduced. The dietary strategy also increased intake of $\omega$-3 and $\omega$-6 fatty acids. Plant-derived soluble fibre was also added. Weight did not change significantly. In addition to encouraging results obtained in plasma lipids, improved angiographic appearances were seen in patients treated with diet alone or diet plus cholestyramine in this study[52].

The STARS study gives a clue to what is perhaps an important feature of successful dietary intervention studies. Not only may it be important to reduce saturated fat intake, but it might also be necessary to modify the composition of the ingested fats. A number of studies have examined this possibility. In the DASH study, the effect of dietary patterns on blood pressure was examined[53]. A diet rich in fruits, vegetables, and low fat dairy products reduced blood pressure more than a control diet in 459 subjects with mild hypertension, independent of sodium or caloric intake. Similarly, in the Lyon Diet Heart Study, after approximately 4 years in a post-myocardial population, a 'Mediterranean' diet result in reduced cardiac events compared with control diet, though the numbers were relatively small[54]. The Diet And Reinfarction Trial (DART) also modified diet, the most important component being the introduction of fatty fish, with beneficial results[55]. It is notable that modest, if any, changes in the usual measured plasma lipids occurred in these studies, demonstrating the shortcomings of conventional lipid risk factor measurement. The very substantial GISSI-Prevenzione trial, in 11,324 post-myocardial infarction subjects in Italy investigated the addition of vitamin E and/or n-3 poly-unsaturated fatty acids (PUFA) to the diet. Dietary supplementation with n-3 PUFA led to reduction in death or cardiac events by 10–20%[56]. There is some evidence that the effects of n-3 ($\omega$-3) fatty acids may be mediated by an electrophysiological effect in suppressing malignant ventricular arrhythmias[57]. Finally, and most recently, a report from US women in the Breast Cancer Detection and Demonstration Project (BCDDP) indicated that women with better Recommended Food Score (RFS) have a lower than expected all-cause mortality, despite adjustment for confounding reductions in known coronary risk factors. Although not a clinical trial, this study is powerful because of the large number of events recorded (2065 deaths after a median follow-up of 5.6 years) from a total of 42,554 women who completed a food frequency questionnaire[58]. The contrasting results of trials of saturated fat reduction and trials where intake of unsaturated fats has been the aim have been reviewed by Oliver[59].

Hypertension is an important risk factor for coronary artery disease. Although multiple studies attest to the importance of lowering blood pressure by pharmacological means in hypertensive subjects, salt restriction has a potentially important role to play in lowering blood pressure. The DASH study mentioned above has also studied the effects of modest salt restriction in lowering blood pressure. Even modest sodium restriction – to less than 100 mmol/day had significant beneficial effects on blood pressure, which were enhanced with the DASH diet for any given sodium intake over the control diet population[60].

## Multifactorial intervention studies

Schuler and colleagues performed a randomised multifactorial intervention trial with an intensive physical exercise programme and a low-fat diet in 113 patients with coronary artery disease[61]. They used the American Heart Association Phase 3 diet with fat intake <20% of energy. Lipid lowering drugs were not prescribed. Intensive cardiac investigations were performed at 1 year of intervention. Coronary artery disease progressed at a slower pace in the intervention group. In the intervention group, body weight decreased by 5%, total cholesterol by 10%, LDL by 8%, and triglycerides by 24%. All changes were highly significant[61]. There are some inconsistencies here with regard to triglyceride levels, which fell in some studies, but failed to do so in others. This issue is partly addressed by Lavie and Milani[62]. In 313 patients not taking any lipid modifying therapy undertaking an exercise programme and an American Heart Association Phase I diet[63], the reductions seen in triglyceride levels were restricted to patients with high baseline triglycerides. This could, however, be an example in part of regression toward the mean.

## Dietary additives

### Phytosterols in the diet

Chisholm *et al*[64] studied the effect of replacing butter with margarine of canola (rape-seed like) oil. Concentrations of LDL cholesterol fell by about 10%. No adverse lipoprotein patterns were found. In addition to substitution of one fat by another, new approaches have been taken with the introduction of proprietary brands of margarine containing plant stanol esters. Plant stanol esters reduce cholesterol absorption and when incorporated into diets low in saturated fat and cholesterol have achieved reductions in LDL cholesterol of up to 24%[65]. When plant fatty acids are added to the diet of animals, they can in turn modify the body composition of those animals. This approach has been applied to egg production and to some meats. When consumed by humans, these products appear to have the same beneficial effects as when the original plant fatty acids are eaten. Although entire populations have been treated with plant sterols (in Finland), it remains possible that adverse effects may occur in the long-term. Phytosterols, as these compounds are called, are remarkably similar to human sterols, and could potentially interact with steroid hormone biosynthesis[66].

### Antioxidant vitamins

Considerable interest has been shown in dietary supplementation, particularly with antioxidant vitamins. Although oxygen is essential for life, it has been known for many years that excess oxygen has harmful effects. Oxidation of intrinsic structural molecules in the body may result in irreversible change, and there are numerous enzyme systems which protect against oxidation. It has been hypothesized that low density lipoprotein cholesterol, when oxidized, is particularly atherogenic, and that antioxidant vitamins might protect against this[67]. Preliminary studies using $\alpha$-tocopherol and $\beta$-carotene have been disappointing[68]; although one study using vitamin E supplementation gave positive results, neither the GISSI-Prevenzione trial[56], nor the recent very large HOPE study showed benefit in patients at high risk for coronary artery disease events[69]. The National Academy of Sciences Institute of Medicine has recently re-evaluated the Dietary Reference Intakes (DRIs) for antioxidant vitamins, selenium, and carotenoids and concluded that definite upper intake levels for these compounds exist, with lack of benefit for pharmacological levels of supplementation[70].

### Alcohol

High levels of alcohol ingestion are directly damaging to myocardium, possibly through a mechanism involving the non-oxidative metabolism of ethanol to fatty acid ethyl esters[71]. In contrast, moderate alcohol consumption is associated with a lower risk of coronary heart disease[72]. Although there are potentially confounding reasons for this (in some Westernized countries higher alcohol intake is associated with greater wealth and higher socio-economic status), there is a plausible biological mechanism. Alcohol increases the serum concentration of high density lipoprotein cholesterol (HDL). The effect does not appear to be specific for any type of alcoholic beverage[73]. It is unclear how much of the effect relates to the ethanol itself, or to congeners in alcoholic drinks, which have other potentially beneficial effects such as antioxidant activity. One interesting study from Copenhagen indicates that the association between alcohol ingestion and risk of an ischaemic heart disease event is highly dependent on concentration of LDL cholesterol. In other words, those with the highest baseline risk (high LDL cholesterol) benefit more from the effect of alcohol than those with lower LDL concentrations[74].

## Weight reduction

Western populations continue to increase in weight. In the US, the 1990s saw the prevalence of obesity rise to one-third of the population. In the 1997 *Health Survey for England*[75], it was reported that 17% of men and 20% of women in the UK were obese. Obesity correlates with higher mortality and a higher incidence of chronic disease. Concerns have been raised, however, about the risks of losing weight, particularly rapidly. Dattilo has reviewed 70 studies on almost 1300 subjects and concluded that per kilogram excess weight loss the total cholesterol falls by 0.05 mmol/l, and that favourable influences are seen on glycaemic control in diabetes, lipid oxidizability status, haemostatic factors, left ventricular hypertrophy and blood pressure[76]. Care should be taken to ensure that there is not just substitution of carbohydrate for fat. When study subjects are fed isocaloric diets in which the fat has been substituted by carbohydrate, serum triglycerides tend to increase, and HDL cholesterol levels tend to decrease[77]. Where weight reduction accompanies changes in the energy source in the diet, any adverse changes appear to be lost. One of the clearest indications of the beneficial effects of weight reduction within a single trial is seen in the correlation observed in the MRFIT trial. Weight reduction showed a clear graded relation with total cholesterol reduction[78]. Weight reduction and blood pressure reduction can also be seen in the context of a 3 year clinical trial[79]. Control of obesity in itself has not been shown to lower morbidity or mortality in cardiac patients though the changes above clearly reduce risk, and reduction of excess body fat improves symptoms and lessens fatigue[80].

# Psychosocial intervention

Most patients (and indeed relatives of patients) when interviewed attribute their coronary artery disease event to stress. There is some evidence to support this view in terms, for example, of accumulation of stressful events such as divorce, bereavement, or unemployment[81]. Once coronary artery disease is established, there is firm evidence to indicate that stress is deleterious and may provoke ischaemic events[82,83]. The most well recognized psychological component of coronary artery disease risk is the type A behaviour. The type A personality is hard-driving, competitive, aggressive and impatient. Following a number of studies with null findings in respect of this personality overall, adherents of type A behaviour as a coronary risk factor have pursued the possibility that the hostility element of such behaviour is the most dangerous, in that it promotes rebellion against advice, and continuation of adverse lifestyle traits such as cigarette smoking. The assessment of true type A personality is a skilled task, however[81]. Modification of life-long behaviour patterns is difficult, but there is some evidence that a programme of stress management incorporated within a cardiac rehabilitation programme may be beneficial[84]. It is important to realise that, though type A behaviour may be a risk factor for coronary artery disease, once the disease is present, type A personality may predict a better survival, at least for some categories of patients who are at the highest risk. This paradox probably stems from the 'driven' characteristic of such patients, which may improve their adherence to treatment regimens[85]. Exercise training *per se* does not appear to influence psychosocial functioning, though depressed patients improve[86]. The literature on psychosocial interventions is extremely confused with passionately held views on all sides. A useful overview of cardiac rehabilitation, published by the NHS Centre for Reviews and Dissemination, University of York, discusses this issue[87]. Drawing the threads of multiple papers together, it would appear that psychosocial and educational intervention might correct potentially harmful misconceptions about cardiac disease, improve compliance with recommended regimens such as non-smoking, dietary modification, and increase physical activity. It appears particularly important to include both patient and spouse or partner. Steptoe[83] has stated: 'the recognition that an individual's circumstances and personality interact with biological risk factors may provide new opportunities for prevention, and for more refined risk stratification'.

Depression is a manifestation of the most adverse psychosocial reaction to myocardial infarction. In some patients, of course, depression is present beforehand. It is common, with 13–19% of patients exhibiting some features of the disorder. Importantly, it is correlated with substantially increased risk of mortality, angina, arrhythmias, rehospitalisation, prolonged disability and continued smoking[88].

Studies of rehabilitation in depressed patients probably suffer from the dilution of patients with major problems by patients who form the mass of people suffering from, and then recovering from, any major medical disorder. In addition, the interventions applied to the mass of recovering myocardial infarction patients may not be intensive enough or suited to significantly depressed patients[89]. Although the major adverse impact on prognosis of significant depression is well documented by Creed[88], the evidence for benefit is not persuasive – at least in terms of subsequent cardiac morbidity. There can be few, however, who would deny patients adequate care when as many as one in six post-myocardial infarction patients are affected, and specialised help is available, and perhaps too rarely sought. Strategies for correcting the misapprehensions many patients have about their illness have been well reviewed by Thompson and Lewin[90].

# Conclusions

Treatments available for the cardiac patient range from complex surgical procedures to psychosocial interventions. Valuable guidelines exist and have been widely distributed[91], but their real challenge is in their implementation. Although it is clear that some strategies can save more lives or relieve symptoms better than others, only a fully integrated cardiac team can realise the maximum benefits of the appropriate treatments for every patient.

*References*

1   World Health Organization. *Needs and Action Priorities in Cardiac Rehabilitation and Secondary Prevention in Patients with Coronary Heart Disease*. WHO Technical Report Service 831. Geneva: World Health Organization, 1993

2   Wenger NK, Froelicher ES, Smith LK *et al*. *Cardiac Rehabilitation*. Clinical Practice Guideline No. 17. AHCPR Publication No. 96-0672. Rockville, MD: US Department of Health and Human Services, Public Health Service, Agency for Health Care Policy and Research and the National Heart, Lung, and Blood Institute, 1975

3   Hennekens CH, Albert CM, Godfried SL. Adjunctive drug therapy of acute myocardial infarction – evidence from clinical trials. *N Engl J Med* 1996; **335**: 1660–7

4   FRISC II Investigators. Invasive compared with non-invasive treatment in unstable coronary artery disease: FRISC II prospective randomised multicentre study. *Lancet* 1999; **354**: 708–15

5   Villella A, Maggioni AP, Villella M *et al*. Prognostic significance of maximal exercise testing after myocardial infarction treated with thrombolytic agents: the GISSI-2 data-base. Gruppo Italiano per lo Studio della Sopravvivenza Nell'Infarto. *Lancet* 1995; **346**: 523–9

6   Villella M, Villella A, Barlera S, Franzosi MG, Maggioni AP. Prognostic significance of double product and inadequate double product response to maximal symptom-limited exercise stress testing after myocardial infarction in 6296 patients treated with thrombolytic agents. GISSI-2 Investigators. Gruppo Italiano per lo Studio della Sopravvivenza nell-Infarto Miocardico. *Am Heart J* 1999; **137**: 443–52

7   Shaw LJ, Peterson ED, Kesler K *et al*. A meta-analysis of predischarge risk stratification after acute myocardial infarction with stress electrocardiographic, myocardial perfusion, and ventricular function imaging. *Am J Cardiol* 1996; **78**: 1327–37

8    Maggioni AP. Secondary prevention: improving outcomes following myocardial infarction. *Heart* 2000; **84 (Suppl I)**: i5–7

9    McLeod AA, Chamberlain DA. Recent advances in beta-blocking therapy: clinical indications and pharmacology. In: Goodwin JF, Yu PN. (eds) *Progress in Cardiology*, vol 13. Philadelphia, PA: Lea and Febiger, 1985; 145–78

10   Singh BN. The coming of age of the Class III antiarrhythmic principle: retrospective and future trends. *Am J Cardiol* 1996; **78 (Suppl 4A)**: 17–27

11   Anand S, Yusuf S. Oral anticoagulant therapy in patients with coronary artery disease: a meta-analysis. *JAMA* 1999; **282**: 2058–67

12   Mehta SR, Eikelboom JW, Yusuf S. Long-term management of unstable angina and non-Q-wave myocardial infarction. *Eur Heart J Suppl* 2000; **2 (Suppl E)**: E6–12

13   Scandinavian Simvastatin Survival Study Group. Randomised trial of cholesterol lowering in 4444 patients with coronary heart disease. *Lancet* 1994; **344**: 1383–9

14   Tonkin AM, Colquhoun D, Emberson J *et al*. Effects of pravastatin in 3260 patients with unstable angina: results from the LIPID study. *Lancet* 2000; **356**: 1871–5

15   Rubins HB, Robins SJ, Collins D *et al*. Gemfibrozil for the secondary prevention on coronary heart disease in men with low levels of high-density lipoprotein cholesterol. *N Engl J Med* 1999; **341**: 410–8

16   Scott T, Thompson D, Lewin R. *Information for Post-myocardial Infarction Patients and Families* (protocol for a Cochrane Review). Oxford: The Cochrane Library, issue 4, 2000

17   Burke LE. Adherence to a heart-healthy lifestyle – what makes the difference? In: Wenger NK, Smith LK, Froelicher ES, Comoss PM (eds). *Cardiac Rehabilitation. A Guide to Practice in the 21st Century*. Basel: Marcel Dekker, 1999; 385–93

18   Prochaska JO, Congdon K. In: Wenger NK, Smith LK, Froelicher ES, Comoss PM (eds). *Cardiac Rehabilitation. A Guide to Practice in the 21st Century*. Basel: Marcel Dekker, 1999; 361–70

19   Brubaker PH, Warner JG, Rejeski WJ *et al*. Comparison of standard- and extended-length participation in cardiac rehabilitation on body composition, functional capacity and blood lipids. *Am J Cardiol* 1996; **78**: 769–73

20   Kuczmarski RJ, Flegal KM, Campbell SM, Johnson CL. Increasing prevalence of overweight among US adults: the National Health and Nutrition Examination Surveys, 1960–1991. *JAMA* 1994; **272**: 205–11

21   Powell KE, Pratt M. Physical activity and health. *BMJ* 1996; **313**: 126–7

22   Miller Jr HS, Paffenbarger Jr RS. The prevention and treatment of coronary disease: the case for exercise. In: Shephard RJ, HS Miller Jr HS. (eds) *Exercise and the Heart in Health and Disease*, 2nd edn. Basel: Marcel Dekker, 1999; 295–301

23   Shaw LW. Effects of a prescribed supervised exercise program on mortality and cardiovascular morbidity in patients after myocardial infarction: the National Exercise and Heart Disease Project. *Am J Cardiol* 1981; **48**: 39–46

24   Oldridge N, Guyatt GH, Fischer ME, Rimm AA. Cardiac rehabilitation after myocardial infarction: combined experience of randomized clinical trials. *JAMA* 1988; **260**: 945–50

25   O'Connor GT, Buring JE, Yusuf S *et al*. An overview of randomized clinical trials of rehabilitation with exercise after myocardial infarction. *Circulation* 1989; **80**: 234–44

26   Jolliffe J, Rees K, Taylor RS, Thompson D, Oldridge N, Ebrahim. Cochrane collaboration. 2001; In press

27   Wannamethee SG, Shaper AG, Walker M. Physical activity and mortality in older men with diagnosed coronary heart disease. *Circulation* 2000; **102**: 1358–63

28   Ganz P, Braunwald E. Coronary blood flow and myocardial ischaemia. In: Braunwald E. (ed) *Heart Disease. A Textbook of Cardiovascular Medicine*, 5th edn. Philadelphia, PA: WB Saunders, 1997; 1161–3

29   Ehsani, Martin WH, Heath GW, Coyle EF. Cardiac effects of prolonged and intense training in patients with coronary artery disease. *Am J Cardiol* 1982; **50**: 246–54

30   Clausen JP. Circulatory adjustments to dynamic exercise and effect of physical training in normal subjects and in patients with coronary artery disease. *Prog Cardiovasc Dis* 1976; **18**: 459–95

31   Todd IC, Ballantyne D. The antianginal efficacy of exercise training: a comparison with beta blockade. *Br Heart J* 1990; **64**: 14–9

32  Todd IC, Ballantyne D. Effect of exercise training on the total ischaemic burden: an assessment by 24 hour ambulatory electrocardiographic monitoring. *Br Heart J* 1992; **68**: 560–6

33  Larson EB, Bruce RA. Exercise and aging. *Ann Intern Med* 1986; **106**: 783–5

34  Young A, Dinan S. Fitness for older people. *BMJ* 1994; **309**: 331–4

35  Fiatarone MA, O'Neill EF, Ryan ND *et al*. Exercise training and nutritional supplementation for physical frailty in very elderly people. *N Engl J Med* 1994; **330**: 1769–75

36  Campbell AJ, Robertson MC, Gardner MM, Norton RN, Tilyard MW, Buchner DM. Randomised controlled trial of a general practice programme of home based exercise to prevent falls in elderly women. *BMJ* 1997; **315**: 1065–9

37  Hardman AE. Role of exercise and weight loss in maximizing LDL cholesterol reduction. *Eur Heart J Suppl* 1999; *1 (Suppl S)*: S123–31

38  Lewis T. *Diseases of the Heart*. London: Macmillan, 1942; 26

39  European Heart Failure Training Group. Experience from controlled trials of physical training in chronic heart failure. Protocol and patient factors in effectiveness in the improvement in exercise tolerance. *Eur Heart J* 1998; **19**: 466–75.

40  NIH Consensus Development Panel. Physical activity and cardiovascular health. *JAMA* 1996; **276**: 241–6

41  Goodman JM. Sudden cardiac death and exercise in healthy adults. In: Shephard RJ, Miller Jr HS. (eds) *Exercise and the Heart in Health and Disease*. Basel: Marcel Dekker, 1999; 303–18

42  Curfman GD. Is exercise beneficial – or hazardous – to your heart? *N Engl J Med* 1993; **329**: 1730–1

43  Correspondence. Triggering of acute myocardial infarction by exercise. *N Engl J Med* 1994; **330**: 1156–7

44  Bartecchi CE, Mackenzie TD, Schrier RW. The human costs of tobacco use (Part 1). *N Engl J Med* 1994; **330**: 907–12

45  Kottke TE, Battista RN, DeFriese GH, Brekke ML. Attributes of successful smoking cessation interventions in medical practice. A meta-analysis of 39 controlled trials. *JAMA* 1988; **259**: 2883–9

46  Department of Health. *Smoking Kills. A White Paper on Tobacco*. Cm 4177. London: Stationery Office, 1998

47  Raw M, McNeill A, Wet R. Smoking cessation guidelines for health professionals. A guide to effective smoking cessation interventions for the health care system. *Thorax* 1998; **53 (Suppl 5)**: S1–19

48  Tang JL, Armitage JM, Lancaster T, Silagy CA, Fowler GH, Neil HA. Systematic review of dietary intervention trials to lower blood total cholesterol in free-living subjects. *BMJ* 1998; **316**: 1213–9

49  Davey Smith G, Ebrahim S. Commentary: dietary change, cholesterol reduction, and the public health – what does meta-analysis add? *BMJ* 1998; **316**: 1220

50  Ornish D, Brown SE, Scherwitz LW *et al*. Can lifestyle changes reverse coronary heart disease? *Lancet* 1990; **336**: 129–33

51  Fair JM. Lipid lowering for coronary risk reduction. In: Wenger NK Smith LK, Froelicher ES, Comoss PM (eds). Cardiac Rehabilitation. A Guide to Practice in the 21st Century. Basel: Marcel Dekker, 1999; 223–33

52  Watts GF, Lewis B, Brunt JN *et al*. Effects on coronary artery disease of lipid-lowering diet, or diet plus cholestyramine, in the St Thomas' Atherosclerosis Regression Study (STARS). *Lancet* 1992; **339**: 563–9

53  Appel LJ, Moore TJ, Obarzanek E. A clinical trial of the effects of dietary patterns on blood pressure. *N Engl J Med* 1997; **336**: 1117–24

54  De Lorgeril M, Salen P, Martin JL, Monjaud I, Delaye J, Mamelle N. Mediterranean diet, traditional risk factors, and the rate of cardiovascular complications after myocardial infarction: final report of the Lyon Diet Heart Study. *Circulation* 1999; **99**: 779–85

55  Burr ML et al. Effects of changes in fat, fish, and fibre intakes on death and myocardial infarction: Diet and Reinfarction Trial (DART). Lancet 1989; **2**: 757–61

56  GISSI-Prevenzione Investigators (Gruppo Italiano per lo Studio della Sopravivenza nell'infarto miocardico). Dietary supplementation with n-3 polyunsaturated fatty acids and vitamin E after myocardial infarction: results of the GISSI-Prevenzione trial. Lancet 1999; **354**: 447–55

57   O'Keefe JH, Harris WS. Omega-3 fatty acids: time for clinical implementation? *Am J Cardiol* 2000; **85**: 1239–41

58   Kant AK, Schatzkin A, Graubard BI, Schairer C. A prospective study of diet quality and mortality in women. *JAMA* 2000; **283**: 2109–15

59   Oliver MF. It is more important to increase the intake of unsaturated fats than to decrease the intake of saturated fats: evidence from clinical trials relating to ischemic heart disease. *Am J Clin Nutr* 1997; **66 (Suppl)**: 980S–986S

60   Sacks FM, Svetkey LP, Vollmer WM *et al*. Effects on blood pressure of reduced dietary sodium and the dietary approaches to stop hypertension (DASH) diet. *N Engl J Med* 2001; **344**: 3–10

61   Schuler G, Hambrecht R, Schlierf G *et al*. Regular physical exercise and low-fat diet. Effects on progression of coronary artery disease. *Circulation* 1992; **86**: 1–11

62   Lavie CJ, Milani RV. Effects of cardiac rehabilitation and exercise training on low-density lipoprotein cholesterol in patients with hypertriglyceridemia and coronary artery disease. *Am J Cardiol* 1994; **74**: 1192–5

63   Anonymous. Report of the National Cholesterol Education Program Expert Panel on Detection, Evaluation, and Treatment of High Blood Cholesterol in Adults. *Arch Intern Med* 1988; **148**: 36–69

64   Chisholm A, Mann J, Sutherland W, Duncan A, Skeaff M, Frampton C. Effect on lipoprotein profile of replacing butter with margarine in a low fat diet: randomised crossover study with hypercholesterolaemic subjects. *BMJ* 1996; **312**: 931–4

65   Cater NB. Historical and scientific basis for the development of plant stanol ester foods as cholesterol-lowering agents. *Eur Heart J Suppl* 1999; **1 (Suppl S)**: S36–44

66   Moghadasian MH, Frohlich JJ. Effects of dietary phytosterols on cholesterol metabolism and atherosclerosis: clinical and experimental evidence. *Am J Med* 1999; **107**: 588–94

67   Steinberg D *et al*. Beyond cholesterol: modifications of low-density lipoprotein that increase its atherogenicity. *N Engl J Med* 1989; **320**: 915–24

68   Hennekens CH, Burin JE, Peto R. Antioxidant vitamins – benefits not yet proved. *N Engl J Med* 1994; **330**: 1080–1

69   The Heart Outcomes Prevention Evaluation Study Investigators. Vitamin E supplementation and cardiovascular events in high-risk patients. *N Engl J Med* 2000; **342**: 154–60

70   Standing Committee on the Scientific Evaluation of Dietary Reference Intakes (DRIs). *Dietary Reference Intakes for Vitamin C, Vitamin E, Selenium, and Carotenoids*. Washington, DC: National Academy Press, 2000

71   Beckemeier ME, Bora PS. Fatty acid ethyl esters: potentially toxic products of myocardial ethanol metabolism. *J Mol Cell Cardiol* 1998; **30**: 2487–94

72   Maclure M. Demonstration of deductive meta-analysis: ethanol intake and risk of myocardial infarction. *Epidemiol Rev* 1993; **15**: 328–51

73   Rimm EB, Klatsky A, Grobbee D, Stampfer MJ. Review of moderate alcohol consumption and reduced risk of coronary heart disease: is the effect due to beer, wine, or spirits? *BMJ* 1996; **312**: 731–6

74   Hein HO, Suadicani P, Gyntelberg F. Alcohol consumption, serum low density lipoprotein cholesterol concentration, and risk of ischaemic heart disease: six year follow up in the Copenhagen male study. *BMJ* 1996; **312**: 736–41

75   Prescott-Clarke P, Primatesta P. *Health Survey for England 1997*. London: HMSO, 1999

76   Dattilo A. Weight management and exercise in the treatment of obesity. In: Wenger NK, Smith LK, Froelicher ES, Comoss PM (eds). *Cardiac Rehabilitation. A Guide to Practice in the 21st Century*. Basel: Marcel Dekker, 1999; 247–56

77   Clinical Debate. Should a low-fat, high-carbohydrate diet be recommended for everyone? *N Engl J Med* 1997; **337**: 562–7

78   Blackburn H, Leon AS. Preventive cardiology in practice: Minnesota studies on risk factor reduction. In: Pollock ML, Schmidt DH. (eds) *Heart Disease and Rehabilitation*, 2nd edn. New York: John Wiley, 1986; 265–301

79   Stevens VJ, Obarzanek E, Cook NR *et al*. Long-term weight loss and changes in blood pressure: results of the trials of hypertension prevention, phase II. *Ann Intern Med* 2001; **134**: 1–11

80   Squires RW *et al*. Cardiovascular rehabilitation: status 1990. *Mayo Clin Proc* 1990; **65**: 731–55

81  Blumenthal JA. Psychologic assessment in cardiac rehabilitation. *J Cardiopulm Rehabil* 1985; **5**: 208–15

82  Gullette EC, Blumenthal JA, Babyak M *et al*. Effects of mental stress on left ventricular and peripheral vascular performance in patients with coronary artery disease. *JAMA* 1997; **277**: 1521–6

83  Steptoe A. Psychosocial factors in the aetiology of coronary heart disease. *Heart* 1999; **82**: 258–9

84  Blumenthal JA, Emery CF, Rejeski WJ. Stress management and exercise training in cardiac patients with myocardial ischaemia. *Arch Intern Med* 1997; **157**: 2213–23

85  Barefoot JC, Peterson BL, Harrell FE *et al*. Type A behavior and survival: a follow-up study of 1,467 patients with coronary artery disease. *Am J Cardiol* 1989; **64**: 427–32

86  Blumenthal JA *et al*. The effects of exercise training on psychosocial functioning after myocardial infarction. *J Cardiopulm Rehabil* 1988; **8**: 183–93

87  Dinnes J, Droogan J, Glanville J, et al.  Cardiac Rehabilitation. *Effective Health Care* 1998; **4** (No 4): 1-12

88  Creed F. The importance of depression following myocardial infarction. *Heart* 1999; **82**: 406–8

89  Taylor C Barr, Houston-Miller N, Ahn DK *et al*. The effects of exercise training programs on psychosocial improvement in uncomplicated postmyocardial infarction patients. *J Psychosom Res* 1986; **30**: 581–7

90  Thompson DR, Lewin RJP. Management of the post-myocardial infarction patient: rehabilitation and cardiac neurosis. *Heart* 2000; **84**: 101–5

91  Wood D, Durrington P, Poulter N *et al*. Joint British recommendations on prevention of coronary heart disease in clinical practice. *Heart* 1998; **80** (**Suppl 2**): S1–29

# What is the optimal medical management of ischaemic heart failure?

**John G F Cleland\*, Joseph John†, Jatinder Dhawan† and Andrew Clark\***

*\*Department of Cardiology, Castle Hill Hospital and Hull Royal Infirmary, Kingston upon Hull, UK and †Department of Cardiology, Scunthorpe General Hospital, Scunthorpe, UK*

Ischaemic heart disease is probably the most important cause of heart failure. All patients with heart failure may benefit from treatment designed to retard progressive ventricular dysfunction and arrhythmias. Patients with heart failure due to ischaemic heart disease may also, theoretically, benefit from treatments designed to relieve ischaemia and prevent coronary occlusion and from revascularisation. However, there is little evidence to show that effective treatments, such as angiotensin converting enzyme (ACE) inhibitors and β-blockers, exert different effects in patients with heart failure with or without coronary disease. Moreover, there is no evidence that treatment directed specifically at myocardial ischaemia, whether or not symptomatic, or coronary disease alters outcome in patients with heart failure. Some agents, such as aspirin, designed to reduce the risk of coronary occlusion appear ineffective or harmful in patients with heart failure. There is no evidence, yet, that revascularisation improves prognosis in patients with heart failure, even in patients who are demonstrated to have extensive myocardial hibernation. On current evidence, revascularisation should be reserved for the relief of angina.

Large-scale, randomised controlled trials are currently underway investigating the role of specific treatments targeted at coronary syndromes in patients who have heart failure. The CHRISTMAS study is investigating the effects of carvedilol in a large cohort of patients with and without hibernating myocardium. The WATCH study is comparing the efficacy of aspirin, clopidogrel and warfarin. The HEART-UK study is assessing the effect of revascularisation on mortality in patients with heart failure and myocardial hibernation. Smaller scale studies are currently assessing the safety and efficacy of statin therapy in patients with heart failure.

Only when the results of these and other studies are known will it be possible to come to firm conclusions about whether patients with heart failure and coronary disease should be treated differently from other patients with heart failure due to left ventricular systolic dysfunction.

*Correspondence to:*
*Prof John G F Cleland,*
*Department of*
*Cardiology, University of*
*Hull, Castle Hill Hospital,*
*Castle Road, Cottingham,*
*Kingston upon*
*Hull HU16 5JQ, UK*

Ischaemic heart disease is the commonest cause of left ventricular systolic dysfunction leading to heart failure in industrialised societies. The prognosis of newly diagnosed heart failure is poor. More than 30%

of patients will die within 3 months and the subsequent annual mortality is around 10%, although much worse in patients with severe heart failure[1,2]. Most importantly, clinical trials show that the prognosis of heart failure can be modified substantially by a number of pharmacological therapies[3–12]. However, many treatments for heart failure subjected to randomised trials failed to show benefit or have shown harm[13], despite being based on plausible hypotheses. If we should learn one lesson from the randomised controlled trials, it is that treatments cannot be assumed to be beneficial based on theory alone. Formal scientific evaluation of all treatments is essential.

## Targets for therapy in patients with heart failure

Three major cardiovascular pathways leading to progression of heart failure or death are obvious (Fig. 1).

1. Left and/or right ventricular function may slowly deteriorate, either due to progressive ventricular remodelling, due to decline in the contractile properties of cardiac myocytes or due to an increased load on the heart due to changes in neuro-endocrine, peripheral vascular and/or renal function

2. Left ventricular function may decline abruptly due to coronary vascular occlusion

3. Cardiac function may decline abruptly due to the onset of an arrhythmia, usually atrial fibrillation when the event is not fatal

This is a simple scenario and is a useful starting point, but reality is likely to be much more complex. Ventricular remodelling does occur after myocardial infarction and may be extensive in the first year[14]; thereafter, changes are small[15]. Long-term changes in ventricular volume

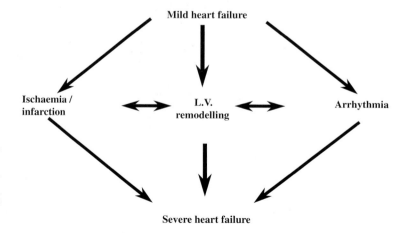

**Fig. 1** Interaction of likely common cardiovascular pathways for the progression of heart failure.

in patients with chronic heart failure in response to ACE inhibitors are poorly documented, with studies incorporating few patients[16] or showing only small changes[17]. The benefits of β-blockers may develop over a longer period and may be more substantial[18-20], but long-term data are still sparse. The mechanisms of ventricular remodelling are poorly understood and likely to reflect a complex array of hypertrophy, cell death and myocardial fibrosis[21] in response to neuro-endocrine and haemodynamic factors[22].

A number of 'ischaemic' syndromes could make an important contribution to ventricular remodelling. Transmural infarcts, without a surviving epicardial rim of myocardium, may be subject to high and unprotected wall stress in the infarcted zone and, therefore, may be much more likely to remodel. Partial thickness infarcts may lead to an acute decline in ventricular function, although be less likely to trigger extensive remodelling. Recurrent myocardial ischaemia will alter systolic function, neuro-endocrine activation, wall stress and probably accelerate apoptosis. Non-functioning but viable (*i.e.* hibernating or stunned) myocardium may also be associated with accelerated apoptosis. Patent infarct related arteries may limit remodelling, by modifying the 'ischaemic' substrate, although it is also possible that the reverse is true because the nature of the myocardial injury may also determine arterial patency[23,24]. Silent occlusion of coronary arteries leading to a progressive decline in ventricular function may manifest as worsening heart failure rather than overt ischaemia[25]. The extent to which exertional breathlessness in heart failure is predominantly a manifestation of myocardial ischaemia is also unknown. We are just beginning to unravel the prevalence of these ischaemic syndromes. They appear to be common[22,26-28], it is likely they are important, but the efficacy and nature of treatment directed at them is uncertain.

Progression of heart failure reflects not a vicious cycle, but a matrix (Fig. 1). Myocardial ischaemic events may lead to ventricular remodelling and arrhythmias. Arrhythmias may lead to a decline in ventricular function and myocardial ischaemia. Ventricular remodelling may predispose to arrhythmia. Ventricular remodelling could even predispose to ischaemic events, including vascular occlusion, because coronary arteries have to remodel over the epicardial surface of the heart, because the metabolic demands of the failing myocardium are increased due to hypertrophy and increased wall tension and because of activation of haemostatic factors[29].

However, the most common manifestation of a vascular event in patients with heart failure may be sudden death[25,30,31]. Epidemiological studies suggest that about 30% of all patients in the community who suffer a myocardial infarction will not reach hospital alive[32,33]. It is likely that patients with heart failure, who have less ventricular reserve and who are more prone to arrhythmias have a much higher rate of sudden death within the first few minutes of a myocardial infarction. The failure of anti-arrhythmic medication to improve survival in patients with heart failure may have more to do with the inappropriateness of the target than the toxicity of the drugs[30,34,35]. This may explain why implantable defibrillators have been shown to reduce mortality, so far, only in highly selected groups of patients with heart failure[10,11,36,37].

In view of the above, management of coronary disease could be the most important target for therapy in order to improve prognosis in the great majority of patients with heart failure, while the potential of therapy directed at the coronary circulation to improve the symptoms of heart failure should also be recognised.

# Diagnostic steps in patients with heart failure and ischaemic heart disease

The over-riding reason for carrying out a diagnostic investigation in any patient, including those with heart failure, is to assist in deciding what treatment is most likely to benefit a patient. Until a treatment has been demonstrated to be effective (preferably cost-effective) then investigations to decide whether it should be deployed cannot be considered mandatory and could be considered undesirable.

European guidelines do not recommend routine coronary arteriography or myocardial viability testing in patients with heart failure[38–41]. This is logical as the only treatments for heart failure secondary to left ventricular systolic dysfunction that are agreed to improve prognosis are ACE inhibitors, β-blockers and, with less certainty, spironolactone[4–9]. There is no evidence that these treatments exert substantially different benefits in patients with or without ischaemic heart disease (IHD) and, therefore, no need to carry out diagnostic stratification for this purpose[42,43]. Many patients with heart failure will have clear clinical evidence of IHD heart disease, usually a myocardial infarction and/or a previous revascularisation procedure. These patients do not require angiography to establish the nature of their left ventricular dysfunction although, some would argue, it is important to establish the pattern of their coronary disease. However, in the absence of disabling symptomatic angina uncontrolled by medical therapy, there is no randomised controlled trial to show that revascularisation improves symptoms or prognosis in heart failure or, indeed, in any patient with a left ventricular ejection fraction <35%. Therefore, there is no mandate for coronary arteriography in such patients. In patients who have no definitive history of ischaemic heart disease, a coronary angiogram is required if it is considered desirable to exclude coronary disease. However, again, in the absence of angina, there is no justification for revascularisation and the recommended medical treatment will be similar whether or not ischaemic heart disease is the cause; therefore, there is no mandate for arteriography. Of course, for prognostic reasons[44], for patient information, for research reasons and to satisfy the curiosity of doctors, coronary arteriography will often be carried out. Similar arguments apply to the use of investigations to detect 'silent' ischaemia, stunning and hibernation. Merely showing that a test predicts a poor outcome does not prove that an intervention is effective or safe. Until it can be shown that angiography and/or myocardial viability testing are useful in selecting treatments that are shown to alter outcome, they cannot be considered to have a routine place in the management of patients.

In summary, current evidence does not support the need for routine investigations for the presence of the pattern of coronary disease in patients with heart failure. However, investigation is justified when concomitant angina unresponsive to medical therapy is present.

# Standard treatments for heart failure in patients with ischaemic heart disease

## Diuretics

Clinical experience and placebo-controlled trials indicate that diuretics improve the symptoms of heart failure, but there are no substantial clinical trials to show whether they alter prognosis. Thiazide diuretics have reduced both the risk of myocardial infarction and left ventricular failure in trials of hypertension[45–47].

## Digoxin

The role of digoxin in the management patients with heart failure in sinus rhythm is uncertain. Studies that helped define a potential role for digoxin were conducted prior to β-blockers entering wide-spread use in heart failure and now need to be repeated (Table 1). Digoxin still

**Table 1** Interaction between aetiology and outcome (death or hospitalisation for worsening heart failure) comparing digoxin with placebo in the DIG trial

| Mean follow-up 3 years | Placebo No. with event/total | Digoxin No. with event/total | Change Absolute/relative |
|---|---|---|---|
| IHD (71%) | 873/2398 (36.4%) | 731/2405 (30.4%) | –6.0%/16% |
| Non-IHD (29%) | 413/996 (41.5%) | 306/983 (31.1%) | –10.4%/25% |

Statistical tests for heterogeneity of action between IHD and non-IHD were not significant.

appears to have an important role in the control of atrial fibrillation in heart failure even in the presence of a β-blocker[48,49].

A combined analysis of the PROVED[50] and RADIANCE[51] trials suggested that withdrawal of digoxin from patients with dilated cardio-myopathy led to a decline in exercise capacity and ejection fraction and markedly increased the risk of worsening heart failure[52]. However, there was no increased risk of deterioration on withdrawing digoxin from patients with heart failure due to IHD. The large DIG trial showed a trend to excess mortality with digoxin due to myocardial infarction and sudden death, both potential manifestations of IHD[53]. Subset analysis according to aetiology suggested a smaller impact of digoxin on the combined end-point of worsening heart failure leading to death or hospitalisation in patients with IHD.

β-Blockers might reduce the efficacy of digoxin, if digoxin's benefit is primarily related to heart rate reduction. On the other hand, β-blockers might protect against unwanted side-effects of digoxin, while digoxin could limit the possibly unwanted acute negative inotropic effect of β-blockers, producing a beneficial synergy between agents. More research into the current role of digoxin for the management of patients with heart failure and ischaemic heart disease is required.

## ACE inhibitors and angiotensin receptor antagonists

Clinical trials show that ACE inhibitors improve symptoms and reduce morbidity and mortality in patients with chronic heart failure (Table 2)[54,55] and after myocardial infarction[56–58]. The hypothesis that the principal benefit of ACE inhibitors is mediated through a reduction in ventricular remodelling is widely accepted, but there is little evidence to support this belief (see above)[59].

There is considerable evidence that ACE inhibitors exert benefit by reducing the risk of recurrent vascular events and this may be their most important effect. Perhaps the clearest evidence for the vascular effects of ACE inhibitors comes from a study from which heart failure patients were excluded, the HOPE study[60]. In HOPE, ramipril reduced the risk of death, myocardial, stroke and cardiac arrest among patients with or at high risk of vascular disease. A reduction in sudden death, a common presentation of acute vascular occlusion, was also observed. The SOLVD studies, comparing enalapril and placebo in patients with heart failure or major chronic left ventricular systolic dysfunction, also showed a reduction in myocardial infarction (Table 3)[61]. These data were supported by trends to a reduction in myocardial infarction in all of the landmark studies of ACE inhibitors in patients with post-infarction heart failure or left ventricular systolic dysfunction[56,58,61,62]. It

**Table 2** Trials of ACE inhibitors in chronic heart failure

| Trial: mean follow-up | Placebo<br>Mortality/total | ACE inhibitor<br>Mortality/total | Change in mortality<br>Absolute/relative |
|---|---|---|---|
| Consensus: 0.5 years | | | |
|     IHD (77%) | 49/97 (50.5%) | 23/95 (24.2%) | −26.3%/48% |
|     Non-IHD (23%) | 7/29 (24.1%) | 9/28 (32.1%) | +8.0%/+33% |
| V-HeFT-II: 2.5 years | | | |
|     IHD (53%) | 78/208 (37.5%) | 77/219 (35.2%) | −2.5%/7% |
|     Non-IHD (47%) | 75/193 (38.9%) | 55/184 (29.9%) | −9.0%/23% |
| SOLVD treatment: 3.5 years | | | |
|     IHD (71%) | 362/927* (39.1%) | 322/903* (35.7%) | −3.4%/9% |
|     Non-IHD (29%) | 148/352* (42.1%) | 130/381* (34.1%) | −8.0%/19% |
| Garg & Yusuf meta-analysis | Placebo | ACE Inhibitor | |
| Mortality | | | |
|     IHD (64%) | 488/1757 (27.8%) | 415/1997 (20.8%) | −7.0%/17% |
|     Non-IHD (36%) | 187/1006 (18.6%) | 173/1132 (15.3%) | −3.3%/18% |
| Mortality or hospitalisation | | | |
|     IHD | 704/1757 (40.1%) | 566/1997 (28.3%) | −11.8%/29% |
|     Non-IHD | 292/1006 (29.0%) | 263/1132 (23.2%) | −5.8%/20% |

Statistical tests for heterogeneity of action between IHD and non-IHD were not significant.
*Recalculated from percentages at crude annualised.

is also clear that ACE inhibitors reduce the risk of sudden death in patients with heart failure[30,55,56].

The mechanism by which ACE inhibitors reduce arterial occlusive events is uncertain. ACE inhibitors have been reported to improve coronary endothelial function in patients[63] and the development of fatty streaks in animal models[64,65], although the latter requires toxic doses of ACE inhibitors and the relevance of the animal models are open to question[64]. A recent report indicated no effect of ACE inhibitors on the development of carotid atherosclerosis[66], suggesting that the predominant effect of ACE inhibitors may be due to reducing plaque

**Table 3** Effects of enalapril on myocardial infarction and unstable angina in the SOLVD trials

| | Placebo<br>At risk | Placebo<br>% Events | Enalapril<br>At risk | Enalapril<br>% Events | % Reduction |
|---|---|---|---|---|---|
| IHD | 2683 | 28.1 | 2667 | 24.1 | 18 |
| Non-IHD | 710 | 14.1 | 723 | 8.9 | 43, $P = 0.04$ |
| Prior MI | 2517 | 28.2 | 2552 | 23.7 | 20 |
| No prior MI | 880 | 16.5 | 835 | 12.1 | 34 |
| Angina | 1216 | 39.1 | 1179 | 30.0 | 28 |
| No angina | 2182 | 17.5 | 2214 | 15.9 | 13, $P = 0.01$ |

rupture rather than the development of atherosclerosis. ACE inhibitors also increase endogenous thrombolysis and so could prevent plaque rupture progressing to coronary occlusion[67–69].

A meta-analysis of trials of ACE inhibitors in heart failure showed a trend to greater reduction in mortality and the composite end-point of death or hospitalisation for heart failure among patients with IHD than those without[70]. However, the SOLVD studies showed that ACE inhibitors could reduce the coronary event rate even in patients with heart failure not primarily due to IHD[61]. As coronary disease was not rigorously excluded in the 'non-IHD' population in these studies, it is entirely plausible that most of the benefit observed in patients with heart failure even without overt coronary disease is due to a reduction in coronary occlusion (Table 3).

Recently, the ELITE-II study suggested that angiotensin receptor antagonists were not superior and, indeed, may not be as effective as ACE inhibitors in patients with heart failure[71]. No subgroup data were presented to indicate whether patients with IHD fared differently. However, there were trends to more vascular deaths in the losartan group and a significant excess of sudden, possibly vascular, death[30]. Also, among patients treated with β-blockers, a possible therapeutic marker for IHD, there was a significant excess of deaths among those randomised to losartan compared to captopril. These data lend support to the view that increases in vascular wall bradykinin and prostaglandin may be an important mechanism of ACE inhibitor benefit[59].

In summary, ACE inhibitors form one of the mainstays of the treatment of heart failure secondary to IHD. Overall, when analysed on an intention to treat basis, studies suggest that ACE inhibitors reduce mortality by about 23% and death or hospitalisation for worsening heart failure by 37% in patients with IHD[70]. Intention-to-treat studies ignore cross-over effects, which are often substantial, leading to an underestimate of the real magnitude of a treatment's benefit. The true benefit of ACE inhibitors may be twice as great as the studies suggest. With the exception of a history of angio-oedema, there are no absolute contra-indications. A few patients will not tolerate ACE inhibitors because of renal dysfunction or hypotension.

## Beta-blockers

Clinical trials show that β-blockers improve symptoms and reduce morbidity and mortality in patients with heart failure (Table 4)[9,65,72]. As with ACE inhibitors the mechanism of benefit is uncertain. Compared to ACE inhibitors, studies have shown much more striking effects of β-blockers on left ventricular systolic function[22]. This marked reverse

**Table 4** Trials of β-blockers in heart failure

| | Placebo Mortality/total | Carvedilol Mortality/total | Reduction in mortality Absolute/relative |
|---|---|---|---|
| USCT: 6.7 months | | | |
| IHD (48%) | 17/189 (9.0%) | 13/332 (3.9%) | −5.1%/57% |
| Non-IHD (52%) | 14/208 (6.7%) | 9/362 (2.5%) | −4.2%/63% |
| CIBIS-II: 1.3 years | | | |
| IHD | 121/654 (18.5%) | 75/662 (11.3%) | −7.2%/39% |
| Non-IHD | 15/157 (9.6%) | 13/160 (8.1%) | −1.5%/16% |
| MERIT: 1 year | | | |
| IHD | 161*/1312 (12.3%) | 103*/1294 (8.0%) | −4.3%/35%* |
| Non-IHD | 56*/689 (8.1%) | 42*/696 (6.0%) | −2.1%/26%* |
| BEST: 2 years | | | |
| IHD | 7/791 | 7/796 | Non-significant 10% |
| Non-IHD | ?/563 | ?/558 | reduction in mortality. No heterogeneity between IHD/non-IHD |
| COPERNICUS: 0.9 year | | | |
| IHD | 140/760 (18.4%) | 103/778 (13.2%) | −5.2%/31% |
| Non-IHD | 50/373 (13.4%) | 27/378 (7.1%) | −6.3% / 48% |

Statistical tests for heterogeneity of action between IHD and non-IHD were not significant for all studies.
Divide absolute benefit by duration of follow-up to compare absolute benefits across trials.
*Recalculated from figure.

remodelling might be due to prevention of ischaemia and stunning or the resuscitation of myocardial hibernation[22]. At first sight, the fact that most studies show that ventricular function improves to a greater extent and more consistently in patients with heart failure due to dilated cardiomyopathy than in those with IHD appears to confound this hypothesis[73–76], but on further consideration perhaps the reverse is true[22]. Subendocardial ischaemia has been documented in patients with dilated cardiomyopathy in the absence of epicardial coronary disease, possibly reflecting microvascular disease and a low arterial-subendocardial pressure gradient during diastole when blood flow occurs[77,78]. Thus, dilated cardiomyopathy may be a model of chronic myocardial ischaemia without infarction. In contrast, most patients with heart failure and IHD have had a myocardial infarction and, therefore, a myocardial scar that will not respond, at least in the short-or medium-term, to therapy. This could account for the lesser response in patients with IHD. Relief of stunning and or hibernation could account for those cases with IHD who respond, in terms of ventricular function, like a patient with dilated cardiomyopathy. Extensive scar without ischaemia could account for why some patients with IHD do not respond, in terms of ventricular function, to a β-blocker. β-Blockers may be the best available test for the presence of myocardial stunning or hibernation, it may also be the best therapy[22,79,80]. These issues are currently being addressed in a substantial ($n$ = 400) clinical trial, the CHRISTMAS study[22], in which patients, stratified by the volume of hibernating myocardium, are randomised to placebo or carvedilol. The study will report in 2001.

Despite a potentially greater and more consistent effect of β-blockers on ventricular function in patients with dilated cardiomyopathy, these agents appear to have similar or greater effects on mortality in patients with IHD[65,81,82]. This suggests that β-blockers have an additional mechanism of benefit in patients with IHD that compensates for their less consistent effects on ventricular function. The obvious candidate mechanism for this effect is coronary protection. β-Blockers have not been shown to reduce restenosis after atherectomy, a process that may be somewhat related to endogenous atherosclerosis[83]. β-Blockers may modify vascular wall permeability to lipid particles, while drugs such as carvedilol, that can retard oxidation of LDL, may reduce lipid accumulation in plaque[64]. β-Blockers may also reduce the risk of plaque rupture or increase endogenous thrombolysis[84].

At first sight, the studies of heart failure have generally not shown a reduction in myocardial infarction with β-blockers. This is contrast with previous and recent studies of β-blockers post-infarction, where a substantial effect on recurrent myocardial infarction was observed[12,85,86]. The reason for the difference probably reflects differences in the presentation of myocardial infarction. It is likely that most recurrent infarctions in studies of heart failure present as sudden death[30] and studies of β-blockers show that, numerically, this is their most important effect[3,7,8]. β-Blockers could not only reduce the rate of infarction, but also reduce the risk of subsequent arrhythmia; therefore it would not be surprising to see an increase in non-fatal myocardial infarction with β-blockers in patients with heart failure.

The evidence that $\beta_1$-selective and non-selective agents exert different effects is inconclusive[65,87]. Only non-selective agents have been shown to reduce mortality, long-term, after myocardial infarction, although meta-analysis failed to show conclusive evidence of heterogeneity[86,88]. Similarly, there are trends to a greater effect with non-selective agents in heart failure but only in some analyses have these shown a significant effect[89,90]. Confirmation of the hypothesis that there are differences in the effect of β-blockers in heart failure is being sought in a study (COMET) comparing metoprolol with carvedilol in patients with heart failure[87].

In summary, β-blockers are part of the first-line treatment for all patients with heart failure secondary to left ventricular systolic dysfunction regardless of the underlying aetiology and, apart from a few patients with recent severe decompensation, severity. The only absolute contra-indication is asthma but use may be limited by low arterial pressure (*e.g.* systolic <90 mmHg) and bradycardia. Initial exacerbation of symptoms is not uncommon but, with persistence, this is usually reversed. More than 85% of patients initiated on a β-blocker can be maintained on them[3,7,8].

## Spironolactone

One substantial randomised controlled study, unsupported by any smaller trials, has shown that the combination of spironolactone and an ACE inhibitor, compared to ACE inhibitor alone, reduced mortality substantially in patients with severe heart failure[6]. Patients taking β-blockers or digoxin in addition to their ACE inhibitor appeared to obtain even greater benefits from spironolactone. Spironolactone also appeared to improve symptoms. Reductions in both sudden death and death from progressive heart failure were observed. Non-significant reductions in hospitalisation due to myocardial infarction and stroke were also noted on spironolactone despite the improvement in prognosis, which exposed patients to a longer period at risk of non-fatal events. Patients with and without IHD benefited equally.

In summary, spironolactone should be considered in all patients with heart failure secondary to left ventricular systolic dysfunction who remain severely symptomatic despite treatment with ACE inhibitors, β-blockers and a substantial dose of conventional diuretic. Further clinical trials of aldosterone receptor antagonists in post-infarction ventricular dysfunction and in milder degrees of heart failure are expected.

## Hydrallazine and nitrates

Compared to other available treatments, the efficacy of this combination is not well established and it is often poorly tolerated[91,92]. Only 186 patients were randomised to this combination in V-HEFT-I study and up to 50% failed to tolerate one or other component[92]. Its use, even as an alternative to ACE inhibitors where they are not tolerated, is open to doubt. There is little evidence that adding either of these agents to a standard regimen of diuretics, ACE inhibitors and β-blockers confers any benefit on symptoms or prognosis[93,94]. However, nitrates may be useful in the management of angina. Whether short- or long-acting nitrates are preferred is open to question.

## Amiodarone

Trials of amiodarone after myocardial infarction have shown no major impact on mortality. Two randomised trials have been conducted in patients with heart failure; one open-label[95], the other double-blind[96,97].

The open-label, GESSICA study suggested a substantial reduction in mortality. 30% of patients had dilated cardiomyopathy or Chaga's disease and a substantial number had a history of alcoholism. Only 39% of patients had had a myocardial infarction. However, there was a trend to greater benefit in those with IHD[98]. In CHF-STAT, over 70% of patients had IHD as the cause for heart failure. This double-blind trial showed no overall effect on mortality, but patients **without** IHD did have a substantial prognostic benefit and a reduced need for hospitalisation[96,97].

A meta-analysis of trials of amiodarone suggested an overall mortality benefit[99], but the validity of the analysis must be questioned as there was clear heterogeneity between the effect observed in GESSICA and the other trials, in which case meta-analysis is an inappropriate way to assess effect.

### Calcium antagonists

Substantial trials of amlodipine[100,101], felodipine[102,103] and diltiazem[104] have been reported none of which showed an overall effect on mortality. The PRAISE trial showed a 60% reduction in mortality in patients **without** IHD but no effect in those with IHD[100]. However, it is possible that control of hypertension in those with hypertensive heart disease was largely responsible for the result. A second trial with much more stringent diagnostic entry criteria for dilated cardiomyopathy has been conducted to test the validity of the results of the first PRAISE trial[101]. This showed no mortality benefit. The neutral effect of amlodipine on mortality suggests that this agent is safe for use in patients with heart failure.

The DiDi trial[104], conducted exclusively in patients with dilated cardiomyopathy, suggested that diltiazem improved symptoms and exercise capacity but had no effect on prognosis. In view of the propensity of diltiazem to precipitate heart failure after myocardial infarction, it would seem wise to avoid this agent whenever possible in patients with heart failure[105]. Post-infarction trials with verapamil have suggested either no benefit or harm in patients with heart failure[106,107].

In summary, amlodipine has been established as a safe agent for use in heart failure and may be used to manage angina in this setting. Whether it is of benefit to add amlodipine to diuretics, spironolactone, ACE inhibitors and β-blockers in patients who have persistent hypertension is untested.

## Standard treatments for coronary disease in patients with heart failure

β-Blockers, calcium antagonists and nitrates have been dealt with above. Detailed discussion about the merits and risks of treatments directed at coronary vascular disease are dealt with in this section

## Smoking cessation

There is no substantial study investigating the effects of smoking cessation in heart failure. Smoking causes sympathetic activation, increases carboxy-haemoglobin thereby reducing oxygen transport in the circulation and has been implicated as a risk factor for atherosclerotic plaque rupture. For these reasons, it would seem wise to support cessation.

## Antithrombotic measures

Heart failure is a prothrombotic state and patients with heart failure are at high risk of fatal and non-fatal vascular events. However, the evidence that antithrombotic treatment is beneficial, or indeed safe, in patients with heart failure is limited and controversial.

Warfarin has been shown, in randomised controlled trials, to reduce the long-term risk of re-infarction and death after myocardial infarction[29,106] and observational data suggest that patients with heart failure treated with warfarin fare better, after adjustment for baseline variables[29,108]: At least 20% of patients with heart failure have atrial fibrillation and these patients should certainly receive warfarin[109]. However, whether warfarin is required in patients in sinus rhythm, regardless of the severity of ventricular dysfunction, remains in doubt[29]. Treatment guidelines in Europe and the US do not currently recommend routine prophylaxis with warfarin unless atrial fibrillation is present[39–41] or even discourage its use[110].

Aspirin is widely considered to be part of the routine treatment of patients with coronary disease although the quality of the data on which this advice is based is increasingly open to question, as is the safety of aspirin in patients with heart failure[29,111]. Individual long-term post-infarction trials have uniformly failed to show a reduction in mortality with aspirin (Fig. 2)[29,112,113] and the validity of the meta-analysis of the aspirin trials is now seriously in doubt[111]. It is only within the first 6 weeks after myocardial infarction that a reduction in mortality with aspirin has been proven[111]. In contrast to the lack of effect on mortality, several studies suggest that aspirin might reduce the risk of myocardial infarction, which is a paradox given the high mortality of myocardial infarction. Aspirin has consistently been associated with increases in sudden death in secondary prevention studies, leading to the suggestion that chronic aspirin therapy may modify the presentation of vascular events rather than prevent them[111,113].

Trends to an adverse effect of aspirin on mortality amongst patients with heart failure were noted in subset analyses of two large long-term, postinfarction aspirin trials (Table 5)[112,113]. The circumstantial evidence

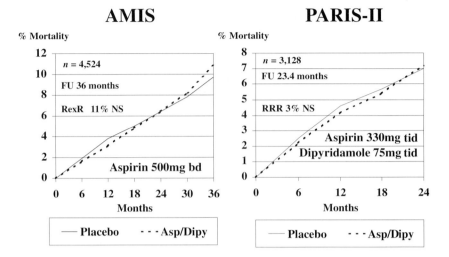

**Fig. 2** Large, long-term mortality trials of aspirin after myocardial infarction.

supporting the use of aspirin in patients with heart failure due to IHD is contradictory and inconclusive[29,111]. Extensive summaries of the clinical evidence have been published recently[29,111]. There are sound theoretical reasons for being concerned about an adverse effect of aspirin in patients with heart failure. Compared to healthy subjects, patients with heart failure have heightened activation of both vasoconstrictor and counter-regulatory vasodilator systems. There is plenty of opportunity for aspirin to have a negative impact on this delicate balance. Aspirin, in doses as low as 75 mg/day, has been shown both to impair vascular wall prostacyclin production for long periods[114] and enhance the vasoconstrictor response to endothelin[115]. High-dose aspirin can also provoke salt and water retention

**Table 5** Effects of aspirin on total mortality in patients with and without evidence of heart failure after myocardial infarction

|  | Mortality (%) Placebo | PARIS II Aspirin | Mortality (%) Placebo | AMIS Aspirin |
|---|---|---|---|---|
| Total mortality | 114/1565 (7.3%) | 111/1565 (7.1%) | 219/2267 (9.7%) | 246/2267 (10.9%) |
| HF absent | NA | NA | 6.9% | 8.3% |
| HF present | NA | NA | 21.2% | 23.7% |
| NYHA I | 5.8% | 4.9% | 7.3% | 8.6% |
| NYHA II | 8.9% | 9.4% | 14.3% | 14.3% |
| First infarct | 6.2% | 5.9% | 8.1% | 9.2% |
| >1 infarct | 13.5% | 13.5% | 19.6% | 19.2% |
| Digoxin – no | 6.3% | 5.5% | 7.4% | 9.3% |
| Digoxin – yes | 13.7% | 15.6% | 21.0% | 20.8% |

NYHA I was attributed to all patients after myocardial infarction who did not exhibit features of heart failure.

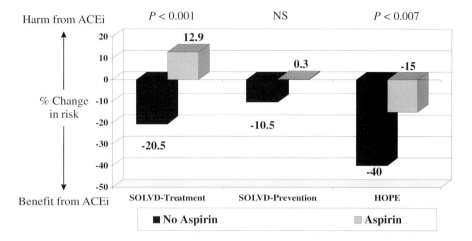

**Fig. 3** Effect of ACE inhibitors on mortality (SOLVD) or mortality/morbidity (HOPE) in the presence and absence of aspirin.

although it is unclear whether doses that are currently employed for cardiovascular prophylaxis do so[116].

The controversy surrounding aspirin in heart failure has been further fuelled by an apparent deleterious interaction between aspirin and ACE inhibitors (Fig. 3)[29,111]. The theoretical basis for this interaction is that ACE inhibitors enhance vasodilator/anti-aggregatory prostaglandin production by enhancing bradykinin production and that this is an important mechanism of ACE inhibitor benefit[29,59]. Aspirin may block this mechanism of benefit. Several small randomised controlled trials have shown that the central haemodynamic effects of ACE inhibitors are grossly attenuated by aspirin[117,118]. The evidence of an interaction in the peripheral forearm or renal beds is less conclusive[29]. The SOLVD studies[29] and the HOPE study[5] showed striking evidence of an aspirin/ACE inhibitor interaction. Worryingly, the SOLVD-treatment study suggested a higher mortality on enalapril compared to placebo amongst patients taking aspirin (Fig. 3). The postinfarction studies did not show a consistent interaction between aspirin and ACE inhibitors, perhaps reflecting the instability of baseline treatment in these studies[29,119]. There is clear evidence that many patients cease to take their aspirin within a few months of infarction while many patients who developed heart failure were placed on open-label ACE inhibitors confounding any chance of observing an interaction[120]. A recent meta-analysis blurred these differences between different sets of trials, and failed to support an interaction[119]. However, randomised controlled trials on over 15,000 stable patients in SOLVD and HOPE suggests a highly significant interaction between aspirin and ACE inhibitors.

A recent, substantial randomised-controlled pilot study showed a trend to an excess of deaths and vascular events in patients with heart failure taking aspirin compared to no antithrombotic treatment or warfarin[5,121]. Aspirin was associated with a significant excess in hospitalisation, largely due to an increase in worsening heart failure. Warfarin appeared to reduce markedly the frequency of non-fatal vascular events but, compared to no antithrombotic treatment did not exert a beneficial trend in mortality. Patients randomised to warfarin had the least days in hospital and lowest risk of adverse events among the three groups. A large ($n$ = 4500), randomised controlled trial comparing warfarin, aspirin and clopidogrel in patients with heart failure is currently being conducted[5,121].

In summary, it is not clear that aspirin or warfarin should be used routinely in patients with heart failure and coronary disease. Treatment guidelines in Europe and the US generally do not recommend routine use of aspirin in patients with heart failure[39–41] or even discourage its use[110]. Clopidogrel, an antiplatelet agent that does not interfere with prostaglandin production may prove the agent of choice in the majority of patients.

## Lipid lowering therapy

Patients with heart failure have been uniformly excluded from studies of lipid lowering therapy. This may be appropriate, as there is evidence that patients with heart failure who have a low cholesterol may have a worse prognosis[12,122,123]. Low cholesterol may only be a marker of more severe disease but the possibility that, in patients with heart failure, that it is intrinsically undesirable should also be considered.

The 4S study provided some evidence that in patients with ventricular dysfunction simvastatin can retard progression to heart failure[124]. However, conclusive evidence that cholesterol-lowering therapy is appropriate in heart failure awaits appropriate trial evidence. There are theoretical concerns about the use of statins in heart failure. Statins reduce the naturally occurring antioxidant ubiquinone, an effect both on the metabolic pathway for ubiquinone production and due to a reduction in plasma LDL, a ubiquinone-rich particle[125]. Patients with heart failure are under increased oxidant stress[126] and ubiquinone supplements have been shown in some well controlled studies to improve symptoms, cardiac function and quality of life in patients with heart failure[127,128] as well as reduce the risk of hospitalisation[129]. Uncontrolled studies have also suggested favourable effects on ventricular function and prognosis[130]. The exclusion of patients with heart failure from trials and the above theoretical concerns means that statins cannot yet be assumed to be safe or effective for routine use in patients with heart failure, coronary disease and hyperlipidaemia. Randomised clinical trials are underway.

## Coronary revascularisation

Randomised controlled trials comparing revascularisation with medical therapy have effectively excluded patients with heart failure and patients with an ejection fraction less than 35% (Tables 6–8)[131–133]. Subgroup analyses of patients with mild left ventricular dysfunction have included only small numbers of patients and these have suggested only trends to overall benefit[134]. Indeed, the CASS study only observed a significant benefit in a subgroup of patients with 3-vessel disease within the subgroup with left ventricular dysfunction (ejection fraction 35–50%)[135]. Although the relative benefit in this sub-subgroup appeared large. it represented a total of only 18 deaths. There are no randomised controlled trials of angioplasty in heart failure, but studies comparing

**Table 6** Exclusion criteria for randomised controlled trials of coronary artery bypass grafting

| | |
|---|---|
| VA | LV aneurysm |
| | 'Serious cardiac disease' |
| | Uncompensated CHF |
| CASS | EF < 35% |
| ECSS* | EF < 50% |

*The only study to reach its primary end-point.

**Table 7** CASS randomised study – summary of results[135]

EF 34–50% in 160 0f 780 (21%) randomised

6% of the 160 had heart failure

60% had angina

78 had 3 vessel disease of whom 7% had CHF

| | Medical | Surgical |
|---|---|---|
| 1–2 vessel disease | 46 | 36 |
| 3 vessel disease | 36 | 42 |
| Mortality at 7 years | | |
| Overall | 25 (30%) | 11 (16%) |
| 3 vessel disease | 13 (36%) | 5 (12%) |

**Table 8** VA randomised study – summary of results

EF 34–50% in 325 of 686 (21%) randomised

Low prevalence of CHF

| | Medical n = 175 | Surgical n = 150 | |
|---|---|---|---|
| Mortality | | | |
| 5 years | 47 (27%) | 30 (20%) | NS |
| 7 years | 65 (37%) | 39 (26%) | P < 0.05 |
| 11 years | 89 (51%) | 71 (47%) | NS |

medical treatment and angioplasty in patients with chronic stable angina have suggested that a medical strategy may be superior[136,137] and may lead to better outcomes, reserving intervention only for when medical therapy has failed to control angina.

The combined effect of ACE inhibitors, β-blockers and spironolactone is probably to reduce mortality by > 50% which matches or exceeds the expectations of benefit with revascularisation. National databases and observational reports are consistent with a 30-day operative mortality from coronary artery bypass surgery of about 7%[138]. Only observational studies and anecdote exist to support the selection of patients with heart failure for revascularisation using myocardial 'viability' testing. Considering the paucity of evidence to support revascularisation for heart failure, the relatively high postoperative morbidity and mortality and the costs generated by revascularisation, it is difficult to justify investigating patients with heart failure with a view to revascularisation.

A study comparing a strategy of whether or not to proceed to coronary investigation leading to revascularisation among patients with heart failure and evidence of a substantial volume of myocardium affected by reversible ischaemia or myocardial stunning/hibernation has been initiated in the UK[138]. All patients will receive optimal medical therapy for heart failure. The study intends to recruit 800 patients to determine whether this strategy of management can reduce all-cause mortality by 25%. A high rate of cross-over between treatment arms has been allowed for.

## Conclusions

There is evidence that ACE inhibitors and β-blockers improve prognosis in patients with heart failure and ischaemic heart disease by enhancing ventricular function and by reducing coronary events. It is also likely that β-blockers, and possibly ACE inhibitors, have favourable effects on other ischaemic syndromes. In contrast, treatments directed primarily against coronary disease, including aspirin, statins and revascularisation, have not yet been shown to be effective or safe in patients with heart failure. There is little clinical imperative to investigate patients with heart failure for the presence and pattern of IHD until such time as these tests are shown to improve therapy for patients.

### References

1 Cleland JGF, Gemmel I, Khand A, Boddy A. Is the prognosis of heart failure improving? *Eur J Heart Failure* 1999; **1**: 229–41

2 Khand A, Gemmel I, Clark A, Cleland JGF. Is the prognosis of heart failure improving? *J Am Coll Cardiol* 2000; **36**: 2284–6

3 Packer M, Bristow MR, Cohn JN *et al*. The effect of carvedilol on morbidity and mortality in patients with chronic heart failure. *N Engl J Med* 1996; **334**: 1349–55

4 Cleland JGF, Swedberg K, Poole-Wilson PA. Successes and failures of current treatment of heart failure. *Lancet* 1998; **352**: st19–28

5 Jones CG, Cleland JGF. Meeting report – LIDO, HOPE, MOXCON and WASH Studies. *Eur J Heart Failure* 1999; **1**: 425–31

6 Pitt B, Zannad F, Remme WJ *et al*. The effect of spironolactone on morbidity and mortality in patients with severe heart failure. *N Engl J Med* 1999; **341**: 709–17

7 MERIT-HF Study Group. Effect of metoprolol CR/XL in chronic heart failure: Metoprolol CR/XL Randomised Intervention Trial in Congestive Heart Failure (MERIT-HF). *Lancet* 1999; **333**: 2001–7

8 CIBIS-II Investigators and Committee. The Cardiac insufficiency Bisoprolol Study II (CIBIS-II): a randomised trial. *Lancet* 1999; **353**: 9–13

9 Witte K, Thackray S, Clark A, Cooklin M, Cleland JGF. Clinical trials update. IMPROVEMENT-HF, COPERNICUS, MUSTIC, ASPECT-II and APRICOT. *Eur J Heart Failure* 2000; **2**: 455–61

10 Thackray S, Witte KK, Khand A, Dunn A, Clark AL, Cleland JGF. Clinical trials update: highlights of the scientific sessions of the American Heart Association year 2000: Val HeFT, COPERNICUS, MERIT, CIBIS-II, BEST, AMIOVIRT, V-MAC, BREATHE, HEAT, MIRACL, FLORIDA, VIVA and the first human cardiac skeletal muscle myoblast transfer for heart failure. *Eur J Heart Failure* 2001; **3**: 117–24

11 Dargie HJ, The CAPRICORN Steering Committee. Design and methodology of the CAPRICORN trial – a randomised double-blind, placebo-controlled study of the impact of carvedilol on morbidity and mortality in patients with left ventricular dysfunction after myocardial infarction. *Eur J Heart Failure* 2000; **2**: 325–32

12 Louis A, Cleland JGF, Crabbe S, Ford S, Thgackray S, Houghton T, Clark AL. Clinical trials update: CAPRICORN, COPERNICUS, MIRACLE, STAF, RITZ-2, RECOVER and RENAISSANCE and cachexia and cholesterol in heart failure. Highlights of the Scientific Sessions of the American College of Cardiology, 2001. *Eur J Heart Failure* 2001; **3**:

13 Massie BM. 15 years of heart failure trials: what have we learned? *Lancet* 1998; **352**: I29–33

14 Sutton MSJ, Pfeffer MA, Plappert T *et al*. Quantitative two-dimensional echocardiographic measurements are major predictors of adverse cardiovascular events after acute myocardial infarction: the protective effects of captopril. *Circulation* 1994; **89**: 68–75

15 Sutton MSJ, Pfeffer MA, Moye L *et al*. Cardiovascular death and left ventricular remodeling two years after myocardial infarction. Baseline predictors and impact of long-term use of captopril: Information from the survival and ventricular enlargement (SAVE) trial. *Circulation* 1997; **96**: 3294–9

16 Konstam MA, Rousseau MF, Kronenberg MW *et al*. Effects of the angiotensin converting enzyme inhibitor enalapril on the long-term progression of left ventricular dysfunction in patients with heart failure. *Circulation* 1992; **86**: 431–8

17 Greenberg B, Quinones MA, Koilpillai C *et al*. Effects of long-term enalapril therapy on cardiac structure and function in patients with left ventricular dysfunction: results of the SOLVD echocardiography substudy. *Circulation* 1995; **91**: 2573–81

18 Doughty RN, Whalley GA, Gamble G, MacMahon S, Sharpe N, on behalf of the Australia-New Zealand Heart Failure Research Collaborative Group. Left ventricular remodelling with carvedilol in patients with congestive heart failure due to ischemic heart disease. *J Am Coll Cardiol* 1997; **29**: 1060–6

19 MacMahon S, Sharpe N, Doughty R *et al*. Randomised, placebo-controlled trial of carvedilol in patients with congestive heart failure due to ischaemic heart disease. *Lancet* 1997; **349**: 375–80

20 Hall SA, Cigarroa CG, Marcoux L, Risser RC, Grayburn PA, Eichhorn EJ. Time course of improvement in left ventricular function, mass and geometry in patients with congestive heart failure treated with beta-adrenergic blockade. *J Am Coll Cardiol* 1995; **25**:1154–61

21 Ferrari R, Sharpe N, Cohn JN. Cardiac remodeling –concepts and clinical implications: a consensus paper from an international forum on cardiac remodeling. Behalf of an International Forum on Cardiac Remodeling. *J Am Coll Cardiol* 2000; **35**: 569–82

22 Cleland JGF, Pennell DJ, Murray GD *et al*. The Carvedilol Hibernation Reversible Ischaemia Trial; Marker of Success (CHRISTMAS). *Eur J Heart Failure* 1999; **1**: 191–6

23 Lamas GA, Flaker GC, Mitchell G *et al*. Effect of infarct artery patency on prognosis after acute myocardial infarction. *Circulation* 1995; **92**: 1101–9

24 Cleland JGF, Puri S. How do ACE inhibitors reduce mortality in patients with left ventricular dysfunction with and without heart failure: remodelling, resetting, or sudden death? *Br Heart J* 1994; **72**: S81–6

25 Uretsky B, Thygesen K, Armstrong PW *et al*. Acute coronary findings at autopsy in heart failure patients with sudden death: results from the assessment of treatment with lisinopril and survival study (ATLAS) trial. *Circulation* 2000; **102**: 611–6

26 DiCarli M, Sherman T, Khanna S *et al*. Myocardial viability in asynergic regions subtended by occluded coronary arteries: relation to the status of collateral flow in patients with chronic coronary artery disease. *J Am Coll Cardiol* 1994; **23**: 860–8

27 Senior R, Glenville B, Basu S *et al*. Dobutamine echocardiography and thallium-201 imaging predict functional improvement after revascularisation in severe ischaemic left ventricular dysfunction. *Br Heart J* 1995; **74**: 358–64

28 Lee KS, Marwick TH, Cook SA *et al*. Prognosis of patients with left ventricular dysfunction, with and without viable myocardium after myocardial infarction. *Circulation* 1994; **90**: 2687–94

29 Cleland JGF. Anticoagulant and antiplatelet therapy in heart failure. *Curr Opin Cardiol* 1997; **12**: 276–87

30 Cleland JGF, Massie BM, Packer M. Sudden death in heart failure: vascular or electrical? *Eur J Heart Failure* 1999; **1**: 41–5

31 Cleland JGF, Thackray S, Goodge L, Kaye GC, Cooklin M. Outcome studies with device therapy in patients with heart failure. *J Clin Pacing* 2001; In press

32 Tunstall-Pedoe H, Kuulasmaa K, Amouyel P, Arveiler D, Rajakangas A, Pajak A. Myocardial infarction and coronary deaths in the World Health Organization MONICA project. *Circulation* 1994; **90**: 583–612

33 Davies MJ, Thomas A. Thrombosis and acute coronary artery lesions in sudden cardiac death. *N Engl J Med* 1984; **310**:1137–40

34 Greenberg HM, Dwyer Jr EM, Hochman JS, Steinberg JS, Echt DS, Peters RW. Interaction of ischaemia and encainide/flecainide treatment: a proposed mechanism for the increased mortality in CAST I. *Br Heart J* 1995; **74**: 631–5

35 Hallstrom AP, Anderson JL, Carlson M *et al*. Time to arrhythmic, ischemic, and heart failure events: exploratory analyses to elucidate mechanisms of adverse drug effects in the Cardiac Arrhythmia Suppression Trial. *Am Heart J* 1995; **130**: 71–9

36 The Antiarrhythmics Versus Implantable Defibrillators (AVID) Investigators. A comparison of antiarrhythmic drug therapy with implantable defibrillators in patients resuscitated from near-fatal ventricular arrhythmias. *N Engl J Med* 1997; **337**: 1576–83

37 Bigger JT, for the Coronary Artery Bypass Graft (CABG) Patch Trial Investigators. Prophylactic use of implanted cardiac defibrillators in patients at high risk for ventricular arrhythmias after coronary-artery bypass graft surgery. *N Engl J Med* 1997; **337**: 1569–75

38 Cleland JGF, Erdmann E, Ferrari R *et al*. Guidelines for the diagnosis of heart failure. *Eur Heart J* 1995; **16**: 741–51

39 Konstam M. AHCPR Guidelines. Heart failure: management of patients with left ventricular systolic dysfunction. *Prim Cardiol* 1994; **20**:41-44-49.

40 ACC/AHA Task Force. Guidelines for the evaluation and management of heart failure. *J Am Coll Cardiol* 1995; **26**: 1376–98

41 The Task Force of the Working Group on Heart Failure of the European Society of Cardiology. The treatment of heart failure. *Eur Heart J* 1997; **18**: 736–53

42 Follath F, Cleland JGF, Klein W, Murphy R. Etiology and response to drug treatment in heart failure. *J Am Coll Cardiol* 1998; **32**: 1167–72

43 Cleland JGF, McGowan J. Heart failure due to ischaemic heart disease: epidemiology, pathophysiology and progression. *J Cardiovasc Pharmacol* 1999; **33**: S17–29

44 Cowburn PJ, Cleland JGF, Coats AJS, Komajda M. Risk stratification in chronic heart failure. *Eur Heart J* 1998; **19**: 696–710

45 SHEP Cooperative Research Group. Prevention of stroke by anti-hypertensive drug treatment in older persons with isolated systolic hypertension. Final results of the Systolic Hypertension in the Elderly Program (SHEP). *JAMA* 1991; **265**: 3255–64

46 Dahlof B, Lindholm LH, Hansson L, Schersten B, Ekbom T, Wester PO. Morbidity and mortality in the Swedish Trial in Old Patients with Hypertension (STOP-Hypertension). *Lancet* 1991; **338**: 1281–5

47  Cleland JGF. Progression from hypertension to heart failure. Mechanisms and management. *Cardiology* 1999; **92 (Suppl 1)**: 10–9

48  Khand AU, Rankin AC, Martin W, Taylor J, Cleland JGF. Digoxin or carvedilol for the treatment of atrial fibrillation in patients with heart failure? *Heart* 2000; **83 (Suppl 1)**: P30

49  Khand A, Rankin AC, Kaye GC, Cleland JGF. Systematic review of the management of atrial fibrillation in patients with heart failure. *Eur Heart J* 2000; **21**: 614–32

50  Uretsky BF, Young JB, Shahidi E *et al*. Randomized study assessing the effect of digoxin withdrawal in patients with mild to moderate chronic congestive heart failure: results of the PROVED trial. *J Am Coll Cardiol* 1993; **22**: 955–62

51  Packer M, Gheorghiade M, Young JB *et al*. Withdrawal of digoxin from patients with chronic heart failure treated with angiotensin-converting-enzyme inhibitors. *N Engl J Med* 1993; **329**: 1–7

52  Gheorghiade M, Young JB, Uretsky BF, Packer M. The effects of digoxin withdrawal in patients with stable heart failure due to coronary artery disease compared to primary cardiomyopathy; insights from the PROVED and RADIANCE studies. *Circulation* 1995; **92**: I-142

53  The Digitalis Investigation Group. The effect of digoxin on mortality and morbidity in patients with heart failure. *N Engl J Med* 1997; **336**: 525–33

54  Cleland JGF, Swedberg K, Poole-Wilson PA. Successes and failures of current treatment of heart failure. *Lancet* 1998; **352**: I19–28

55  Cleland JGF, Cowburn PJ, McMurray JJV. In: Cleland JGF (ed). *Heart Failure: A Systematic Guide to Clinical Practice*. London: Science Press, 1997

56  Kober L, Torp Pedersen C, Carlsen JE *et al*. A clinical trial of the angiotensin-converting-enzyme inhibitor trandolapril in patients with left ventricular dysfunction after myocardial infarction. *N Engl J Med* 1995; **333**: 1670–6

57  Ball SG, Hall AS, Mackintosh AF *et al*. Effect of ramipril and morbidity of survivors of acute myocardial infarction with clinical evidence of heart failure. *Lancet* 1993; **342**: 821–8

58  Pfeffer MA, Braunwald E, Moye LA *et al*. Effect of captopril on mortality and morbidity in patients with left ventricular dysfunction after myocardial infarction – results of the survival and ventricular enlargement trial. *N Engl J Med* 1992; **327**: 669–77

59  Cleland JGF, Witte K, Thackray S. Bradykinin and ventricular function. *Eur Heart J* 2000; **Suppl H**: H20–9

60  The Heart Outcomes Prevention Evaluation Study Investigators. Effects of angiotensin-converting-enzyme inhibitor, ramipril, on cardiovascular events in high risk patients. *N Engl J Med* 2000; **342**: 145–53

61  Yusuf S, Pepine CJ, Garces C *et al*. Effect of enalapril on myocardial infarction and unstable angina in patients with low ejection fractions. *Lancet* 1992; **340**: 1173–8

62  Cleland JGF, Erhardt L, Murray G, Hall AS, Ball SG. Effect of ramipril on morbidity and mode of death among survivors of acute myocardial infarction with clinical evidence of heart failure. *Eur Heart J* 1997; **18**: 41–51

63  Mancini GBJ, Henry GC, Macaya C *et al*. Angiotensin-converting enzyme inhibition with quinapril improves endothelial vasomotor dysfunction in patients with coronary heart disease – the TREND (Trial on Reversing Endothelial Dysfunction) Study. *Circulation* 1996; **94**: 258–65

64  Cleland JGF, Krikler D. Modification of atherosclerosis by agents that do not lower cholesterol. *Br Heart J* 1993; **69**: 54–62

65  Cleland JGF, Bristow M, Erdmann E, Remme WJ, Swedberg K, Waagstein F. Beta-blocking agents in heart failure. Should they be used and how? *Eur Heart J* 1996; **17**: 1629–39

66  MacMahon S, Sharpe N, Gamble G *et al*. Randomized, placebo controlled trial of the ACE inhibitor, ramipril, in patients with coronary or other occlusive arterial disease. PART-2 Collaborative Research Group (Prevention of Atherosclerosis with Ramipril Trial). *J Am Coll Cardiol* 2000; **36**: 438–43

67  Wright RA, Flapan AD, Alberti KGMM, Ludlam CA, Fox KAA. Effects of captopril therapy on endogenous fibrinolysis in men with recent, uncomplicated myocardial infarction. *J Am Coll Cardiol* 1994; **24**: 67–73

68  Lonn EM, Yusuf S, Jha P *et al*. Emerging role of angiotensin converting enzyme inhibitors in cardiac and vascular protection. *Circulation* 1994; **90**: 2056–69

69  Ridker PM, Gaboury CL, Conlin PR, Seely EW, Williams GH, Vaughan DE. Stimulation of plasminogen activator inhibitor *in vivo* by infusion of angiotensin II: evidence of a potential interaction between the renin-angiotensin system and fibrinolytic function. *Circulation* 1993; **87**: 1969–73

70  Garg R, Yusuf S. Overview of randomized trials of angiotensin-converting enzyme inhibitors on mortality and morbidity in patients with heart failure. *JAMA* 1995; **273**: 1450–6

71  Pitt B, Poole Wilson PA, Segal R *et al*. Effect of losartan compared with captopril on mortality in patients with symptomatic heart failure: randomised trial – the Losartan Heart Failure Survival Study ELITE II. *Lancet* 2000; **355**: 1582–7

72  Cleland JGF, Freemantle N, McGowan J, Clark A. The evidence for beta-blockers equals or surpasses that for ACE inhibitors in heart failure. *BMJ* 1999; **318**: 824–5

73  Woodley SL, Gilbert EM, Anderson JL *et al*. B-blockade with bucindolol in heart failure caused by ischemic versus idiopathic dilated cardiomyopathy. *Circulation* 1991; **84**: 2426–41

74  Fisher ML, Gottlieb SS, Plotnick G *et al*. Beneficial effects of metoprolol in heart failure associated with coronary artery disease: a randomized trial. *J Am Coll Cardiol* 1994; **23**: 943–50

75  Waagstein F. Metoprolol in addition to ACE-inhibitors causes regression of left ventricular dilatation and increases exercise ejection fraction in ischemic cardiomyopathy. *J Am Coll Cardiol* 1997; **29**: 206A

76  Bristow MR, Gilbert EM, Abraham WT *et al*. Carvedilol produces dose-related improvements in left ventricular function and survival in subjects with chronic heart failure. *Circulation* 1996; **94**: 2807–16

77  Unverferth DV, Magorien RD, Lewis RP, Leier CV. The role of subendocardial ischemia in perpetuating myocardial failure in patients with non-ischemic congestive cardiomyopathy. *Am Heart J* 1983; **105**: 176–9

78  van der Heuvel AF, van Veldhuisen DJ, Van der Wall EE, Blanksma PK, Siebelink HM, van Gilst, Crijns HJ. Regional myocardial blood flow reserve impairment and metabolic changes suggesting myocardial ischemia in patients with idiopathic dilated cardiomyopathy. *J Am Coll Cardiol* 2001; **35**: 19–38

79  O'Keefe J, Magalski A, Stevens TL *et al*. Predictors of improvement in left ventricular ejection fraction with carvedilol for congestive heart failure. *J Nucl Cardiol* 2000; **7**: 3–7

80  Chen C, Aksenov S, Hong H, Liu J, Marak J, Fallon J *et al*. Protective effects of a beta-blocker on progressive left ventricular remodeling in chronic ischemic cardiomyopathy with hibernating myocardium. *J Am Coll Cardiol* 2001; **37** (**Suppl A**): 353A. Abstract

81  Lechat P, Jaillon P, Fontaine ML *et al*. A randomized trial of beta-blockade in heart failure: the Cardiac Insufficiency Bisoprolol Study (CIBIS). *Circulation* 1994; **90**: 1765–73

82  Waagstein F, Bristow MR, Swedberg K *et al*. Beneficial effects of metoprolol in idiopathic dilated cardiomyopathy. *Lancet* 1993; **342**: 1441–6

83  Serruys PW, Foley DP, Hofling B *et al*. Carvedilol for prevention of restenosis after directional coronary atherectomy: final results of the European carvedilol atherectomy restenosis (EUROCARE) trial. *Circulation* 2000; **101**: 1512–8

84  Andreotti F, Kluft C, Davies GJ, Huisman LGM, De-Bart ACW, Maseri A. Effect of propranolol (long acting) on the circadian fluctuation of tissue plasminogen activator and plasminogen activator inhibitor 1. *Am J Cardiol* 1991; **68**: 1295–9

85  Von der Lippe G, Hansen HS, Lund-Johansen P *et al*. The Norwegian Multicentre Study Group. Timolol induced reduction in mortality and reinfarction in patients surviving acute myocardial infarction. *N Engl J Med* 1981; **304**: 801–7

86  Freemantle N, Cleland JGF, Young S, Mason J, Harrison J. What is the current place of beta blockade in secondary prevention after myocardial infarction: systematic overview and meta regression analysis? *BMJ* 1999; **318**: 1730–7

87  McGowan J, Murphy R, Cleland JGF. Carvedilol for heart failure; clinical trials in progress. *Heart Failure Rev* 1999; **4**: 89–95

88  Cleland JGF, McGowan J, Cowburn PJ. β-blockers for chronic heart failure: from prejudice to enlightenment. *J Cardiovasc Pharmacol* 1998; **32**: S52–60

89  Doughty RN, Rodgers A, Sharpe N, MacMahon S. Effects of beta-blocker therapy on mortality in patients with heart failure – a systematic overview of randomised controlled trials. *Eur Heart J* 1997; **18**: 560–5

90  Heidenreich PA, Lee TT, Massie BM. Effect of beta-blockade on mortality in patients with heart failure: a meta-analysis of randomised trials. *J Am Coll Cardiol* 1997; **30**: 27–34

91  Cleland JGF, McMurray JJF, Cowburn PJ. (eds) *Heart Failure: A Systematic Approach for Clinical Practice*. London: Science Press, 1997

92  Cohn JN, Archibald DG, Ziesche S *et al*. Effect of vasodilator therapy on mortality in chronic congestive heart failure: results of a Veterans Administration Cooperative Study. *N Engl J Med*

1986; **314**: 1547–52

93 Lewis BS, Rabinowitz B, Schlesinger Z. Effect of isosorbide-5-mononitrate on exercise performance and clinical status in patients with congestive heart failure. results of the nitrates in congestive heart failure (NICE) study. *Cardiology* 1999; **91**: 1–7

94 Elkayam U, Johnson JV, Shotan A *et al*. Double-blind, placebo-controlled study to evaluate the effect of organic nitrates in patients with chronic heart failure treated with angiotensin-converting enzyme inhibition. *Circulation* 1999; **99**: 2652–7

95 Doval HC, Nul DR, Grancelli HI, Perrone SV, Bortman GR, Curiel R. Randomised trial of low-dose amiodarone in severe congestive heart failure. *Lancet* 1994; **344**: 493–8

96 Singh SN, Fletcher RD, Fisher SG *et al*. Amiodarone in patients with congestive heart failure and asymptomatic ventricular arrhythmia. *N Engl J Med* 1995; **333**: 77–82

97 Massie BM, Fisher SG, Deedwania PC, Singh BN, Fletcher RD, Singh SN. Effect of amiodarone on clinical status and left ventricular function in patients with congestive heart failure. *Circulation* 1996; **93**: 2128–34

98 Nul DR, Grancelli HI, Varini SD *et al*. No etiologic differences in survival benefits from amiodarone in severe congestive heart failure. *J Am Coll Cardiol* 1997; **29**: 247A

99 Amiodarone Trials Meta-analysis Investigators. Effect of prophylactic amiodarone on mortality after acute myocardial infarction and in congestive heart failure: meta-analysis of individual data from 6500 patients in randomised trials. *Lancet* 1997; **350**: 1417–24

100 Packer M, O'Connor CM, Ghali JK *et al*. Effect of amlodipine on morbidity and mortality in severe chronic heart failure. *N Engl J Med* 1996; **335**: 1107–14

101 Thackray S, Witte K, Clark AL, Cleland JGF. Clinical trials update: OPTIME-CHF, PRAISE-2, ALL-HAT. *Eur J Heart Failure* 2000; **2**: 209–12

102 Cohn JN, Ziesche SM, Loss LE, Anderson GF, and the V-HeFT Study Group. Effect of felodipine on short-term exercise and neurohormones and long-term mortality in heart failure: results of V-HeFT-III. *Circulation* 1995; **92**: I-143

103 Littler WA, Sheridan DJ. Placebo controlled trial of felodipine in patients with mild to moderate heart failure. *Br Heart J* 1995; **73**: 428–33

104 Figulla HR, Gietzen F, Zeymer U *et al*. Diltiazem improves cardiac function and exercise capacity in patients with idiopathic dilated cardiomyopathy: results of the diltiazem in dilated cardiomyopathy trial. *Circulation* 1996; **94**: 346–52

105 Goldstein RE, Boccuzzi SJ, Cruess D *et al*. Diltiazem increases late-onset congestive heart failure in postinfarction patients with early reduction in ejection fraction. *Circulation* 1991; **83**: 52–60

106 Cleland JGF, Ray SG, McMurray JJV. Overview of post infarction trials. In: Cleland JGF. (ed) *Prevention Strategies after Myocardial Infarction*. London: Science Press, 1994; 37–73

107 Hansen JF. Effect of verapamil on mortality and major events after acute myocardial infarction (The Danish Verapamil Infarction Trial II – DAVIT II). *Am J Cardiol* 1990; **66**: 779–85

108 Al-Khadra AS, Salem DN, Rand WM, Udelson JE, Smith JJ, Konstam MA. Warfarin anticoagulation and survival: a cohort analysis from the studies of left ventricular dysfunction. *J Am Coll Cardiol* 1998; **31**: 749–53

109 Cleland JGF, Cowburn PJ, Falk RH. Should all patients with atrial fibrillation receive warfarin? Evidence from randomised clinical trials. *Eur Heart J* 1996; **17**: 674–81

110 Baker DW, Wright RF. Management of heart failure: IV. Anticoagulation for patients with heart failure due to left ventricular systolic dysfunction. *JAMA* 1994; **272**: 1614–8

111 Cleland JGF, Bulpitt CJ, Falk RH *et al*. Is aspirin safe for patients with heart failure? *Br Heart J* 1995; **74**: 215–9

112 Aspirin Myocardial Infarction Study Research Group. A randomised, controlled trial of aspirin in persons recovered from myocardial infarction. *JAMA* 1980; **243**: 661–8

113 Klimt CR, Knatterud GL, Stamler J, Meier P. Persantine-Aspirin Reinfarction Study. Part II. Secondary coronary prevention with persantine and aspirin. *J Am Coll Cardiol* 1986; **7**: 251–69

114 Davie AP, Love MP, McMurray JJV. Even low-dose aspirin inhibits arachidonic acid-induced vasodilatation in heart failure. *Clin Pharmacol Ther* 2000; **67**: 530–7

115 Haynes G, Webb DJ. Endothelium-dependent modulation of responses to endothelin-1 in human veins. *Clin Sci* 1993; **84**: 427–33

116 Riegger GAJ, Kahles HW, Elsner D, Kromer EP, Kochsiek K. Effects of acetylsalicylic acid on renal function in patients with chronic heart failure. *Am J Med* 1991; **90**: 571–5

117 Hall D, Zeitler H, Rudolph W. Counteraction of the vasodilator effects of enalapril by aspirin in severe heart failure. *J Am Coll Cardiol* 1992; **20**: 1549–55

118 Spaulding C, Charbonnier B, Cohen-Solal A *et al*. Acute hemodynamic interaction of aspirin and ticlopidine with enalapril. Results of a double-blind, randomised comparative trial. *Circulation* 1998; **98**: 757–65

119 Flather MD, Yusuf S, Kober L *et al*. Long term ACE-inhibitor therapy in patients with heart failure or left ventricular dysfunction: a systematic overview of data from individual patients. *Lancet* 2000; **355**: 1575–81

120 Stafford RS. Aspirin use is low among United States outpatients with coronary artery disease. *Circulation* 2000; **101**: 1097–101

121 WASH Steering Committee & Investigators. The WASH study (Warfarin/Aspirin Study in Heart Failure) rationale, design and end-point. *Eur J Heart Failure* 1999; **1**: 95–9

122 Richartz BM, Radovancevic B, Frazier OH, Vaughn WK, Taegtmeyer H. Low serum cholesterol levels predict high perioperative mortality in patients supported by a left-ventricular assist system. *Cardiology* 1998; **89**: 184–8

123 Rauchhaus M, Doehner W, Davos CH *et al*. Serum total cholesterol, high density lipoprotein, and prognosis in patients with chronic heart failure. *J Am Coll Cardiol* 2001; **37** (**Suppl A**): 156A

124 Kjekshus J, Pedersen TR, Olsson AG, Faergeman O, Pyorala K. The effects of simvastatin on the incidence of heart failure in patients with coronary disease. *J Cardiac Failure* 1997; **3**: 249–54

125 Mabuchi H, Haba T, Tatami R *et al*. Effects of an inhibitor of HMG CoA reductase on serum lipoproteins and ubiquinone 10 levels in patients with familial hypercholesterolaemia. *N Engl J Med* 1981; **305**: 478–82

126 McMurray J, McLay J, Chopra M, Bridges A, Belch JJF. Evidence for enhanced free radical activity in chronic congestive heart failure secondary to coronary artery disease. *Am J Cardiol* 1990; **65**: 1261–2

127 Hofman-Bang C, Rehnquist N, Swedberg K, Wiklund I, Astrom H, for the Q10 study group. Coenzyme Q10 as an adjunctive in the treatment of chronic congestive heart failure. *J Cardiac Failure* 1995; **1**: 101–7

128 Langsjoen PH, Vadhanavikit S, Folkers K. Response of patients in classes III and IV of cardiomyopathy to therapy in blind and crossover trial with coenzyme Q10. *Proc Natl Acad Sci USA* 1985; **82**: 4240–4

129 Morisco C, Trimarco B, Condorelli M. Effect of coenzyme Q-10 therapy in patients with congestive heart failure: a long-term multicenter randomized study. *Clin Invest Suppl* 1993; **71**: S134–6

130 Langsjoen PH, Langsjoen PH, Folkers K. Long-term efficacy and safety of coenzyme Q10 therapy for idiopathic dilated cardiomyopathy. *Am J Cardiol* 1990; **65**: 521–3

131 Varnauskas E, European Coronary Surgery Study Group. Twelve-year follow-up of survival in the randomized European Coronary Surgery Study. *N Engl J Med* 1988; **319**: 332–7

132 Peduzzi P, Detre K, Murphy M *et al*. Ten year incidence of myocardial infarction and prognosis after infarction. *Circulation* 1991; **83**: 747–55

133 CASS Principal Investigators and their Associates. Coronary Artery Surgery Study (CASS): a randomised trial of coronary artery bypass surgery. *Circulation* 1983; **68**: 939–50

134 Yusuf S, Zucker D, Peduzzi P *et al*. Effect of coronary artery bypass graft surgery on survival: overview of 10 year results from randomised trials by the Coronary Artery Bypass Graft Surgery Trialists Collaboration. *Lancet* 1994; **344**: 563–70

135 Passamani E, Davis KB, Gillespie MJ, Killip T, and the CASS Principal Investigators and their Associates. A randomized trial of coronary artery bypass surgery. Survival of patients with a low ejection fraction. *N Engl J Med* 1985; **312**: 1665–71

136 RITA-2 Trial Participants. Coronary angioplasty versus medical therapy for angina: the second randomised intervention treatment of angina (RITA-2) trial. *Lancet* 1997; **350**: 461–8

137 Pitt B, Waters D, Brown WV, van Boven AJ, Schwartz L, Title LM *et al*. for the Atovastatin versus Revascularisation Treatment Investigators. Aggressive lipid lowering therapy compared with angioplasty in stable coronary artery disease. Atorvastatin Versus Revascularization Treatment Investigators. *N Engl J Med* 1999; **341**: 70–6

138 Cleland JGF on behalf of the HEART UK Investigators and Committees. The Heart Failure Revascularisation Trial (HEART): rationale, design and methodology. *Eur J Heart Failure* 2002; In press

# Diabetes

**Adam D Timmis**

*Department of Cardiology, London Chest Hospital, London, UK*

The causes of accelerated atherogenesis in diabetes are unclear but the consequences in terms of cardiovascular morbidity and mortality are profound. Thus diabetes not only increases the risk of coronary heart disease but also increases the case fatality rate, ensuring that the majority of patients die of cardiovascular causes, often before the age of 50 years. The problem is compounded by autonomic neuropathy which alters the perception of cardiac pain, attenuating symptoms which are often atypical or absent. This may delay presentation or lead to inappropriate triage decisions such that access to defibrillators and specific treatment is denied. Central to the cardio-vascular management of diabetes is vigorous risk factor modification although clear evidence that this leads to extra protection against coronary heart disease beyond that achieved in non-diabetic individuals has not been forthcoming. In other respects too, the management of diabetic patients with heart disease is underpinned by the same evidence-base as applies to non-diabetic patients, and it is noteworthy that 15–20% of the patients in most of the landmark clinical trials have been diabetic. Recently, however, trials such as the United Kingdom Prospective Diabetes Study (UKPDS), the Heart Outcomes Prevention Evaluation (HOPE) study, and the Diabetes Mellitus, Insulin Glucose Infusion in Acute Myocardial Infarction (DIGAMI) study have identified novel strategies for reducing cardiovascular risk in diabetes. These trials have already had a major impact on cardiological practice, emphasising the prime import-ance of blood pressure control and converting enzyme inhibition for reducing cardio-vascular risk in diabetes as well as the value of insulin therapy for reducing mortality in diabetic myocardial infarction. Additional trials, already in progress, are expected to refine further the cardiovascular management of patients with diabetes in order to provide an effective challenge for a problem that shows no signs of going away.

Much of the excess morbidity and mortality among diabetic patients is attributable to accelerated atherogenesis. Indeed, 75% of all deaths in patients with diabetes are from this cause[1]. With our ageing, sedentary and increasingly obese population, the number of affected individuals will continue to rise with major knock-on effects for cardiological practice.

## Accelerated atherogenesis

Conventional risk factors, particularly hypertension and dyslipidaemia, occur more commonly in diabetes, but account for less than 25% of the

Correspondence to:
Mr Adam D Timmis,
Department of
Cardiology, London Chest
Hospital, Banner Road,
London E2 9JX, UK

excess risk of coronary heart disease[2]. Thus, most of the excess risk is attributable directly or indirectly to diabetes itself. Mechanisms are unclear although it is generally accepted that, in common with all other major risk factors, diabetes promotes atherogenesis by increasing oxidative stress and lipid peroxidation in the arterial endothelium.

## Hyperglycaemia

Because hyperglycaemia is a late event in the process leading from insulin resistance to frank diabetes, it is often regarded as a minor player in the pathogenesis of accelerated atherosclerosis[3]. Nevertheless, it has recently been implicated in mechanisms of increased oxidative stress by reversible glycosylation of protein amino groups. This has no direct pathological consequences, but leads to irreversible oxidation of fructoselysine which produces a variety of advanced glycation end products (AGEs)[4]. These react with a specific receptor (RAGE) at the vascular endothelium, increasing vascular endothelial production of superoxide anion and other oxidative products which accelerate atherogenesis[5]. Recent data indicate that reducing vascular exposure to AGEs by injection of soluble RAGE (which 'mops up' circulating AGEs) suppresses accelerated atherosclerosis in diabetic mice. Whether RAGE scavenging drugs will have a clinical role, however, is not known[6].

## Hyperinsulinaemia, and insulin resistance

Metabolic characteristics of the cardiovascular dysmetabolic syndrome include hyperinsulinaemia and insulin resistance[7]. Hyperinsulinaemia promotes smooth muscle proliferation in the vessel wall and stimulates production of plasminogen activator inhibitor. These adverse proliferative and thrombogenic actions, however, must be set against the vasculo-protective effects of insulin which include stimulation of endothelial nitric oxide production, such that net effects on atherogenesis are hard to quantify[8]. Epidemiological studies have been contradictory[9], and taken together suggest that hyperinsulinaemia is only weakly predictive of accelerated atherogenesis without necessarily implying a causal relation-ship[10]. Insulin resistance correlates better with coronary artery disease, and in the Insulin Resistance Atherosclerosis Study had an independent effect on carotid intimal medial wall thickness that persisted following adjustment for smoking, lipid levels, hypertension, diabetes and gender[11].

## Dyslipidaemia

In type 2 diabetes, chylomicrons and atherogenic very low density lipoprotein (VLDL) remnants accumulate[12-14]. Hypertriglyceridaemia causes high density lipoprotein (HDL) levels to diminish and low density lipoprotein (LDL) particles to become smaller and denser, increasing their ability to penetrate the arterial intima and their susceptibility to oxidation. Thus, while total cholesterol levels may be normal, the atherogenicity of LDL and VLDL is enhanced, and circulating levels of protective HDL are reduced. Nevertheless, dyslipidaemia probably accounts for only a part of the increased susceptibility to coronary heart disease in diabetes, since treatment does not reduce risk to the level seen in patients without diabetes.

*Procoagulant factors*

Oxidative stress and endothelial dysfunction in diabetes results in deficient production of prostacyclin and plasminogen activator inhibitor, and is also responsible for increased platelet production of thromboxane $A_2$[15]. The net effect of these changes is to enhance vasoconstrictor and thrombotic responses to plaque rupture in diabetes, increasing plaque burden and the risk of myocardial infarction.

# Cardiovascular risk

The Framingham study showed that diabetes independently increased the relative risk of coronary heart disease by 66% in men and 203% in women followed-up for 20 years[2]. The heightened risk in women has since been confirmed by a large volume of clinical data, most recently the report that diabetes abolishes gender differences in coronary calcification measured by ultrafast computed tomography[16]. The Whitehall study of male civil servants extended the Framingham observations by showing that sub-clinical glucose intolerance, in addition to frank diabetes, also increased coronary risk[17]. The Multiple Risk Factor Interventional Trial (MRFIT) with its very large population of middle-aged men was able to provide more detailed information about the interaction between diabetes and other risk factors in determining coronary risk[18]. This trial confirmed the heightened risk attributable to diabetes, and also the independent effects of serum cholesterol, blood pressure and smoking in men with and without diabetes. MRFIT showed that in men with diabetes, 12-year cardiovascular mortality was much higher at every level of these major risk factors considered singly and in combination, and that with progressively more unfavourable risk factor status the mortality rate rose much more steeply than in men without diabetes.

# Protecting against coronary heart disease

The MRFIT investigators recommended 'rigorous sustained intervention in people with diabetes to control blood pressure, lower serum cholesterol, and abolish cigarette smoking...', recommendations that remain central to the cardiovascular management of diabetes today. Disappointingly, however, there is not yet clear evidence that these recommendations lead to extra protection against coronary heart disease beyond that achieved in non-diabetic individuals, although important protection against microvascular complications (retinopathy, renal disease) does occur. Nevertheless, as practice evolves from single to multifactorial risk assessment, in which absolute coronary risk can be readily assessed from colour-coded charts, the clinical impact of risk factor modification can be expected to increase[19].

## Lowering blood pressure

Hypertension commonly occurs in type 2 diabetes, and contributes importantly to the heightened risk of macrovascular and microvascular disease[20–23]. Trial data have suggested that the benefits of treating hypertension apply equally to diabetic and non-diabetic patients, a suggestion emphatically confirmed in the hypertensive cohort of the UK Prospective Diabetes Study (UKPDS)[24]. Comparison of patients allocated either to tight blood pressure control (<150/85 mmHg) using captopril or atenolol, or to less-tight control showed that tight control for a mean of 8.4 years was associated with significant reduction in the risk of death related to diabetes, and with reductions in all microvascular end-points. Predictably, reductions in the risk of heart failure and stroke also occurred, but the 21% reduction in the risk of myocardial infarction was not significant. The Hypertension Optimal Treatment (HOT) study also reported reductions in myocardial infarction in patients treated to a target diastolic blood pressure of $\leq 80$ mmHg compared with targets of $\leq 85$ or $\leq 90$ mmHg, but again the changes were not significant[25]. Based largely on these recent trial data, a target blood pressure of < 130 mmHg systolic and <80 mmHg diastolic is now recommended for diabetic patients[26]. Lower targets might be appropriate for diabetic patients with micro-albuminuria, in whom considerable data support the use of ACE inhibitors for protecting against deterioration of renal function, a beneficial effect that occurs independently of blood pressure reduction[27,28]. However, UKPDS reported that captopril or atenolol was similarly effective in reducing the incidence of diabetic complications and concluded that for most patients blood pressure reduction itself is more important than the agent used[29].

## Lipid modification

Hypertriglyceridaemia with reductions in HDL cholesterol are the typical abnormalities detected on routine laboratory testing in type 2 diabetes[12]. This provides a logic for fibrate therapy in addition to exercise and weight reduction. The Helsinki study suggested a trend towards reduced coronary events in diabetic patients treated with gemfibrozil for 5 years[30], but data from other fibrate studies have generally been inconclusive. Nevertheless, a recent secondary prevention trial of gemfibrozil in men with low HDL cholesterol (<1 mmol/l) followed-up for 5 years, showed that a 6% increase in HDL plus a 31% reduction in triglyceride concentrations were associated with a 22% relative risk reduction in non-fatal myocardial infarction or coronary death[31]. It is expected that fibrates will have increasing application in diabetic coronary disease but further trials are needed and meanwhile statins will have the major role based on subgroup analyses of major trials[32-34] which have shown convincingly that hypercholesterolaemic diabetic patients gain similar relative benefit as non-diabetic patients in the secondary prevention of coronary artery disease, and greater absolute benefit due to their higher event rate. Thus, statin therapy for all diabetics with known atherosclerotic disease (secondary prevention) is now recommended to lower total cholesterol concentrations below 5.0 mmol/l (LDL <3.0 mmol/l) or by 20–25%, whichever is lower. Additional fibrate therapy to correct hyper-triglyceridaemia and increase HDL should also be considered as necessary. In diabetic patients without overt atherosclerotic disease (primary prevention), an absolute risk = 30% of developing coronary heart disease over the next 10 years, as deduced from colour-coded risk prediction charts, is sufficiently high to justify drug treatment[26].

## Smoking cessation

Observational data suggest that the risk of myocardial infarction is reduced by up to 50% within 1 year of quitting smoking. Since the cardiac risk attributable to smoking is magnified considerably in diabetes, as indeed is the risk attributable to all other risk factors, the benefits of quitting are likely to be as great, if not greater in diabetic then non-diabetic patients[18].

## Glycaemic control

Strict glycaemic control has long been recommended in diabetes, based on epidemiological surveys that have reported more favourable clinical outcomes for groups with lower plasma glucose and glycosylated haemoglobin concentrations[35-37]. However, whether these more favourable outcomes reflected less severe underlying disease rather than the benefits of glycaemic control remained unresolved until publication of UKPDS in which 3867 newly diagnosed patients with type 2 diabetes were randomly assigned to an intensive (sulphonylurea or insulin) or conventional treatment policy[38]. After follow-up for 10 years, glycosylated haemoglobin concentrations in the two groups were 7.0% and 7.9%, respectively, a difference of only 11%. Nevertheless, this trial confirmed the close relation between glycaemia and the risk of microvascular and macrovascular complications[39], including coronary heart disease, and also dispelled concerns about the potential adverse cardiovascular effects of sulphonylureas. Importantly, in the group randomised to intense glycaemic control, significant protection against microvascular complications occurred although macrovascular complications were not similarly affected, the 16% reduction in the risk of myocardial infarction being of only borderline statistical significance. In short, therefore, UKPDS has confirmed the importance of strict glycaemic control (glycosylated haemoglobin 7% or lower) for protection against microvascular, but not macrovascular, complications of diabetes. Whether the newly available thiazolidinediones (glitazones) prove more effective for reducing cardiovascular risk remains to be seen, but there are grounds for optimism. These drugs improve long-term glycaemic control by increasing insulin sensitivity[40]. They may, therefore, have a special role for correcting insulin resistance in the cardiovascular dysmetabolic syndrome which is thought to play an important pathogenic role in the accelerated atherogenesis that affects South Asians among others[41]. Glitazones are well tolerated with good side-effect profiles, problems with hepatotoxicity seen with troglitazone (now withdrawn) not occurring with rosiglitazone or pioglitazone. Their insulin sensitizing effects may also benefit other manifestations of the dysmetabolic syndrome, and preliminary studies with rosiglitazone have shown small reductions in diastolic blood pressure and late increases in HDL cholesterol[92,93].

## Antiplatelet therapy

An overview of randomised trials has shown that the benefits of antiplatelet therapy for secondary prevention of coronary heart disease are similar for groups with and without diabetes[42]. Thus patients with diabetic coronary heart disease should all receive a daily aspirin. Though not strictly evidence-based, aspirin is now recommended for diabetic adults without clinical manifestations of atheromatous disease (primary prevention) since platelet dysfunction is common and the prevalence of subclinical disease high. Evidence for non-aspirin platelet inhibitors in diabetic subgroups is unavailable. However, as an adjunct to coronary stenting, glycoprotein IIb/IIIa receptor antagonists have a useful role[43], reducing the rate of adverse events in patients with diabetes to a level comparable to that of patients without diabetes.

## ACE inhibition

ACE inhibition can protect against the development of atherosclerotic plaque in experimental animals fed lipid-rich diets[44–46]. Potential for similar benefit in humans was reported by the TREND investigators who showed that treatment with quinapril improved coronary endothelial function in patients with coronary disease[47]. This potential has now been confirmed by the Heart Outcomes Prevention Evaluation (HOPE) study in which significant reductions in the risk of the combined primary outcome (death, myocardial infarction and stroke) occurred in high-risk patients randomised to treatment with ramipril[48]. Among these high-risk patients were 3577 with diabetes who had a previous cardiac event or at least one other cardiovascular risk factor, but not heart failure or proteinuria. Within this diabetic subgroup, randomisation to ramipril reduced the risk of the combined primary outcome by 25%, with an additional reduction in the risk of overt nephropathy[49]. Further large trials of ACE inhibition for protecting against cardiovascular end-points are in progress, but meanwhile there is clear indication for ACE inhibition with ramipril in any diabetic patient with multiple risk factors, established vascular disease, or micro-albuminuria.

# Screening for coronary heart disease

The prevalence of subclinical coronary artery disease in the diabetic population is high[50,51] as reflected by a long-term rate of myocardial infarction and cardiovascular death comparable to that of non-diabetic patients with a documented history of myocardial infarction[52]. Subclinical disease is commonly non-obstructive due to outward remodelling of the coronary artery[53]. However, obstructive disease may also be clinically silent, particularly in diabetes when autonomic neuropathy may interfere with the perception of cardiac pain such that symptoms take longer to develop after the onset of myocardial ischaemia (prolonged anginal perceptual threshold[54]) or do not occur at all (silent ischaemia[55]).

There has been recent debate about the value of screening programmes to detect subclinical coronary artery disease in patients with diabetes using non-invasive tests[56,57]. As a universal principal this can scarcely be justified, because there is only a 5–10% incidence of obstructive lesions (> 50% luminal narrowing at angiography) among asymptomatic diabetic cohorts, ensuring that the sensitivity of stress testing (electrocardiographic or perfusion imaging) is very low[58–60]. Moreover, the mere demonstration of obstructive coronary disease does not usually affect management, there being no evidence to support angioplasty in asymptomatic cases, while the potential prognostic benefits of surgery in the minority with 3 vessel or left main disease needs to be balanced against the heightened procedural risk and less favourable longer term outcome in patients with diabetes (see below). Nevertheless, in certain subgroups, screening for coronary artery disease is recommended because it can lead to treatment strategies that favourably affect prognosis. These include diabetic patients needing renal transplantation or major non-cardiac vascular surgery in whom coronary revascularisation may reduce the procedural risk[61-63].

## Angina and revascularisation

Angina in diabetes is commonly atypical, perhaps because of abnormalities in the perception of angina caused by autonomic neuropathy[54,55], but a positive stress test indicates a high probability of underlying coronary disease and the need for specific anti-anginal treatment, often with additional angiographic assessment. The disease is typically diffuse affecting both proximal and distal coronary segments and this makes revascularisation by angioplasty or bypass surgery more difficult and more hazardous. Indeed, diabetes has long been recognised as one of the major independent predictors of long-term mortality after surgery[64]. The results of angioplasty also tend to be less good in diabetic compared with non-diabetic patients. Again, diffuse disease makes for technically more difficult angioplasty procedures and, in addition, re-stenosis rates are consistently higher[65]. In the recent BARI trial of angioplasty versus bypass surgery, subgroup analysis showed that patients without diabetes had comparable results with either revascularisation modality, in contrast to patients with diabetes who fared significantly worse with angioplasty[66]. The investigators concluded that, for most diabetics requiring revascularisation, coronary bypass surgery was preferable. More recently, however, a predefined subgroup analysis from the EPISTENT trial showed that angioplasty and stenting combined with infusion of abciximab (a glycoprotein IIb/IIIa receptor inhibitor) improved the long-term outcome in diabetic patients substantially, with a 6 month incidence of ischaemic end-points comparable to that achieved in non-diabetic patients[43]. The data suggest, therefore, that stenting and IIb/IIIa receptor blockade may have an important role in diabetic angioplasty.

## Acute myocardial infarction

The risk of acute myocardial infarction is 50% greater in diabetic men and 150% greater in diabetic women than in non-diabetic individuals[2]. Autonomic dysfunction and increased platelet activation combine to attenuate circadian and seasonal rhythms, increasing the risk of acute myocardial infarction throughout the day and the year[67]. Autonomic dysfunction, by altering the perception of ischaemic cardiac pain, predisposes to 'silent' myocardial infarction[68] which has the potential to delay access to emergency facilities early after coronary events, increasing the risk of out-of-hospital sudden death[69,70]. All the major complications of myocardial infarction occur more commonly in diabetes, particularly heart failure which affects nearly 50% of diabetics compared with under 30% of non-diabetics[71]. This difference is not accounted for by infarct size, but may reflect the more severe and diffuse disease in diabetes that limits coronary reserve and intensifies ischaemia in non-infarcted segments by a watershed effect[72]. Diabetes-specific myocardial disease may also have a role, and contractile dysfunction remote from the infarct zone has been reported[72]. Hospital and long-term mortality rates are increased[68,71,72].

Insulin and glucose infusion for 24 h followed by subcutaneous insulin for at least 3 months improves survival in patients with myocardial infarction and a presenting blood glucose concentration ≥11.0 mmol/l, with or without frank diabetes[73]. This protects against ischaemic injury and improves left ventricular function[74] by preserving the shift to anaerobic myocardial glucose metabolism during acute ischaemia, an insulin-dependent adjustment that may be deficient in diabetes due to absolute or relative lack of insulin[75,76].

In other respects, the treatment of acute myocardial infarction in diabetes should be conventional, responses to thrombolytic therapy – judged by patency of the infarct-related artery and mortality reduction – being similar to patients without diabetes[72]. Similarly, diabetes does not appear to affect the benefits of aspirin[42], nor that of β-blockers[77] and statins[32]. ACE inhibitors, in particular, have a special role and should be given to all diabetic patients with acute myocardial infarction, not only because of the heightened risk of left ventricular failure, for which these drugs are of proven benefit, but also because of the protection they afford against microvascular and macrovascular complications (see previously).

# Sudden death

The increased risk of plaque events in patients with diabetes predisposes to sudden death. However, other mechanisms also contribute[78,79], particularly autonomic neuropathy which may be arrhythmogenic through prolongation of QT interval and selective reductions in vagal tone which increases sympathetic activity[80–82]. Moreover, altered perception of ischaemic cardiac pain may deprive diabetic patients of the signal to stop exercising allowing ischaemia to intensify to the point that arrhythmias are triggered[83]. Autonomic neuropathy may also interfere with pain perception during plaque events, delaying presentation to hospital or leading to inappropriate triage decisions such that access to defibrillators and specific treatment is denied[84]. This emphasises the importance of retaining low diagnostic thresholds for coronary heart disease in the diabetic patient presenting with atypical symptoms.

# Heart failure

Epidemiological, pathological and haemodynamic data provide the evidence-base for diabetes-specific myocardial disease, commonly called 'diabetic cardiomyopathy'. Thus the Framingham investigators reported that the annual incidence of heart failure was substantially greater across all age groups in diabetic than non-diabetic individuals, even after controlling for underlying coronary and rheumatic heart disease[85]. The inference that diabetes itself might predispose to heart failure was supported by postmortem reports in diabetics with heart failure describing normal coronary arteries and heart valves[86]. Myocardial histology in diabetic heart failure (myocyte hypertrophy, interstitial fibrosis, increased PAS-positive material and intramyocardial micro-angiopathy[87]) is similar to changes found in hypertensive left ventricular disease, emphasising the importance of effective antihypertensive therapy as reported in UKPDS[24]. Analysis of systolic time intervals has provided evidence of both systolic and diastolic left ventricular dysfunction in diabetic individuals in whom there was no clinical evidence of coronary artery disease[88].

The pathogenesis of diabetic cardiomyopathy is unclear, although possible mechanisms include the synergistic impact of hypertension plus chronic derangement of myocardial metabolism, with increased free fatty acid oxidation and decreased glucose utilization[89]. Treatment strategies are the same as for non-diabetic patients with heart failure, and are directed at controlling provocative factors, particularly arrhythmias and hypertension. Diuretics may adversely influence metabolic control in diabetes but are mandatory for symptomatic treatment, while the efficacy of ACE-inhibition is undiminished, judging by subgroup analyses of the Studies Of Left Ventricular Dysfunction (SOLVD) prevention and treatment trials[90,91]. β-Blockers too are recommended, although this is based on generalisation from randomised trials rather than specific data for patients with diabetes.

## References

1   Bierman EL. Atherogenesis in diabetes. *Atheroscler Thromb* 1992; **12**: 647–59
2   Kannel WB, McGee DL. Diabetes and cardiovascular risk factors: the Framingham Study. *Circulation* 1979; **59**: 8–13

3 Haffner SM, Stern MP, Hazuda HP, Mitchell BD, Patterson JK. Cardiovascular risk factors in confirmed prediabetic individuals: does the clock for coronary heart disease start ticking before the onset of clinical diabetes? *JAMA* 1990; **263**: 2893–8

4 Chappey O, Dosquet C, Wautier M-P, Wautier JL. Advanced glycation end products, oxidant stress and vascular lesions. *Eur J Clin Invest* 1977; **27**: 97–108

5 Yan SD, Stern D, Schmidt AM. What's the RAGE? The receptor for advanced glycation end products (RAGE) and the dark side of glucose. *Eur J Clin Invest* 1997; **27**: 179–81

6 Park L, Raman KG, Lee KJ *et al*. Suppression of accelerated diabetic atherosclerosis by the soluble receptor for advanced glycation endproducts. *Nat Med* 1998; **4**: 1025–31

7 Reaven GM. Role of insulin resistance in human disease. *Diabetes* 1988; **37**: 1595–607

8 Hsueh WA, Law RE. Cardiovascular risk continuum: implications of insulin resistance and diabetes. *Am J Med* 1998; **105 (Suppl 1A)**: 4S-14S

9 Wingard DL, Barret-Connor EL, Ferrara A. Is insulin really a heart disease risk factor? *Diabetes Care* 1995; **18**: 1299–304

10 Ruige JB, Assendelft WJJ, Dekker JM *et al*. Insulin and risk of cardiovascular disease: a meta-analysis. *Circulation* 1998; **97**: 996–1001

11 Howard G, O'Leary DH, Zaccaro D *et al*. Insulin sensitivity and atherosclerosis. *Circulation* 1996; **93**: 1809–17

12 Kreisberg RA. Diabetic dyslipidemia. *Am J Cardiol* 1998; **82**: 67U–73U

13. Haffner SM. Diabetes, hyperlipidemia, and coronary artery disease. *Am J Cardiol* 1999; **83**: 17F–21F

14 Feher MD, Elkeles RS. Lipid modification and coronary heart disease in type 2 diabetes: different from the general population. *Heart* 1999; **81**: 10–1

15 Davi G, Ciabottoni G, Consoli A *et al*. *In vivo* formation of 8-iso-prostaglandin F2a and platelet activation in diabetes mellitus: effects of improved metabolic control. *Circulation* 1999; **99**: 224–9

16 Colhoun HM, Rubens MB, Underwood R, Fuller JH. The effects of type 1 diabetes mellitus on the gender differences in coronary artery calcification. *J Am Coll Cardiol* 2000; **36**: 2160–7

17 Fuller JH, Shipley MJ, Rose G, Jarrett RJ, Keen H. Mortality from coronary heart disease and stroke in relation to degree of glycaemia: the Whitehall study. *BMJ* 1983; **287**: 867–70

18 Stamler J, Vaccaro O, Neaton J *et al*. Diabetes, other risk factors, and 12-yr cardiovascular mortality for men screened in the Multiple Risk Factor Intervention Trial. *Diabetes Care* 1993; **16**: 434–44

19 Wood D, De Backer G, Faergeman O *et al*. *Clinician's Manual on Total Risk Management*. London: Science Press, 2000

20 Hypertension in Diabetes Study Group. HDS 1: prevalence of hypertension in newly presenting type 2 diabetic patients and the association with risk factors for cardiovascular and diabetic complications. *J Hypertens* 1993; **11**: 309–17

21 Hypertension in Diabetes Study Group. HDS. 2: increased risk of cardiovascular complications in hypertensive type 2 diabetic patients. *J Hypertens* 1993; **11**: 319–25

22 United Kingdom Prospective Diabetes Study (UKPDS) Group. Risk factors for coronary artery disease in non-insulin dependent diabetes (UKPDS 23). *BMJ* 1998; **316**: 823–8

23 United Kingdom Prospective Diabetes Study (UKPDS) Group. Diabetic retinopathy at diagnosis of type 2 diabetes and associated risk factors (UKPDS 30). *Arch Ophthalmol* 1998; **116**: 297–303

24 United Kingdom Prospective Diabetes Study (UKPDS) Group. Tight blood pressure control and risk of macrovascular and microvascular complications in type 2 diabetes (UKPDS 38). *BMJ* 1998; **317**: 703–13

25 Hansson L, Zanchetti A, Carruthers SG *et al*. Effects of intensive blood pressure lowering and low-dose aspirin in patients with hypertension : principal results of the Hypertension optimal treatment (HOT) randomised trial. *Lancet* 1998; **352**: 1252–68

26 Wood D, Durrington P, Poulter N, McInnes G, Rees A, Wray R. Joint British recommendations on prevention of coronary heart disease in clinical practice. *Heart* 1998; **80 (Suppl 2)**: 1–26

27 Lewis EJ, Hunsicker LG, Bain RP, Rohde RD. The effect of angiotensin-converting-enzyme inhibition on diabetic nephropathy. *N Engl J Med* 1993; **329**: 1456–62

28 Kasiske BL, Kalil RSN, Ma JZ, Liao M, Keane WK. Effect of antihypertensive therapy on the kidneys in patients with diabetes: a meta-regression analysis. *Ann Intern Med* 1993; **118**: 129–38

29    United Kingdom Prospective Diabetes Study (UKPDS) Group. Efficacy of atenolol and captopril in reducing risk of macrovascular and microvascular complications in type 2 diabetes (UKPDS 39). *BMJ* 1998; **317**: 713–20

30    Koskinen P, Manttari M, Manninen V *et al*. Coronary heart disease incidence in NIDDM patients in the Helsinki Heart Study. *Diabetes Care* 1992; **15**: 820–5

31    Rubins HB, Robins SJ, Collins D *et al*. Gemfibrozil for the secondary prevention of coronary heart disease in men with low levels of high density lipoprotein cholesterol. *N Engl J Med* 1999; **341**: 410–8

32    Pyorala K, Pederson T, Kjekshus J *et al*, and the Scandinavian Simvastatin Survival Study (4S) Group. Cholesterol lowering with simvastatin improves prognosis of diabetic patients with coronary heart disease: a subgroup analysis of the Scandinavian Simvastatin Survival Study (4S). *Diabetes Care* 1997; **20**: 614–20

33    Sacks FM, Pfeffer MA, Moye LA *et al*. The effect of pravastatin on coronary events after myocardial infarction in patients with average cholesterol levels. *N Engl J Med* 1996; **335**: 1001–9

34    Long-term Intervention with Pravastatin in Ischaemic Disease (LIPID) Study Group. Prevention of cardiovascular events and death with pravastatin in patients with coronary heart disease and a broad range of initial cholesterol levels. *N Engl J Med* 1998; **339**: 1349–57

35    Klein R. Hyperglycemia and microvascular and macrovascular disease in diabetes. *Diabetes Care* 1995; **18**: 258–68

36    Moss SE, Klein R, Klein BEK *et al*. The association of glycemia and cause-specific mortality in a diabetic population. *Arch Intern Med* 1994; **154**: 2473–9

37    Gaster B, Hirsch IB. The effects of improved glycemic control on complications in type 2 diabetes. *Arch Intern Med* 1998; **158**: 134–40

38    United Kingdom Prospective Diabetes Study (UKPDS) Group. Intensive blood-glucose control with sulphonylureas or insulin compared with conventional treatment and risk of complications in patients with type 2 diabetes (UKPDS 33). *Lancet* 1998; **352**: 837–53

39    United Kingdom Prospective Diabetes Study (UKPDS) Group. Association of glycaemia with macrovascular and microvascular complications of type 2 diabetes (UKPDS 35). *BMJ* 2000; **321**: 405–12

40    Fuchtenbusch M, Standl E, Schatz H. Clinical efficacy of new thiazolidinediones and glinides in the treatment of type 2 diabetes mellitus. *Exp Clin Endocrinol Diabetes* 2000; **108**: 151–63

41    Chisholm DJ, Campbell LV, Kraegen EW. Pathogenesis of the insulin resistance syndrome (syndrome X). *Clin Exp Pharmacol Physiol* 1997; **24**: 782–4

42    Antiplatelet Trialists' Collaboration. Collaborative overview of randomised trials of randomised trials of antiplatelet therapy. 1: prevention of death, myocardial infarction, and stroke by prolonged antiplatelet therapy in various categories of patients. *BMJ* 1994; **308**: 81–106

43    Marso SP, Lincoff AM, Ellis SG *et al*. Optimizing the percutaneous interventional outcomes for patients with diabetes mellitus: results of the EPISTENT (Evaluation of platelet IIb/IIIa inhibitor for stenting trial) diabetic substudy. *Circulation* 1999; **100**: 2477–84

44    Chobanian AV, Haudenschild CC, Nickerson C, Drago R. Anti-atherogenic effect of captopril in the Watanabe heritable hyperlipidaemic rabbit. *Hypertension* 1990; **15**: 327–31

45    Aberg G, Ferrer P. Effects of captopril on atherosclerosis in Cynomolgus monkeys. *J Cardiovasc Pharmacol* 1990; **15** (**Suppl**): S65–72

46    Rolland PH, Charpiot P, Friggi A *et al*. Effects of angiotensin-converting enzyme inhibition with perindolol on hemodynamics, arterial structures, and wall rheology in the hindquarters of atherosclerotic mini-pigs. *Am J Cardiol* 1993; **71**: 22E–27E

47    Mancini GB, Henry GC, Macaya C *et al*. Angiotensin-converting enzyme inhibition with quinapril improves endothelial vasomotor dysfunction in patients with coronary artery disease. The TREND (Trial on Reversing ENdothelial Dysfunction) Study. *Circulation* 1996; **94**: 258–65

48    Yusuf S, Sleight P, Pogue J, Bosch J, Davies R, Dagenais G, for The Heart Outcomes Prevention Evaluation (HOPE) Study Investigators. Effects of an angiotensin-converting-enzyme inhibitor, ramipril, on cardiovascular events in high-risk patients. *N Engl J Med* 2000; **342**: 145–53

49    Heart Outcomes Prevention Evaluation (HOPE) Study Investigators. Effects of ramipril on cardiovascular and microvascular outcomes in people with diabetes mellitus: result of HOPE study and MICRO-HOPE substudy. *Lancet* 2000; **355**: 253-9

50  Enos WF, Holmes RH, Beyer J. Coronary disease among United States soldiers killed in action in Korea: preliminary report. *JAMA* 1953; **152**: 1090–3

51  McGill Jr HC, McMahan A, Zieske AW *et al*. Association of coronary heart disease risk factors with microscopic qualities of coronary atherosclerosis in youth. *Circulation* 2000; **102**: 374–9

52  Haffner SM, Lehto S, Ronnemoa T *et al*. Mortality from coronary heart disease in subjects with type 2 diabetes and in nondiabetic subjects with and without prior myocardial infarction. *N Engl J Med* 1998; **339**: 229–34

53  Glagov S, Weisenberg E, Zarins CK *et al*. Compensatory enlargement of human atherosclerotic coronary arteries. *N Engl J Med* 1987; **316**: 1371–5

54  Ambepityia G, Kopelman PG, Ingram D, Swash M, Mills PG, Timmis AD. Exertional myocardial ischemia in diabetes: a quantitative analysis of anginal perceptual threshold and the influence of autonomic function. *J Am Coll Cardiol* 1990; **15**: 72–7

55  Nesto R, Phillips R, Kett K *et al*. Angina and exertional myocardial ischemia in diabetic and non-diabetic patients: assessment by exercise thallium scintigraphy. *Ann Intern Med* 1988; **108**: 170–5

56  Sayer JW, Timmis AD. Investigation of coronary artery disease in diabetes; is screening of asymptomatic patients necessary? *Heart* 1997; **78**: 525–6

57  Nesto RW. Screening for asymptomatic coronary artery disease in diabetes. *Diabetes Care* 1999; **22**: 1393–5

58  Janaqnd-Delenne B, Savin B, Habib G, Bory M, Vague P, Lassman-Vague V. Silent myocardial ischemia in patients with diabetes: who to screen? *Diabetes Care* 1999; **22**: 1396–400

59  Milan Study on Atherosclerosis and Diabetes (MiSAD) Group. Prevalence of unrecognised silent myocardial ischemia and its association with atherosclerotic risk factors in non insulin-dependent diabetes mellitus. *Am J Cardiol* 1997; **79**: 134–9

60  Koistinen MJ. Prevalence of asymptomatic myocardial ischaemia in diabetic subjects. *BMJ* 1990; **301**: 92–5

61  Manske CL, Wilson RF, Wang Y, Thomas W. Atherosclerotic vascular complications in diabetic transplant candidates. *Am J Kidney Dis* 1997; **29**: 601–7

62  Nesto RW, Watson FS, Kowalchuk GJ *et al*. Silent myocardial ischemia and infarction in diabetics with peripheral vascular disease: assessment by dipyridamole thallium-201 scintigraphy. *Am Heart J* 1990; **120**: 1073–7

63  Younis LT, Miller DD, Chaitman BR. Preoperative strategies to assess cardiac risk before noncardiac surgery. *Clin Cardiol* 1995; **18**: 447–54

64  Adler DS, Goldman L, O'Neil A *et al*. Long-term survival of more than 2,000 patients after coronary artery bypass grafting. *Am J Cardiol* 1986; **58**: 195–202

65  Carrozza JP, Kuntz RE, Fishman RF, Baim DS. Restenosis after arterial injury caused by coronary stenting in patients with diabetes mellitus. *Ann Intern Med* 1993; **118**: 344–9

66  The Bypass Angioplasty Revascularization Investigation (BARI) Investigators. comparison of coronary bypass surgery with angioplasty in patients with multivessel disease. *N Engl J Med* 1996; **335**: 217–25

67  Sayer JW, Wilkinson P, Ranjadayalan K, Ray S, Marchant B, Timmis AD. Attenuation or absence of circadian and seasonal rhythms of acute myocardial infarction. *Heart* 1997; **77**: 325–9

68  Jacoby RM, Nesto RW. Acute myocardial infarction in the diabetic patient: pathophysiology, clinical course and prognosis. *J Am Coll Cardiol* 1992; **20**: 736–44

69  Sayer JW, Archbold RA, Wilkinson P, Ray S, Ranjadayalan K, Timmis AD. Prognostic implications of ventricular fibrillation in acute myocardial infarction: new strategies required for further mortality reduction. *Heart* 2000; **84**: 258–61

70  Uretsky BF, Farquhar D, Berezin A, Hood W. Symptomatic myocardial infarction without chest pain: prevalence and clinical course. *Am J Cardiol* 1977; **40**: 498–503

71  Stevenson R, Ranjadayalan K, Wilkinson P, Roberts R, Timmis AD. Short and long term prognosis of acute myocardial infarction since introduction of thrombolysis. *BMJ* 1993; **307**: 349–53

72  Granger CB, Califf RM, Young S *et al*, and The Thrombolysis and Angioplasty in Myocardial Infarction (TAMI) Study Group. Outcome of patients with diabetes mellitus and acute myocardial infarction treated with thrombolytic agents. *J Am Coll Cardiol* 1993; **21**: 920–5

73 Malmberg K, Ryden L, Efendic S *et al*, for the Diabetes Mellitus, Insulin Glucose Infusion in Acute Myocardial Infarction (DIGAMI) Study Group. Randomized trial of insulin-glucose infusion followed by subcutaneous insulin treatment in diabetic patients with acute myocardial infarction: effects on mortality at 1 year. *J Am Coll Cardiol* 1995; **26**: 57–65

74 Sasso FC, Carbonara O, Cozzolino D *et al*. Effects of insulin-glucose infusion on left ventricular function at rest and during dynamic exercise in healthy subjects and noninsulin dependent diabetic patients: a radionuclide ventriculographic study. *J Am Coll Cardiol* 2000; **36**: 219–26

75 Opie LH. Glucose and the metabolism of ischaemic myocardium. *Lancet* 1995; **345**: 1520–1

76 McGuire DK, Granger CB. Diabetes and ischemic heart disease. *Am Heart J* 1999; **138**: S336–75

77 Malmberg K, Herlitz J, Hjalmarson A, Ryden L. Effects of metoprolol on mortality and late infarction in diabetics with suspected acute myocardial infarction. retrospective data from two large studies. *Eur Heart J* 1989; **10**: 423–8

78 Watkins P, Mackay J. Cardiac denervation in diabetic neuropathy. *Ann Intern Med* 1980; **92**: 304–7

79 Ewing D, Campbell I, Clarke B. Assessment of cardiovascular effects in diabetic autonomic neuropathy and prognostic implications. *Ann Intern Med* 1980; **92**: 308–11

80 Bellavere F, Ferri M, Guarini L *et al*. Prolonged QT period in diabetic autonomic neuropathy: a possible role in sudden cardiac death? *Br Heart J* 1988; **59**: 379–83

81 Ewing D, Boland O, Neilson J, Cho C, Clarke B. Autonomic neuropathy, QT interval lengthening, and unexpected deaths in male diabetic patients. *Diabetologia* 1991; **34**: 182–5

82 Marchant B, Umachandran V, Stevenson R, Kopelman PG, Timmis AD. Silent myocardial ischaemia: the role of subclinical neuropathy in patients with and without diabetes. *J Am Coll Cardiol* 1993; **22**: 1433–7

83 Ranjadayalan K, Umachandran V, Ambepitiya G, Kopelman PG, Mills PG, Timmis AD. Prolonged anginal perceptual threshold in diabetes: effects on exercise capacity and myocardial ischemia. *J Am Coll Cardiol* 1990; **16**: 1120–4

84 Soler N, Bennet M, Pentecost B, Fitzgerald M, Malins J. Myocardial infarction in diabetics. *Q J Med* 1975; **173**: 125–32

85 Kannel WB, Hjortland M, Castelli WP. Role of diabetes in congestive heart failure: the Framingham study. *Am J Cardiol* 1974; **34**: 29–34

86 Rubler S, Dlugash J, Yucheology Y. New types of cardiomyopathy associated with diabetic glomerulosclerosis. *Am J Cardiol* 1972; **30**: 595–60

87 Hardin N. The myocardial and vascular pathology of diabetic cardiomyopathy. *Coron Artery Dis* 1996; **17**: 99–108

88 Zarich S, Nesto R. Diabetic cardiomyopathy. *Am Heart J* 1989; **118**: 1000–5

89 Solang L, Malmberg K, Ryden L. Diabetes mellitus and congestive heart failure: further knowledge needed. *Eur Heart J* 1998; **20**: 789–95

90 The Studies Of Left Ventricular Dysfunction (SOLVD) Investigators. Effect of enalapril on survival in patients with reduced left ventricular ejection fractions and congestive heart failure. *N Engl J Med* 1991; **325**: 293–302

91 The Studies Of Left Ventricular Dysfunction (SOLVD) Investigators. Effect of enalapril on mortality and the development of heart failure in asymptomatic patients with reduced left ventricular ejection fractions. *N Engl J Med* 1992; **327**: 685–91

92 Bakris GL. Rosiglitazone improves blood pressure in patients with type 2 diabetes mellitus. *Diabetologia* 1999; **42** (**Suppl 1**): 228 (Abstrat 858, EASD)

93 Wollfenbuttel BHR, Gomist R, Squatrito S et al. Addition of low-dose rosiglitazone to sulphonylurea therapy improves glycaemic control in type 2 diabetic patients. *Diabet Med* 2000; **17**: 40–7

# Non-surgical treatment of patients with peripheral vascular disease

## Christopher J White

*Department of Cardiology, Ochsner Heart and Vascular Institute, New Orleans, Louisiana, USA*

Dotter first described percutaneous revascularization of peripheral vascular disease (PVD) in 1964[1]. In 1974, Gruentzig developed a balloon catheter for dilation of vascular lesions[2]. Currently, percutaneous transluminal angioplasty (PTA) employs a variety of devices ranging from implantable stents to endovascular radiation devices for re-stenosis and is recognized as a safe and effective alternative to surgery for selected patients.

In addition to the general efficacy of peripheral angioplasty, which is comparable to that of bypass surgery for selected lesions, angioplasty offers several distinct advantages over surgery[3–5]. It is performed under local anaesthesia, making it feasible to treat patients who are at high risk for general anaesthesia. When compared to surgical revascularization, the morbidity from angioplasty is low, generally related to problems at the vascular access site, and mortality is extremely rare. Unlike vascular surgery, there is no recovery period after angioplasty, and most patients can return to normal activity within 24–48 h of an uncomplicated procedure. Finally, angioplasty can be repeated if necessary usually without increased difficulty or increased patient risk compared to the first procedure, and does not preclude surgery as adjunctive or definitive therapy.

## Aorto-iliac disease

### Aortic occlusive disease

Correspondence to:
Christopher J White MD,
Chairman, Department of
Cardiology, Ochsner
Heart and Vascular
Institute, 1514 Jefferson
Highway, New Orleans,
LA 70121, USA

Distal abdominal aortic disease has been conventionally treated with endarterectomy or bypass grafting[6,7]. Frequently, distal aortic occlusive disease is associated with occlusive disease of the iliac arteries. The potential advantages of a percutaneous (non-surgical) technique compared to an aorto-iliac reconstruction are no requirement for general anaesthesia or an abdominal incision, and percutaneous therapy is associated with a shorter hospital stay and lower morbidity[8]. While axillofemoral extra-anatomic bypass offers a lower risk surgical alternative for patients with terminal aorta occlusive disease and severe co-morbidities, it has the disadvantages of a lower patency rate than direct surgical bypass of the lesions and requires that surgical intervention of a normal vessel be performed to achieve inflow.

Since 1980, balloon angioplasty has been used successfully, although not extensively, in the terminal aorta[9–11]. An extension of this strategy has been the use of endovascular stents in the treatment of infrarenal aortic stenoses. While balloon dilation of these lesions has been reported to be effective, the placement of stents offers a more definitive treatment with a larger acute gain in luminal diameter, scaffolding of the lumen to prevent embolization of debris, and theoretically an enhanced long-term patency compared to balloon angioplasty alone[12–15].

Stents are an attractive therapeutic option for the management of large artery occlusive disease to maintain or improve the arterial luminal patency after balloon angioplasty. The utility of stents for infrarenal aortic stenoses has not been demonstrated in randomized trials; however, the clinical results are encouraging.

## Iliac artery intervention

Traditional surgical therapy for iliac obstructive lesions includes aorto-iliac and aortofemoral bypass. They have a 74–95% 5-year patency which is comparable, but not superior, to percutaneous intervention[16]. Ameli and co-workers[17] reported their results for a series of 105 consecutive patients undergoing aortofemoral bypass of whom 58% were treated for claudicating. The operative mortality was 5.7%, the early graft failure rate was 5.7% and the 2-year patency was 92.8%.

Balloon angioplasty of the iliac arteries is a well-accepted therapy for selected patients meeting defined clinical and anatomic criteria (Tables 1–3). The availability of endovascular stents has dramatically affected the results of balloon angioplasty of the iliac arteries[18,19]. Due to the large diameter of the iliac vessels, the risk of thrombosis or re-stenosis after iliac placement of stents is quite low (Fig. 1).

The overall clinical benefit of iliac stent placement has been demonstrated using a meta-analysis of more than 2000 patients from 8 reported angioplasty (PTA) series and 6 stent series[20]. The patients who

**Table 1** Ideal iliac balloon angioplasty lesions

Stenotic lesion
Non-calcified
Discrete (≤ 3 cm)
Patent run-off vessels (≥ 2)
Non-diabetic patients

**Table 2** Contra-indications to iliac balloon angioplasty

Occlusion
Long lesions (≥ 5 cm)
Aorto-iliac aneurysm
Athero-embolic disease
Extensive bilateral aorto-iliac disease

**Table 3** Patency after iliac PTA by clinical and lesion variables[15]

|  | 1 year (%) | 3 year (%) | 5 year (%) |
| --- | --- | --- | --- |
| ST/CL/GR | 81 | 70 | 63 |
| ST/LS/GR | 65 | 48 | 38 |
| OC/CL/PR | 61 | 43 | 33 |
| OC/LS/PR | 56 | 17 | 10 |

CL, claudication; LS, limb-threatening ischaemia; ST, stenosis; OC, occlusion; GR, good run-off; PR, poor run-off.

received iliac stents had a statistically higher procedural success rate and a 43% reduction in late (4 year) failures in patients treated with stents compared to those treated with balloon angioplasty.

Clinical results for provisional iliac stent placement with the Palmaz stent in 184 iliac lesions demonstrated a 91% procedural success rate and a 6-month patency rate of 99%[21]. Long-term follow-up of these iliac lesions demonstrated a 4 year primary patency rate of 86% and a secondary patency rate of 95%. Results for provisional iliac stent placement with the self-expanding Wallstent have demonstrated patency rates at 1 year of 95%; 2 years of 88% and 4 years of 82% in 118 treated lesions[22].

The immediate post-procedure results of a randomized trial of PTA with provisional stenting (stent placement for unsatisfactory balloon angioplasty results) versus *de novo* stenting in iliac arteries demonstrated that pressure gradients across the lesions after primary stent placement

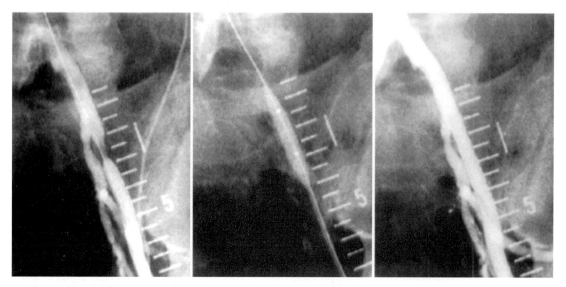

**Fig. 1** Left: baseline angiogram of left external iliac lesion. Middle: deployment of a balloon expandable Palmaz stent. Right: post-stent angiogram.

**Table 4** Randomized trial of iliac PTA *versus* stents[25]

| Procedure | Stent (*n* = 123) | PTA (*n* = 124) |
|---|---|---|
| Technical success (%) | 98.4 | 91.9 |
| Haemodynamic success (%) | 97.6 | 91.9 |
| Clinical success (%) | 97.6 | 89.5 |
| Complication rate (%) | 4.1 | 6.5 |
| Patency (4-year) | 91.6 | 74.3 |

$(5.8 \pm 4.7$ mmHg) were significantly lower after stent placement than after PTA alone $(8.9 \pm 6.8$ mmHg) but not after provisional stenting $(5.9 \pm 3.6$ mmHg)[23]. The primary technical success rate, defined as a post-procedural gradient less than 10 mmHg, revealed no difference between the two treatment strategies, (primary stent = 81% *versus* PTA plus provisional stenting = 89%). By using provisional stenting, the authors avoided stent placement in 63% of the lesions, and still achieved an equivalent acute haemodynamic result compared to primary stenting. Longer-term follow-up will be necessary to evaluate the feasibility and safety of this approach and the impact of provisional stenting on late patency.

Primary placement of Palmaz balloon expandable stents has been evaluated in a multicentre trial for iliac placement in 486 patients followed for up to 4 years (mean $13.3 \pm 11$ months)[24]. Using life-table analysis, clinical benefit was present in 91% at 1 year, 84% at 2 years, and 69% of the patients at 43 months of follow-up. The angiographic patency rate of the iliac stents was 92%. Complications occurred in 10% and were predominantly related to the arterial access site. Five patients suffered thrombosis of the stent of whom four were recanalized with thrombolysis and balloon angioplasty. A preliminary report from a European randomized trial of primary iliac (Palmaz) stent placement *versus* balloon angioplasty demonstrated a 4-year patency of 92% for the stent group *versus* a 74% patency for the balloon angioplasty group (Table 4)[25].

Iliac stent placement may be also be used as an adjunctive procedure to surgical bypass procedures. Clinical results of using iliac angioplasty with or without stent placement to preserve inflow for a femorofemoral bypass over a 14 year period in 70 consecutive patients have been very encouraging[26]. It was found that the patients requiring treatment of the in-flow iliac artery with angioplasty or stent placement did just as well as those without iliac artery disease at 7 years after surgery. These results suggest that percutaneous intervention can provide adequate long-term inflow for femorofemoral bypass as an alternative to aortofemoral bypass in patients at increased risk for a major operation.

Percutaneous therapy of aorto-iliac disease has dramatically changed the standard of care by which these patients are currently treated. It is distinctly unusual in hospitals with qualified interventionists for a patient to undergo aortofemoral bypass surgery for aorto-iliac occlusive disease.

## Abdominal aortic aneurysm exclusion

It is estimated that more than 100,000 abdominal aortic aneurysms are diagnosed each year in the US and approximately 40,000 require surgical correction. It is generally accepted that there is clinical benefit in electively repairing aneurysms larger than 5.0 cm, and in patients with hypertension and chronic obstructive lung disease aneurysms larger than 3.0 cm should be repaired[27]. In low-risk subsets, the operative mortality is 5% compared to 10% in higher risk patients. The experience with covered stent grafts to exclude abdominal aortic and aorto-iliac aneurysms is still early in its clinical experience, performed with stent grafts requiring surgical access to introduce these large diameter devices.

In one large series, 331 aorto-iliac aneurysms were referred for endovascular repair, but only 154 (47%) were found to be suitable candidates (Table 5)[28]. Successful aneurysm exclusion with the endograft

**Table 5**  Abdominal aortic aneurysm classification

| | |
|---|---|
| * | Type A: proximal and distal neck > 10 mm length and less than 25 mm in diameter without involvement of the iliac arteries |
| * | Type B: proximal neck > 10 mm and less than 25 mm diameter; involvement of aortic bifurcation, and iliac diameter < 12 mm |
| * | Type C: proximal neck > 10 mm and less than 25 mm diameter; involvement of aortic bifurcation and common iliac arteries, and iliac diameter < 12 mm |
| * | Type D: involvement of both internal iliac arteries |
| * | Type E: proximal neck < 10 mm or diameter > 25 mm |

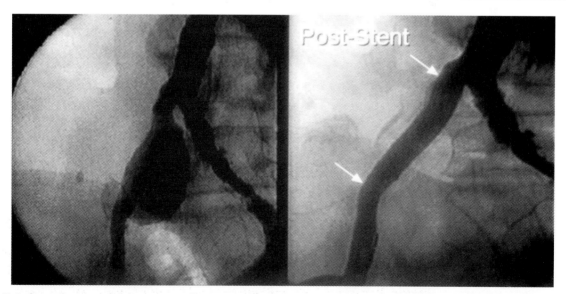

**Fig. 2**  Left: angiogram of right common iliac aneurysm. Right: angiography following placement of a stent graft.

was accomplished in 87% of the patients (Fig. 2). Major complications included death (0.6%), limb amputation (0.6%), emergency surgery (0.6%), vessel occlusion (1.2%), need for dialysis (1.2%), distal embolization (3.3%) and access site complications (3.9%). A total of 17 'endoleaks' were observed, of which 2 fabric tears and one proximal leak closed spontaneously, 13 were sealed with the placement of an additional stent graft, and 2 patients refused further treatment.

At a mean follow-up of 13 months, the secondary patency (including endovascular repair of stent graft leaks) was 87% with an overall mortality rate of less than 1%. Although the initial clinical experience with these devices is encouraging, longer term data will be necessary to determine what role this procedure will have in the management of aneurysmal disease.

The use of covered stent grafts to treat long-segment aorto-iliac occlusive disease has been reported by Marin and co-workers in 42 patients with limb-threatening ischaemia[29]. The stent grafts were hand-made and were constructed using Palmaz stents and 6 mm polytetrafluoroethylene (PTFE) thin-walled grafts. Surgical exposure of the femoral access site was obtained and the lesion crossed with a guidewire. The stent was sewn to the proximal end of the graft and deployed with balloon inflation at the inflow site to the lesion. The distal end of the graft was surgically anastomosed at the outflow site. Procedural success was obtained in 91% (39 of 43 arteries). The 18-month patency rate was 89% and the 2-year limb salvage rate was 94%.

Although no randomized trials comparing stent grafts to conventional surgery have been completed, Cohnert and associates reported the outcome of 37 matched pairs undergoing elective infrarenal abdominal aneurysm repair and stent-graft placement[30]. Interestingly, there was no difference in length of stay in the hospital, there were more deaths in the

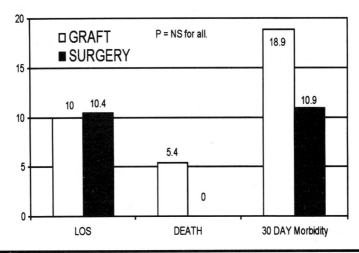

**Fig. 3** Bar graph showing a trend toward higher morbidity and mortality with stent graft placement versus conventional surgery for abdominal aortic aneurysm treatment.[30]

stent-graft group, and the 30-day mortality and morbidity was trending higher for the stent-graft group (Fig. 3).

# Renal artery stenosis

Renovascular hypertension occurs in response to a significant haemodynamic obstruction to renal blood flow. The physiological response to the increased renin stimulation depends upon the configuration of the disease. If the renal artery stenosis is unilateral, then the normal contralateral kidney is capable of excreting the excess volume and creates a vasoconstrictor mediated hypertension. If, however, the renal artery stenosis is bilateral or affects a solitary kidney, then the lack of a normal kidney causes volume overload with renin, suppression creating a volume dependent hypertension.

Atherosclerotic renal artery stenosis, the most common cause of secondary hypertension, affects fewer than 5% of the general hypertensive population[31]. There are, however, several clinical 'high risk' subsets of patients in which atherosclerotic renal artery stenosis is much more common, such as poorly controlled hypertensives with renal insufficiency[32], and in patients with severe hypertension associated coronary or peripheral vascular disease (Table 6)[33–36].

In patients undergoing coronary angiography for suspected coronary artery disease, the incidence of renal artery stenosis ranges from 15% to 18%. In patients with known aneurysmal or occlusive peripheral vascular disease, associated renal artery stenosis is found in 28%[37]. In patients with renal insufficiency, the incidence of renal artery stenosis is as high as 24%[38].

The natural history of renal artery stenosis is to progress over time. The incidence of progression in angiographic studies ranges from 39% to 49%[39–42]. Many of these lesions progress to complete occlusion with loss of renal function[41]. In a prospective study of patients with renal artery stenosis treated medically, progression occurred in 42% (11% progressed to occlusion) of the patients over a 2-year period[43]. Of particular importance is the realization that progression of renal artery stenosis and

**Table 6** Hypertensive patients at increased risk for having renal artery stenosis

|   |   |
|---|---|
| * | Abdominal bruit (systolic and diastolic) |
| * | Onset of hypertension < 20 years or > 55 years |
| * | Malignant hypertension |
| * | Refractory or difficult to control hypertension |
| * | Azotemia with ACE inhibitors |
| * | Atrophic kidney |
| * | Hypertension and associated atherosclerotic disease |
| * | Elderly with renal insufficiency |

loss of renal function are **independent** of the ability to medically control blood pressure[44]. Renal artery stent placement can significantly improve or slow the progression of renal failure in these patients[45,46].

A consensus is developing that patients with significant renal artery stenosis (≥50% diameter stenosis and/or ≥15 mmHg pressure gradient) in the setting of poorly controlled hypertension or renal insufficiency are appropriate candidates for percutaneous revascularization. Other indications for renal artery revascularization include patients with congestive heart failure (flash pulmonary oedema) and unstable angina. Patients on haemodialysis whose parenchyma is supplied by stenotic renal arteries may also be considered candidates for endovascular stent placement[47,48].

## Screening tests for renal artery stenosis

Screening tests for renal artery stenosis and associated renovascular hypertension are designed to either image the anatomical obstruction to blood flow in the renal arteries or to assess the physiological significance of the obstruction. Screening tests designed to detect differences between the kidneys suffer from decreased sensitivity due to the high incidence (approximately 30%) of bilateral atherosclerotic renal artery stenosis.

Historically, screening tests for renal artery stenosis and renovascular hypertension consisted of intravenous urography and random or stimulated measurements of plasma renin activity. While a normal plasma renin level in an untreated patient is useful to rule out the presence of renovascular hypertension, the sensitivity and specificity of an elevated plasma renin level is too low to be useful as a screening test[49].

Captopril renal scintigraphy is based upon the renal response to a dose of the angiotensin-converting enzyme inhibitor (ACEI), causing a reduction in the glomerular filtration rate of the stenotic kidney, resulting in a delayed clearance of the radioisotope which is compared to the function of the contralateral kidney[50]. Initial studies reported sensitivities and specificities as high as 90% for this test in a highly selected population of patients; however, more recent investigations have demonstrated a wide variation in the test's accuracy. The high incidence of bilateral athero-sclerotic lesions (approximately 30%) and the difficulty in interpreting this test in patients with renal insufficiency are problematic. This combined with the high cost and the duration of the examination (imaging is performed over 2 days in some centres) makes this test unattractive for routine patient screening.

Selective renal vein renin measurements have been shown to correlate with reduction in hypertension following revascularization of a stenotic renal artery[51]. However, the requirement to perform these tests under controlled circumstances, withdrawing confounding medications, and its insensitivity in the presence of bilateral renal artery disease makes it unattractive for routine screening.

Spiral computerized tomography provides three-dimensional reconstructions of the aorta and renal arteries[52,53]. While it may be useful in detecting renal artery stenosis, it requires that a high volume of radiographic contrast be given to the patient. It has not gained acceptance as a standard screening test, but may be useful in selected patients such as those with suspected aneurysmal disease of the abdominal aorta.

Magnetic resonance angiography (MRA) is a promising technique for imaging the abdominal aorta and renal arteries without the use of radiographic contrast[54,55]. Artefactual drop-out of images at sites of increased turbulence (ostia of the renal arteries) and its relative high cost continue to be problems in its general application as a screening tool.

Renal duplex ultrasound imaging has become the non-invasive diagnostic test of choice over the past several years[56]. It does not require the patient to receive a contrast agent, is relatively inexpensive, and is easy to perform. Several investigators have demonstrated sensitivities and specificities in excess of 90% for this test. The major drawback to this test is that it requires a skilled technician to perform the examination and, in some patients, their body habitus makes imaging very difficult.

Renal arteriography remains the 'gold standard' for diagnosing renal artery stenosis. This test can be performed in an out-patient setting and, in skilled hands, has very low risk. In our centre, patients suspected of renal artery stenosis undergo diagnostic angiography with intervention at the same time, which is both cost-effective and efficient for the management of these patients.

## Indications for renal intervention

The clinical indications for percutaneous renal artery revascularization are similar to those for surgical revascularization. Patients with ≥50% diameter stenosis of the renal artery and poorly controlled hypertension are candidates for percutaneous intervention. For aorto-ostial lesions, re-stenosis lesions, or following a suboptimal balloon angioplasty (≥ 30% residual diameter stenosis or dissection) the use of endovascular stents is preferred (Fig. 4)[57]. For patients with fibromuscular dysplasia or renal branch artery lesions, we prefer balloon angioplasty with provisional stenting for unsatisfactory results[58,59].

Patients with renal failure and associated renal artery stenosis may benefit from percutaneous revascularization, although this has not been demonstrated in any systematic study. Traditional teaching requires that both renal arteries be compromised to cause renal failure, but in the

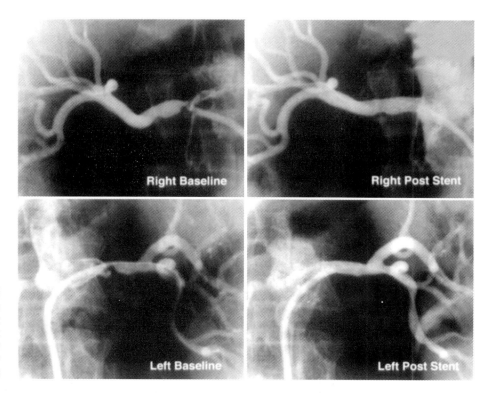

**Fig. 4** Top: right renal angioplasty before (left) and after stent (right). Bottom: left renal angioplasty before (left) and after stent (right)

setting of patients with hypertensive renal insufficiency, a unilateral stenosis may serve to protect the affected kidney from hypertensive damage. This kidney might be expected to respond with improved function if the offending stenotic lesion is treated[60,61].

Finally, treatment of isolated renal artery stenotic lesions which do not cause uncontrolled hypertension or renal insufficiency, has been debated as a means to preserve renal function. The natural history of atherosclerotic renal artery stenosis is to progress with time[39–43]. Timely intervention and correction of these lesions may prevent progressive narrowing of the vessel and loss of renal function. Patients on haemodialysis whose parenchyma is supplied by stenotic renal arteries, and those with renal artery stenosis and refractory congestive heart failure or unstable angina should also be considered candidates for angioplasty or stenting[62–64].

## Contra-indications to renal intervention

Contra-indications to renal angioplasty and stenting are relative and not absolute. The risk *versus* benefit of the procedure must be weighed. Patients with athero-embolic disease or a 'shaggy' aorta are at increased risk of cholesterol emboli with catheter manipulation in the aorta. Patients with renal artery aneurysms are at risk of rupture and surgical correction should be considered.

## Treatment of renovascular hypertension

A randomized trial comparing balloon angioplasty to medical therapy in 106 patients with uncontrolled hypertension and renal artery stenosis (≥50% diameter stenosis) demonstrated failure of medical therapy in 44% (22/50 patients) at 3 months requiring cross-over to angioplasty therapy[65]. At 3 months, there was evidence of improved blood pressure control, a requirement for fewer medications, and improved renal function in the angioplasty group. At 1-year follow-up, 16% ($n = 8$) of the medically treated patients experienced occlusion of the stenotic renal artery versus none in the angioplasty group.

Dorros and colleagues[66] demonstrated that renal artery stent placement was more effective than balloon angioplasty alone in improving or abolishing pressure gradients across renal artery lesions treated. In 76 patients (92 renal arteries) undergoing primary renal artery stent placement, the technical success rate was 100% and the angiographic re-stenosis rate at 6 months was 25%. Clinical follow-up demonstrated that 78% of their patients had stable or improved renal function, with a significant decrease in blood pressure and number of antihypertensive medications for the entire group[67].

A randomized trial comparing balloon angioplasty *versus* stent placement in 85 patients with atherosclerotic renal artery stenosis and hypertension demonstrated a higher success rate and superior long-term patency rate with stent placement compared to balloon angioplasty[68]. At 6 months, the angiographic re-stenosis rate for the balloon angioplasty group was 48% compared to only 14% ($P < 0.01$) for the stent group.

## Treatment of unstable angina and congestive heart failure

We have analyzed the results of renal artery stent placement in another group of 48 patients with unstable angina ($n = 23$) or congestive heart failure ($n = 25$) who had hypertension refractory to medical therapy and ≥70% stenosis of one ($n = 30$) or both ($n = 18$) renal arteries[64]. For the entire cohort of patients, hypertension control was achieved within 24 h in 87% and a sustained benefit was seen in 74% at 6 months.

Our experience with renal stenting in patients with renovascular hypertension and refractory unstable angina or congestive heart failure is very encouraging. These patients were unmanageable with medical therapy alone. The placement of renal stents successfully reduced their afterload and allowed these patients to be managed medically.

## Preservation of renal function

Two reports have demonstrated that renal artery stent placement improved or slowed the progression of renal artery stenosis in a group of patients with impaired renal function and atherosclerotic renal artery stenosis[45,46]. The patients had their renal function analyzed by plotting the slopes of the reciprocal serum creatinine values before and after successful stent placement. The authors found that the progression of renal failure was significantly slowed after stent placement.

# Subclavian artery disease

The treatment of subclavian artery stenosis is a major concern to the physician caring for patients with internal mammary artery coronary bypass grafts which are jeopardized by proximal subclavian stenoses. Significant subclavian stenosis can result in hypoperfusion of the mammary artery graft resulting in angina pectoris, a subclavian steal syndrome which can cause vertebrobasilar insufficiency, or upper extremity claudication.

## Treatment of subclavian artery stenosis

The traditional treatment for symptomatic subclavian stenosis is carotid-to-subclavian artery bypass. Although the immediate clinical success with surgical revascularization is good, complication rates are significant, averaging 13% including stroke in 3% and death in 2%[69–71]. Recent data suggest that angioplasty and stenting may be preferable to surgery in patients with symptomatic subclavian and innominate stenosis[71,72]. The advantages of percutaneous intervention are realized by fewer surgical and anaesthesia-related complications, less procedure related morbidity, and a shorter hospital stay.

Hadjipetrou and colleagues[72] reported a 100% success rate in 18 patients undergoing aortic arch vessel stenosis who were treated with primary stent placement. There were no major complications. The follow-up at 17 months demonstrated no re-stenosis and all patients remained asymptomatic.

Recently, we reported a series of 245 patients undergoing subclavian artery intervention from 6 centres[73]. The overall success rate was 98.5%,

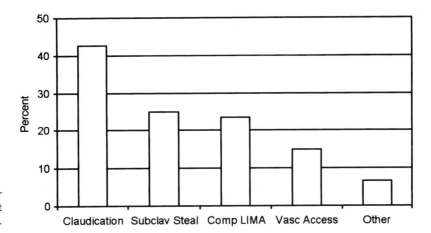

**Fig. 5** Indications for subclavian stent placement.

with a major complication rate of 1%. Clinical symptoms are shown in Figure 5. The mean gradient across the lesions was reduced from 52.5 mmHg to 3.1 mmHg (*P* <0.01). Complications included distal embolization in 3 (1.2%) patients including one transient ischaemic attack. After almost 2 years of follow-up, the primary patency rate was 89% and the secondary patency rate was 98.5% (Fig. 6).

The general consensus is that peripheral vascular stenting of aortic arch vessel disease is equal in efficacy to surgical procedures with less morbidity and mortality than surgery. The long-term patency and symptomatic improvement appear to be excellent, which makes percutaneous stent therapy the treatment of choice in most centres with experienced interventionists.

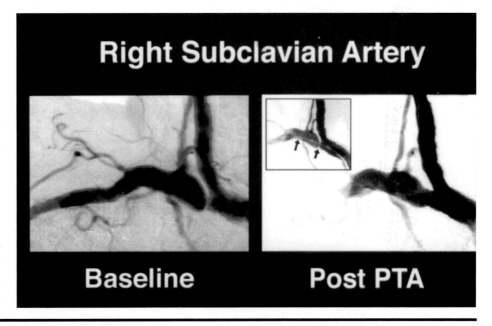

**Fig. 6** Left: baseline subclavian angiogram with tight lesion. Right: post PTA and stent placement.

# Extracranial carotid artery disease

Carotid artery stent placement is a promising technique for stroke prevention (Fig. 7). When compared to surgical endarterectomy, the 'gold standard', percutaneous therapy has the potential to be safer, less traumatic, and more cost-effective. Additionally, percutaneous therapy has the advantage of treating patients at increased surgical risk and is not limited to the cervical portion of the carotid artery. Target event rates for 30-day stroke and death rates are approximately 6% for symptomatic patients and 3% for asymptomatic patients based upon randomized surgical trials.

## Carotid stent trials

The largest single centre series of carotid stents published to date is from Roubin and associates who report the 5 year results for 528 patients and 604 vessels treated with carotid stenting[74]. They reported an excellent

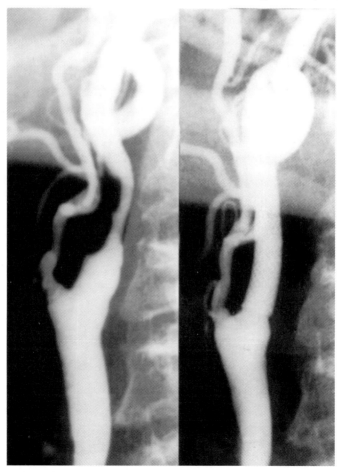

**Fig. 7** Left: baseline angiogram of internal carotid artery stenosis. Right: following deployment of a self-expanding stent.

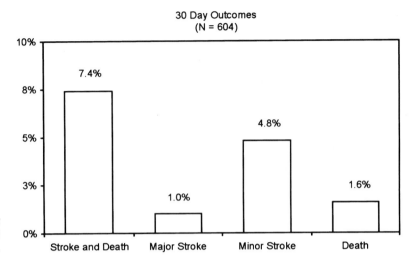

**Fig. 8** Thirty day outcomes of carotid stenting (n = 604)[74].

outcome in both symptomatic and asymptomatic patients with an overall 30-day stroke and death rate of 7.4% (Fig. 8). Of interest, the highest risk group of patients were those over 80 years (Fig. 9).

Patients with extracranial carotid artery disease who require cardiac surgery are difficult management problems due to the increased risk of stroke complicating coronary bypass surgery. Waigand and co-workers treated 50 patients and 53 carotid arteries with ≥ 70% carotid stenoses who were scheduled for coronary bypass surgery or high risk coronary angioplasty[75]. The majority (72%) of the patients had asymptomatic carotid lesions. Periprocedural stroke and death occurred in one (2%) patient. None had a neurological event associated with coronary revascularization. At a mean follow-up of 10 months, there have been

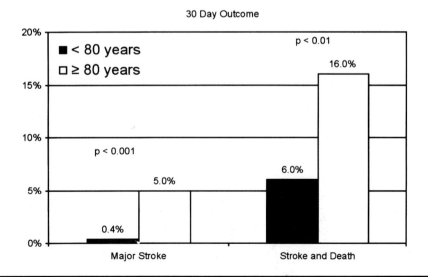

**Fig. 9** Age stratification and outcomes for carotid stent[74].

no major strokes or neurological deaths. Recurrent stenosis was seen in 3 of 46 (6.5%) carotid arteries which were treated successfully with balloon angioplasty. One patient had asymptomatic compression of a balloon expandable stent. The authors concluded that carotid stenting was a reasonable and safe alternative to combined carotid and coronary surgery in patients with severe coronary disease.

The initial results of CAVATAS (Carotid And Vertebral Artery Trans-luminal Angioplasty Study), a randomized trial of carotid intervention versus surgery, have reported favourable results[76]. A total of 504 patients were randomized to either carotid endarterectomy ($n$ = 253) or carotid angioplasty ($n$ = 251) between 1992 and 1997. The majority of the patients (90%) had recent symptomatic lesions. Only 26% of the angioplasty patients received a carotid stent, the remainder were treated with balloon angioplasty alone. The 30-day end-point of disabling stroke or death was equal in both groups (Fig. 10). Complications of cranial nerve injury and myocardial ischaemia were only reported in the surgical group. Long-term follow-up has shown no difference in neurological events between the groups. The authors concluded that angioplasty and surgery were equivalent for safety and efficacy but the angioplasty group experienced less procedural morbidity.

## Carotid stent indications and contra-indications

Currently, in experienced centres, carotid stenting can be recommended as the treatment of choice for selected high risk or unfavourable surgical candidates (Table 7). Once again, the target event (30-day stroke and

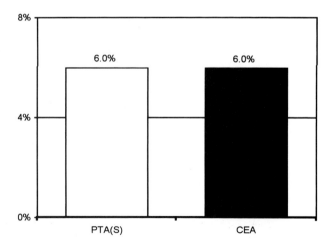

**Fig. 10** CAVATAS: randomized trial of angioplasty *versus* surgery; 30-day stroke and death[76]. PTA(S), angioplasty with or without stent; CEA, carotid endarterectomy.

**Table 7** Indications for carotid stent placement

Increased surgical risk
- \* Medical co-morbidity
  - Severe coronary artery disease
  - Decompensated congestive heart failure
  - Planned coronary bypass surgery
- • Repeat endarterectomy
- • Contralateral carotid occlusion
- • Age ≥ 80 years

Difficult surgical access
- • High cervical lesion
- • Intrathoracic lesion
- • Prior radiation therapy or radical neck surgery

death) rates should be below 6% for symptomatic patients and 3% for asymptomatic patients.

Carotid stenting is contra-indicated in patients with angiographic evidence of intravascular thrombi or filling defects, and in centres where neurovascular rescue is not available. Relative contra-indications include excessive aortic arch vessel tortuosity and inability to dilate the lesion due to calcification.

## References

1  Dotter CI, Judkins MP. Transluminal treatment of arteriosclerotic obstruction. Description of a new technique and a preliminary report of its application. *Circulation* 1964; **30**: 654–70

2  Gruntzig A, Hopff H. Perkutane rekanalisation chronischer arterieller verschlusse mit einem neuen dilatationskatehetr modifikation der Dotter-Technik. *Dtsch Med Wochenschr* 1974; **99**: 2502–7

3  O'Keeffe ST, Woods BO, Beckmann CF. Percutaneous transluminal angioplasty of the peripheral arteries. *Cardiol Clin* 1991; **9**: 519–21

4  Health and Public Policy Committee, American College of Physicians. Percutaneous transluminal angioplasty. *Ann Intern Med* 1983; **99**: 864–9

5  Isner JM, Rosenfeld K. Redefining the treatment of peripheral artery disease. Role of percutaneous revascularization. *Circulation* 1993; **88**: 1534–57

6  Diethrich EB, Santiago O, Gustafson G *et al*. Preliminary observations on the use of the Palmaz stent in the distal portion of the aorta. *Am Heart J* 1993; **125**: 490–501

7  Charlbois N, Saint Geoges G, Hudon G. Percutaneous transluminal angioplasty of the lower abdominal aorta. *Am J Radiol* 1991; **146**: 369–71

8  Tegtmyer CG, Hartwell GD, Selby GB *et al*. Results and complications of angioplasty in aortoiliac diseases. *Circulation* 1991; **83**: 153–60

9  Iyer SS, Hall P, Dorros G *et al*. Brachial approach to management of an abdominal aortic occlusion with prolonged lysis and subsequent angioplasty. *Cathet Cardiovasc Diagn* 1991; **23**: 290–3

10  Long AL, Gaux JC, Raynaud A. Infrarenal aortic stents: initial clinical experience and angiographic follow-up. *Cardiovasc Intervent Radiol* 1993; **16**: 203–8

11,  Diethrich EB. Endovascular treatment of abdominal aortic occlusive disease: the impact of stents and intravascular ultrasound imaging. *Eur J Vasc Surg* 1993; **7**: 228–36

12  Ballard JL, Taylor FC, Sparks SR, Killen JD. Stenting without thrombolysis for aortoiliac occlusive disease: experience in 14 high-risk patients. *Ann Vasc Surg* 1995; **9**: 453–8

13  Roeren T, Post K, Richter N *et al*. Stent angioplasty of the infrarenal aorta and aortic bifurcation. Clinical and angiographic results in a prospective study. *Radiologe* 1994; **34**: 504–10

14  Marin ML, Vieth FJ, Sanchez LA *et al*. Endovascular repair of aortoiliac occlusive disease. *World J Surg* 1996; **20**: 679–86

15  Johnston KW. Iliac arteries: re-analysis of results of balloon angioplasty. *Radiology* 1993; **186**: 207–12

16  Johnston KW. Balloon angioplasty: predictive factors for long-term success. *Semin Vasc Surg* 1989; **3**: 117–22

17  Ameli FM, Stein M, Provan JL *et al*. Predictors of surgical outcome in patients undergoing aortobifemoral bypass reconstruction. *J Cardiovasc Surg* 1990; **30**: 333–9

18  Sullivan TM, Childs MB, Bacharach JM *et al*. Percutaneous transluminal angioplasty and primary stenting of the iliac arteries in 288 patients. *J Vasc Surg* 1997; **25**: 829–39

19  Murphy KD, Encarnacion CE, Le VA, Palmaz JC. Iliac artery stent placement with the Palmaz stent: follow-up study. *J Vasc Intervent Radiol* 1995; **6**: 321–9

20  Bosch JL, Hunink MGM. Meta-analysis of the results of percutaneous transluminal angioplasty and stent placement for aortoiliac occlusive disease. *Radiology* 1997; **204**: 87–96

21  Henry M, Amor M, Thevenot G *et al*. Palmaz stent placement in iliac and femoropopliteal arteries: primary and secondary patency in 310 patients with 2–4 year follow up. *Radiology* 1995; **197**: 167–74

22  Vorwerk D, Gunther RW, Schurmann K, Wendt G. Aortic and iliac stenosis: follow-up results of stent placement after insufficient balloon angioplasty in 118 cases. *Radiology* 1996; **198**: 45–8

23  Tetteroo E, Haaring C, van der Graaf Y *et al*. Intraarterial pressure gradients after randomized angioplasty or stenting of iliac artery lesions. Dutch Iliac Stent Trial Study Group. *Cardiovasc Intervent Radiol* 1996; **19**: 411–7

24  Palmaz JC, Laborde JC, Rivera FJ *et al*. Stenting of the iliac arteries with the Palmaz stent: experience from a multicenter trial. *Cardiovasc Intervent Radiol* 1992; **15**: 291–7

25  Richter GM, Noeldge G, Roeren T *et al*. First long-term results of a randomized multicenter trial: iliac balloon-expandable stent placement versus regular percutaneous transluminal angioplasty. In: Lierman D. (ed) *State of the Art and Future Developments*. Morin Heights, Canada: Polyscience, 1995; 30–5

26  Perler BA, Williams GM. Does donor iliac artery percutaneous transluminal angioplasty or stent placement influence the results of femorofemoral bypass? Analysis of 70 consecutive cases with long-term follow up. *J Vasc Surg* 1996; **24**: 363–70

27  Cronenwett JL. Infrainguinal occlusive disease. *Semin Vasc Surg* 1995; **8**: 284–8

28  Blum U, Voshage G, Lammer J *et al*. Endoluminal stent grafts for infrarenal abdominal aortic aneurysms. *N Engl J Med* 1997; **336**: 13–20

29  Marin ML, Veith FJ, Sanchez LA *et al*. Endovascular repair of aortoiliac occlusive disease. *World J Surg* 1996; **20**: 679–86

30  Cohnert TU, Oelert F, Wahlers T *et al*. Matched pair analysis of conventional versus endoluminal AAA treatment outcomes during the initial phase of an aortic endografting program. *J Endovasc Ther* 2000; **7**: 94–100

31  Simon N, Franklin SS, Bleifer KH *et al*. Clinical characteristics of renovascular hypertension. *JAMA* 1972; **220**: 1209–18

32  Jacobsen HR. Ischemic renal disease: an overlooked clinical entity ? *Kidney Int* 1988; **34**: 729–43

33  Eyler WR, Clark GJ, Rian RL *et al*. Angiography of the renal areas including a comparative study of renal arterial stenosis with and without hypertension. *Radiology* 1962; **78**: 879–92

34  Jean WJ, Al-Bittar I, Xwicke DL *et al*. High incidence of renal artery stenosis in patients with coronary artery disease. *Cathet Cardiovasc Diagn* 1994; **32**: 8–10

35  Olin JW, Melia M, Young JR *et al*. Prevalence of atherosclerosis renal artery stenosis in patients with atherosclerosis elsewhere. *Am J Med* 1990; **88**: 46N–51N

36  Harding MB, Smith LR, Himmelstein SI *et al*. Renal artery stenosis: prevalence and associated risk factors in patients undergoing routine cardiac catheterization. *J Am Soc Nephrol* 1992; **2**: 1608–16

37 Valentine RJ, Clagett GP, Miller GL *et al*. The coronary risk of unsuspected renal artery stenosis. *J Vasc Surg* 1993; **18**: 433–40

38 O'Neil EA, Hansen KJ, Canzanello VJ *et al*. Prevalence of ischemic nephropathy in patients with renal insufficiency. *Am Surg* 1992; **58**: 485–90

39 Meany TF, Dustan HP, Novick AC. Natural history of renal arterial disease. *Radiology* 1968; **9**: 877–87

40 Greco BA, Breyer JA. The natural history of renal artery stenosis: who should be evaluated for suspected ischemic nephropathy? *Semin Nephrol* 1996; **16**: 2–11

41 Schreiber MJ, Pohl MA, Novick AC. The natural history of atherosclerotic and fibrous renal artery disease. *Urol Clin North Am* 1984; **11**: 383–92

42 Wollenweber J, Sheps SG, Davis GD. Clinical course of atherosclerotic renovascular disease. *Am J Cardiol* 1968; **21**: 60–71

43 Zierler RE, Bergelin RO, Isaacson JA *et al*. Natural history of atherosclerotic renal artery stenosis: a prospective study with duplex ultrasonography. *J Vasc Surg* 1994; **19**: 250–8

44 Dean RH, Kieffer RW, Smith BM *et al*. Renovascular hypertension: anatomic and renal function changes during drug therapy. *Arch Surg* 1981; **116**: 1408–15

45 Harden PN, MacLeod MJ, Rodger RSC *et al*. Effect of renal artery stenting on progression of renovascular renal failure. *Lancet* 1997; **349**: 1133–6

46 Watson PS, Hadjipetrou P, Cox SV *et al*. Effect of renal artery stenting on renal function and size in patients with atherosclerotic renovascular disease. *Circulation* 2000; **102**: 1671–7

47 Novick AC, Pohl MA, Schreiber M *et al*. Revascularization for preservation of renal function in patients with atherosclerotic renovascular disease. *J Urol* 1983; **129**: 907–12

48 Kaylor WM, Novick AC, Ziegelbaum M *et al*. Reversal of end stage renal failure with surgical revascularization in patients with atherosclerotic renal artery occlusion. *J Urol* 1989; **141**: 486–8

48 Pickering TG. Diagnosis and evaluation of renovascular hypertension. *Circulation* 1991; **83** (**Suppl I**): I-147–54

49 Fommei E, Ghione S, Palla L *et al*. Renal scintigraphic captopril test in the diagnosis of renovascular hypertension. *Hypertension* 1987; **10**: 212–20

50 Vaughan Jr ED, Buhler FR, Laragh JH *et al*. Renovascular hypertension: renin measurements to indicate hypersecretion and contralateral suppression, estimate renal plasma flow, and score for surgical curability. *Am J Med* 1973; **55**: 402–14

51 Olbricht CJ, Paul K, Prokop M *et al*. Minimally invasive diagnosis of renal artery stenosis by spiral computed tomography angiography. *Kidney Int* 1995; **48**: 1332–7

52 Rubin GD. Spiral (helical) CT of the renal vasculature. *Semin Ultrasound CT MR* 1996; **17**: 374–97

53 Kim D, Edelman RR, Kent KC *et al*. Abdominal aorta and renal artery stenosis: evaluation with MR angiography. *Radiology* 1990; **174**: 727–31

54 Bakker J, Beek FJ, Beutler JJ *et al*. Renal artery stenosis and accessory renal arteries: accuracy of detection and visualization with gadolinium-enhanced breath-hold MR angiography. *Radiology* 1998; **207**: 497–504

55 De Cobelli F, Vanzulli A, Sironi S *et al*. Renal artery stenosis: evaluation with breath-hold, three-dimensional, dynamic, gadolinium-enhanced versus three-dimensional, phase-contrast MR angiography. *Radiology* 1997; **207**: 689–95

56 Olin JW, Piedmonte MR, Young JR *et al*. The utility of duplex ultrasound scanning of the renal arteries for diagnosing significant renal artery stenosis. *Ann Intern Med* 1995; **122**: 833–8

57 White CJ, Ramee SR, Collins TJ, Jenkins JS, Escobar A, Shaw D. Renal artery stent placement: utility in difficult lesions for balloon angioplasty. *J Am Coll Cardiol* 1997; **30**: 1445–50

58 Archibald GR, Beckmann CF, Libertino JA. Focal renal artery stenosis caused by fibromuscular dysplasia: treatment by percutaneous transluminal angioplasty. *Am J Radiol* 1988; **151**: 593–6

59 Cluzel P, Raynaud A, Beyssen B, Pagny JV, Gaux JC. Stenosis of renal branch arteries in fibromuscular dysplasia: results of percutaneous transluminal angioplasty. *Radiology* 1994; **193**: 227–32

60 Novick AC, Pohl MA, Schreiber M *et al*. Revascularization for preservation of renal function in patients with atherosclerotic renovascular disease. *J Urol* 1983; **129**: 907–12

61 Kaylor WM, Novick AC, Ziegelbaum M, Vidt DG. Reversal of end stage renal failure with surgical revascularization in patients with atherosclerotic renal artery occlusion. *J Urol* 1989; **141**: 486–8

62   Pickering TG, Devereux RB, James GD *et al*. Recurrent pulmonary oedema in hypertension due to bilateral renal artery stenosis: treatment by angioplasty or surgical revacularisation. *Lancet* 1988; **ii**: 551–2

63   Messina LM, Zelenock GB, Yao KA, Stanley JC. Renal revascularization for recurrent pulmonary edema in patients with poorly controlled hypertension and renal insufficiency: a distinct subgroup of patients with arteriosclerotic renal artery occlusive disease. *J Vasc Surg* 1992; **15**: 73–82

64   Khosla S, White CJ, Collins TJ *et al*. Effects of renal artery stent implantation in patients with renovascular hypertension presenting with unstable angina or congestive heart failure. *Am J Cardiol* 1997; **80**: 363–6

65   van Jaarsveld BC, Krijnen P, Pieterman H *et al*. The effect of balloon angioplasty on hypertension in atherosclerotic renal artery stenosis. *N Engl J Med* 2000; **342**: 1007–14

66   Dorros G, Prince C, Mathiak L. Stenting of a renal artery stenosis achieves better relief of the obstructive lesion than balloon angioplasty. *Cathet Cardiovasc Diagn* 1993; **29**: 191–8

67   Dorros G, Jaff M, Jain A, Dufek C, Mathiak L. Follow-up of primary Palmaz-Schatz stent placement for atherosclerotic renal artery stenosis. *Am J Cardiol* 1995; **75**: 1051–5

68   van de Ven PJ, Kaatee R, Beutler JJ *et al*. Arterial stenting and balloon angioplasty in ostial atherosclerotic renovascular disease: a randomised trial. *Lancet* 1999; **353**: 282–6

69   Beebe HG, Stark R, Johnson ML *et al*. Choices of operation for subclavian vertebral arterial disease. *Am J Surg* 1980; **139**: 616–23

70   Dorros G, Lewin RF, Jamnadas P *et al*. Peripheral transluminal angioplasty of the subclavian and innominate arteries utilizing the brachial approach: acute outcome and follow-up. *Cathet Cardiovasc Diagn* 1990; **19**: 71–6

71   Gershony G, Basta L, Hagan AD. Correction of subclavian artery stenosis by percutaneous angioplasty. *Cathet Cardiovasc Diagn* 1990; **21**: 165–9

72   Hadjipetrou P, Cox S, Piemonte T, Eisenhauer A. Percutaneous revascularization of atherosclerotic obstruction of aortic arch vessels. *J Am Coll Cardiol* 1999; **33**: 1238–45

73   Jain SP, Zhang SY, Khosla S *et al*. Subclavian and innominate arteries stenting: acute and long term results. *J Am Coll Cardiol* 1998; **31**: 63A

74   Roubin GS, New G, Iyer SS *et al*. Immediate and late clinical outcomes of carotid artery stenting in patients with symptomatic and asymptomatic carotid artery stenosis. *Circulation* 2001; **103**: 532–7

75   Waigand J, Gross CM, Uhlich F *et al*. Elective stenting of carotid artery stenosis in patients with severe coronary artery disease. *Eur Heart J* 1998; **19**: 1365–70

76   Brown MM, for the Carotid and Vertebral Artery Transluminal Angioplasty Study Investigators (CAVATAS). Results of the carotid and vertebral artery transluminal angioplasty study. *Br J Surg* 1999; **86**: 710–1

# Ischaemic heart disease presenting as arrhythmias

**A V Ghuran** and **A J Camm**

*Department of Cardiological Sciences, St George's Hospital Medical School, London, UK*

Despite considerable progress in management over the recent years, coronary artery disease (CAD) remains the leading cause of death in the industrialised world. It is estimated that CAD is responsible for causing 152,000 deaths per year in the UK and one in eight deaths world-wide[1]. Many of these deaths are attributed to the development of ventricular tachyarrhythmias during periods of myocardial ischaemia or infarction. Myocardial ischaemia is characterised by ionic and biochemical alterations, creating an unstable electrical substrate capable of initiating and sustaining arrhythmias, and infarction creates areas of electrical inactivity and blocks conduction, which also promotes arrhythmogenesis. The purpose of this chapter is to review some of the metabolic changes associated with cardiac ischaemia, their relevance to electrophysiological instability, and the clinical manifestation and management of some of the more common arrhythmias that follow cardiac ischaemia. Particular attention is given to the peri-infarction period (arbitrarily accepted as within 48 h of the index myocardial infarction) as arrhythmias are most likely to be seen around this time, and are considered to be non-indicative of long-term prognosis. In contrast, arrhythmias developing in the post-infarction period (after 48 h) have been demonstrated to be associated with an adverse outcome. Regardless of the anti-arrhythmic therapy used in treating peri- and post-infarction arrhythmias, it is presumed that patients who had a myocardial infarction or who have left ventricular dysfunction will also receive other appropriate therapies, such as aspirin, β-blockers, cholesterol lowering agents and angiotensin converting enzymes inhibitors.

## Factors contributing to arrhythmias during acute myocardial ischaemia

### Biochemical and electrophysiological factors

Correspondence to:
Dr A V Ghuran,
Department of
Cardiological Sciences,
St George's Hospital
Medical School,
Cranmer Terrace,
London SW17 0RE, UK
aghuran@totalise.co.uk

Acute myocardial ischaemia is accompanied by significant intracellular and extracellular ionic and metabolic alterations of the myocardial syncytium. Extracellular changes include: elevated potassium, lysophosphoglycerides

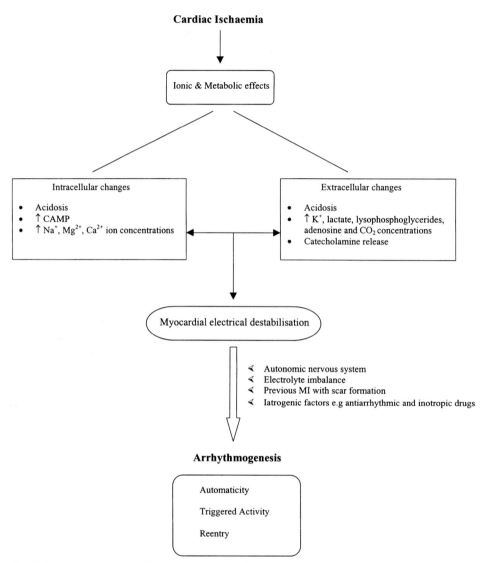

**Fig. 1** Influence of cardiac ischaemia on arrhythmogenesis.

and adenosine concentrations, increased lactate and carbon dioxide production, acidosis, and catecholamine release. Concomitantly, intracellular changes include: acidosis, elevated cyclic adenosine monophosphate (cAMP), and elevated concentrations of calcium, magnesium, and sodium ions[2]. These biochemical and metabolic changes alter inward and outward transmembrane ionic current fluxes, causing profound alterations of the resting membrane and action potential characteristics of the myocyte. Changes such as depolarisation of the resting membrane potential, diminished upstroke velocity, slowed conduction, decreased excitability, shortening of the action potential duration, altered refractoriness, dispersion of repolarisation, and abnormal automaticity, can all occur.

The resultant biochemical and electrical changes do not all occur at once but evolve temporally, providing the electrophysiological trigger and anatomic substrate necessary to induce arrhythmias through virtually all known arrhythmogenic mechanisms (Fig. 1). A history of a previous myocardial infarction with scar formation further contributes to this arrhythmogenic milieu. The presence of myocardial fibrosis causes slowing of cardiac conduction, resulting in re-entry circuits and subsequent ventricular desynchronisation.

## Autonomic nervous system

The pathophysiological role of the autonomic nervous system (ANS) in arrhythmogenesis has been firmly established both experimentally and clinically[3]. Within minutes of myocardial ischaemia there is a striking surge of sympathetic nerve activity caused by a combination of pain, anxiety and reflex activation, which has been demonstrated to be inversely related to left ventricular ejection fraction[4]. A general increase in circulating catecholamines can also aggravate myocardial ischaemia, because of positive chronotropic and inotropic actions, therefore establishing a vicious circle.

A relative excess in sympathetic over vagal activity is generally pro-arrhythmic because of alterations of the electrophysiological properties of the specialised conducting tissue and the cardiac myocyte (Table 1). Consequently, the risk of developing supraventricular and ventricular tachyarrhythmias is increased.

In the early peri-infarction period, cardiac autonomic reflexes can be triggered depending on the site of the myocardial infarction. For instance, acute inferoposterior myocardial ischaemia or infarction often results in bradycardia and hypotension, whereas anterior myocardial ischaemia more frequently evokes tachycardia and hypertension. There is a greater density of vagal afferent receptors in the inferoposterior wall of the left ventricle, which may be responsible for causing an enhanced

**Table 1** Electrophysiological effects of the sympathetic nervous system

- Shifts pacemaker from sinus node to junctional region
- Increases Purkinje fibre automaticity
- Alters P wave morphology and shortens QT interval
- Shortens PR interval
- Increase after-depolarisations (facilitating triggered activity)
- Enhances re-entry during acute myocardial ischaemia
- Decreases ventricular fibrillation threshold

vasopressor and cardio-inhibitory reflex (Benzold-Jarisch reflex). Therefore, a transient increase in vagal activity, is one of the factors implicated in the development of bradyarrhythmias seen during inferior myocardial infarction.

In the post-infarction period, impaired vagal tone, as documented by decreased baroreflex sensitivity and heart rate variability, has been associated with increased inducibility of sustained monomorphic ventricular tachycardia and with sudden death[5].

# Ventricular arrhythmias

The mechanisms of ventricular arrhythmias in acute myocardial ischaemia and infarction have been mainly studied using animal models, and have been shown to occur in several distinct phases[6]. The acute phase, which occurs roughly 2–30 min following coronary artery occlusion when changes are still reversible, demonstrates a bimodal distribution and is divided into phases 1a and 1b. Phase 1a arrhythmias occur between 2–10 min. Although several mechanisms have been proposed to explain these arrhythmias, the pathophysiology is most likely to be related to alterations in cellular electrophysiology and re-entrant mechanisms . Phase 1b arrhythmias occur 10–30 min after acute coronary occlusion and may be related to local accumulation of catecholamines and increased automaticity[6]. The second or delayed phase of ventricular arrhythmias occurs up to 72 h after coronary artery occlusion, with a peak incidence between 12–24 h. These arrhythmias may be caused by abnormal automaticity within surviving Purkinje fibres, triggered activity arising from Purkinje fibres, or re-entry mechanisms involving either the Purkinje fibres or the ischaemic myocardium. Chronic phase arrhythmias developing after 72 h are usually due to re-entry mechanisms.

## Ventricular premature complexes (VPCs)

VPCs commonly develop during periods of ischaemia. In the early peri-infarction period, the incidence of VPCs has been reported to vary between 10–93%[7,8]. They are usually asymptomatic and their presence in the peri-infarction period, regardless of frequency and complexity (bigeminy, multiformity, *etc*) bears no relation to mortality or the development of sustained ventricular tachyarrhythmias. In contrast, their presence in the post-infarction period (usually >10 per h) is a strong predictor of all cause and arrhythmic mortality[9].

**Treatment**

Numerous trials have compared prophylactic anti-arrhythmic drugs with placebo for the treatment of VPCs in the peri-infarction and post-infarction periods following a myocardial infarction. Although there may be a reduction in VPCs' frequency, none of the agents administered (with the exception of β-blockers) have conclusively reduced cardiovascular or all-cause mortality and some anti-arrhythmic drugs may facilitate arrhythmic death[10-14]. VPCs are treated conservatively by alleviation of any on-going cardiac ischaemia, and correction of electrolyte and metabolic disturbances. β-Blockers should be administered as early as possible to avoid the pro-arrhythmic effects of sympathetic stimulation.

## Ventricular arrhythmias

Ventricular tachycardia (VT) is defined as three or more consecutive cardiac depolarisation arising below the atrioventricular node, with an RR interval of less than 500 ms (>120 beats/min). VT is estimated to occur in 3–39% of patients in the peri-infarction period[7,8]. The presentation of ventricular tachycardia during acute myocardial infarction depends on the rate of tachycardia, and on left ventricular function. Significant haemo-dynamic compromise can occur if the tachycardia is fast and sustained, and when there is left ventricular dysfunction. VT increases myocardial oxygen demand, which may result in exacerbation of ischaemia and possible infarct extension. Occasionally, VT is the presenting feature of an otherwise silent myocardial infarction (the presence of a scar provides a stable substrate capable of maintaining a re-entrant tachy-cardia mechanism).

VT is conventionally classified according to its temporal and morphological characteristics. VT is described as non-sustained (NSVT), if the duration is less than 30 s, and sustained if it lasts more than 30 s or requires termination within 30 s because of haemodynamic compromise. VT is described as being 'monomorphic' if the QRS complexes have one morphology; multiple monomorphic if there are two or more runs of different QRS morphologies, but each run has a uniform QRS complex; and polymorphic if the QRS morphology is variable during one episode (Fig. 3).

**Treatment**

The treatment of ventricular tachyarrhythmias should target both the cause of the arrhythmia (upstream approach) as well as the arrhythmic expression of the pathology (downstream approach). In other words, in patients with significant coronary artery disease, revascularisation and haemodynamic optimisation should be considered in the first instance to prevent ventricular arrhythmias and their complications.

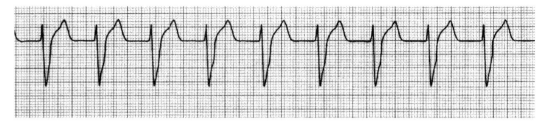

**Fig. 2** Accelerated idioventricular rhythm at a rate of approximately 80 beats per min.

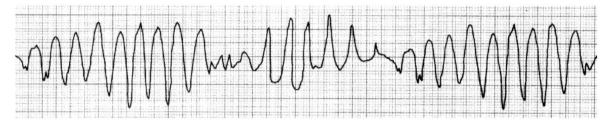

**Fig. 3** Polymorphic VT: note the frequent changes in QRS complex morphology.

## Accelerated idioventricular rhythm (slow ventricular tachycardia)

This rhythm is caused by an abnormally firing ventricular focus, which usurps sinus node pacemaker dominance and further depress sinoatrial node automaticity (Fig. 2). By definition, the heart rate is less than 120 beats/min. It occurs very commonly during myocardial infarction and has been shown to be particularly associated with reperfusion of the myocardium following thrombolytic therapy.

### Treatment

This rhythm is usually benign and has no adverse effect on mortality. Most episodes are transient and require no treatment. If the rhythm causes haemodynamic compromise, for example due to loss of atrio-ventricular synchrony, increasing the atrial rate with atropine or atrial pacing is indicated.

## NSVT

The incidence of NSVT (monomorphic) in the peri-infarction period has generally been reported to occur in 1–7% of patients[15,16]. Limited data are available regarding the prognostic significance of NSVT in the peri-infarction period. Earlier studies have suggested that NSVT had no adverse effect on either in-hospital or 1-year survival[15,17]. However, a recent study by Cheema et al[18] has found that the time of onset of NSVT from admission (≥13 h and ≤24 h) as well as specific NSVT characteristics (association with previous MI or faster heart rates) were significant predictors of long-term survival.

Substantial data have demonstrated that NSVT in the post-infarction period increases the risk of sudden cardiac death by at least 2-fold[19,20]. This risk is further increased to more than 5-fold in patients with left ventricular dysfunction (ejection fraction <0.40)[19,20].

### Treatment

Apart from the early administration of β-blockers (Table 2), the administration of anti-arrhythmic drugs for the treatment of asymptomatic NSVT in the peri-infarction period should generally be avoided. If episodes of NSVT are frequent, rapid, prolonged or associated with significant symptoms, the administration of lidocaine or amiodarone can be considered.

Although the occurrence of NSVT in the post-infarction period is a prognostic marker, its suppression or treatment with anti-arrhythmic drugs has been disappointing[11–14]. CAMIAT was a randomised double-blind placebo control trial designed to investigate the effect of amiodarone on the risk of resuscitated ventricular fibrillation or arrhythmic death among survivors of myocardial infarction with frequent VPCs (≥10 VPCs/h) or at least a short run of NSVT (defined as ≥3 beats at a rate of 100–120 per min , or 3–10 beats at a rate of >120 per min)[13]. Although amiodarone reduced arrhythmic mortality, there was no corresponding reduction in all cause mortality. Subsequent analyses of CAMIAT as well as the European Myocardial Infarct Trial (EMIAT) have demonstrated that the combination of amiodarone plus a β-blocker may have a synergistic interaction with a consequent reduction in all-cause and arrhythmic mortality[21]. Further adequately powered, prospective studies are needed to confirm this interaction.

In the late post-infarction period, the advent of implantable cardioverter defibrillators (ICD) has changed clinical practice. Patients with a history of coronary artery disease, NSVT, left ventricular dysfunction (ejection fraction <0.40) and inducible VT on electrophysiological testing, ICD implantation has been shown to reduce significantly arrhythmic and all-cause mortality[22,23]. The treatment of NSVT outside this carefully selected patient group remains less defined.

## Sustained VT

Peri-infarction sustained VT has an incidence of 0.3–1.9%[15,24]. It is associated with a higher in-hospital mortality, but is not considered to be a prognostic factor among hospital survivors[15]. The occurrence of sustained monomorphic VT is an uncommon arrhythmia in the peri-infarction period. When present, it usually signifies previous myocardial scarring or may be a sign of extensive myocardial damage[24].

**Table 2** Drugs used in the peri-infarction and post-infarction periods to treat arrhythmias

| Drug | Loading dose | Maintenance | Comments | Indications |
|---|---|---|---|---|
| Atropine | Incremental doses of 0.5 mg every 3–5 min up to a maximum of 2 mg. During cardiac arrest (asystole, slow pulseless electrical activity) maximum dose = 3 mg | | Atropine should be used with caution in the setting of acute myocardial infarction because of the protective effects of parasympathetic stimulation against ventricular arrhythmias and infarct extension | Bradyarrhythmias Asystole Slow pulseless electrical activity |
| Metoprolol | IV: 2.5 mg over 2–4 min, may repeat every 5 min up to 15 mg | IV: 5–10 mg every 6 h. Orally: 50 mg every 6 h for 48 h then 100 mg twice daily | Hypotension, bronchospasm, negative inotrope and chronotrope. Acts synergistically with digoxin for rate control in atrial fibrillation. Avoid if heart rate <60 per min or if PR >0.24 s | Treatment of supraventricular, atrial and ventricular tachyarrhythmias |
| Propranolol | IV: 0.5–1 mg every 5 min to a maximum 0.15–0.2 mg/kg | Orally: 40–240 mg/day in 3–4 divided doses | As for metoprolol | As for metoprolol |
| Atenolol | IV: 2.5–10 mg at a rate of 1 mg/min | Orally: 100 mg/day | As for metoprolol | As for metoprolol |
| Esmolol | IV: 0.5 mg/kg/min | IV: 0.05–0.2 mg/kg/min | Very short half-life, as for metoprolol | As for metoprolol |
| Digoxin | IV/orally: 0.25–0.5 mg every 6–8 h up to 1 mg/24 h | IV/orally: 0.125–0.5 mg/day | Peak effects may take up to 2 h | Ventricular rate control for atrial fibrillation, especially if left ventricular dysfunction |
| Verapamil | IV: 2.5–10 mg over 2 min. Can repeat dose after 30 min | IV: 0.125 mg/min Orally: 160–180 mg/day in divided doses | Acts synergistically with digoxin, increase digoxin levels, hypotension, bradycardia, negative inotrope | Treatment of supraventricular and atrial tachyarrhythmias |
| Diltiazem | IV: 0.25–0.35 mg/kg over 2 min | IV: 5–15 mg/h Orally: 90–240 mg/day in divided doses | As for verapamil | As for diltiazem |
| Amiodarone | IV: 300 mg, made up to 20 ml with 5% dextrose (can be given peripherally). A further dose of 150 mg may be given for recurrent or refractory VF/VT | Early infusion of 1 mg/min for 6 h followed by 0.5 mg/min to a maximum daily dose of 2 g. For prolonged infusions administer centrally to avoid thrombophlebis | Can increase digoxin and warfarin levels. Contra-indications: sinus or AV node disease (unless fitted with a pacemaker) iodine sensitivity, pregnancy, breast feeding, thyroid dysfunction (relative) | Treatment of supra-ventricular, atrial and ventricular tachy-arrhythmias, especially if associated left ventricular dysfunction |
| Procainamide | 12–17 mg/kg over 30–60 min (20–30 mg/min) | 2–4 mg/min | Caution in patients with renal insufficiency. Reduce dose or discontinue if QT$_c$ interval is prolonged by 60 ms above baseline or more than 500 ms | Treatment of supra-ventricular, atrial and ventricular tachyarrhythmias |
| Lidocaine | 1–1.5 mg/kg | 1–4 mg/min. Reduce after 24 h to 1–2 mg/min | Additional boluses of 0.5–0.75 mg/kg every 5–10 min as needed, to a maximum of 3 mg/kg | Treatment of ventricular tachyarrhythmias |

In the setting of acute myocardial infarction, polymorphic VT is not usually related to QT interval prolongation, sinus bradycardia, pauses or electrolyte abnormalities. When present, it usually implies recurrent myocardial ischaemia. It has been reported to occur in 0.3–2% of patients in the peri-infarction period[15]. The prognosis is similar to patients with sustained VT.

### Treatment

Rapid treatment of sustained VT is mandatory because of the deleterious effect on cardiac output, the exacerbation of myocardial ischaemia, and the risk of degeneration into ventricular fibrillation. If there is haemodynamic compromise, synchronised direct current cardioversion (DCC) should be implemented. If the patient is haemodynamically stable, pharmacological termination can be attempted. The ACC/AHA has recommended either: amiodarone, procainamide or lidocaine to treat peri-infarction sustained monomorphic VT (Table 2)[25]. Although lidocaine, which has an acceptable safety profile, has been traditionally used for treating stable monomorphic VT, studies have suggested that it is relatively ineffective for termination of VT[26] and less effective against VT than IV procainamide[27] or IV sotalol[28]. Studies investigating the use of amiodarone to treat haemodynamically stable VT are minimal; however, it is effective in treating unstable VT and VF[29] and consequently it is considered an acceptable agent to treat stable VT. The new *Guidelines 2000 for Cardiopulmonary Resuscitation and Emergency Cardiovascular Care*[30] has de-emphasised the use of lidocaine as a first-line agent for the treatment of stable monomorphic VT, recommending either intravenous sotalol or intravenous procainamide as first-line agents in patients with normal left ventricular function. In patients with left ventricular dysfunction, either amiodarone or lidocaine is recommended as a first-line agent as they cause the least additional impairment of LV function[30]. Hypokalaemia and hypomagnesaemia should be corrected by ensuring plasma concentrations ≥ 4 mmol/l and 2 mmol/l, respectively.

If not already administered or contra-indicated, patients with recurrent VT should be established on intravenous amiodarone. In patients who continue to display arrhythmias despite the use of amiodarone at recommended doses, supplemental infusions can be considered[29]. The use of drug combinations (amiodarone plus either β-blocker, lidocaine or procainamide) may be helpful during the early phases of dosing, until amiodarone has reached higher myocardial concentrations[29].

Burst overdrive pacing can also be used to terminate refractory VT. Overdrive pacing is performed by inserting a temporary pacing wire in the right ventricle and pacing 10–20 beats/min faster than the VT rate, for approximately 20–50 beats. Atrial or ventricular pacing at rates marginally higher than the intrinsic sinus rate (physiological overdrive) can help prevent bradycardia-related ventricular arrhythmias.

Peri-infarction polymorphic VT is uncommon and its treatment is the same for sustained VT. However, these arrhythmias are less responsive to class 1 agents and may be suppressed with intravenous amiodarone[31]. As these arrhythmias are usually associated with recurrent ischaemia, treatment should include strategies to reduce ischaemia, such as adequate doses of β-blockers and emergency PTCA/CABG surgery.

## Ventricular fibrillation

Ventricular fibrillation is characterised by rapid, disorganised, multiple re-entrant wavelets in the ventricle, resulting in no uniform ventricular contraction and no cardiac output. Untreated, the arrhythmia is lethal and it is the main mechanism of sudden cardiac death. It has been reported to occur in 3% of acute MI with approximately 60% of episodes occurring within 4 h and 80% within 12 h[32]

### Treatment

The only definitive treatment for VF is defibrillation. Initially, these rhythms are readily treatable; however, the chances of successful defibrillation diminish rapidly with time, declining by 5–10% per min. Therefore, the priority is to minimise any delay between the onset of cardiac arrest and the administration of defibrillation shocks. The treatment of VF is now standardised to local and national resuscitation protocols. Results of the recently published ARREST study, showed that the early use of intravenous amiodarone after 3 failed DC shocks, can increase the number of survivors[33].

In treating peri-infarction ventricular tachyarrhythmias (VT and VF), it is common clinical practice to continue anti-arrhythmic drug infusions for 24–48 h and to discontinue the infusion provided there is no arrhythmic recurrence. In patients with refractory ventricular arrhythmias or electrical storms, high dose β-blockade[34] coupled with atrial or dual chamber pacemaker therapy, light anaesthesia and artificial ventilation may be life-saving. Urgent referral for coronary revascularisation and/or implantable cardioverter defibrillation should be considered for patients who develop ventricular arrhythmias >48 h after the index MI or in whom the arrhythmias persist beyond this point. In patients who are adequately revascularised and who refuse device therapy, pace mapping to identify the arrhythmogenic zone combined with radiofrequency ablation has been shown to be an acceptable strategy in that small proportion of patients with a single tachycardia focus on the endocardial surface[35].

# Sudden cardiac death (SCD) and ICDs

Aborted SCD is, in the majority of cases, caused by life-threatening ventricular tachyarrhythmias. A number of randomised, clinical trials have now demonstrated the superiority of the ICD over anti-arrhythmic drug therapy (mostly or exclusively amiodarone) in survivors of aborted SCD[36]. On the basis of these studies, treatment with an ICD is considered a class 1 indication (available evidence and general agreement that a device or procedure is beneficial and efficacious) for secondary prevention in: (i) survivors of cardiac arrest not accompanied by an acute myocardial infarction or other reversible cause; (ii) patients with syncope of unknown aetiology and inducible haemodynamically significant VT/VF on electrophysiological testing; and (iii) patients with spontaneous, sustained VT[37]. Patients with associated left ventricular dysfunction (≤35%) derive the most benefit from an ICD[36].

Aborted SCD is invariably associated with structural heart disease, which in the adult population is most frequently CAD. Although the exact role of cardiac ischaemia in the pathogenesis of SCD is not clearly defined, it is believed to be the trigger that initiates arrhythmogenesis. Therefore, reversal or prevention of ischaemia should avoid the occurrence of the arrhythmia. A recently published study investigating the effects of coronary artery revascularisation in patients with sustained ventricular arrhythmias in the chronic phase of a myocardial infarction demonstrated that arrhythmia recurrence is still high following revascularisation, particularly in patients with reduced left ventricular function[38]. It is, therefore, recommended that survivors of aborted SCD with obstructive CAD and evidence of an arrhythmic substrate (Q waves, depressed left ventricular function, inducible VT/VF) should not only be revascularised, but should also have an ICD implanted. Controversies in management exist in aborted SCD survivors who are demonstrated to have reversible ischaemia and no arrhythmic substrate (no Q waves, preserved left ventricular function and non-inducible VT/VF). Some electrophysiologists believe that these patients are at low risk, and revascularisation and β-blockers may be all that is required[39], whereas others would recommend implantation of an ICD.

# Supraventricular arrhythmias

## Sinus bradycardia

Sinus bradycardia (< 60 beats/min) is common, occurring in 25–40% of patients within the first hour of a myocardial infarction. It is more common with inferior wall myocardial infarction and is often due to hypervagotonia. Treatment is only necessary when there are symptoms or evidence of haemodynamic compromise. Most cases respond well to intravenous atropine (0.6–1 mg). Persistent symptomatic bradycardia despite atropine is an indication for temporary cardiac pacing.

## Sinus tachycardia

Sinus tachycardia occurs in about 30% of patients with acute myocardial infarction. It can aggravate myocardial ischaemia by increasing myocardial oxygen consumption as well as reducing diastolic coronary artery perfusion time. Sinus tachycardia is also a manifestation of significant ventricular dysfunction, on-going cardiac ischaemia, inadequate analgesia, anxiety, pyrexia and hypovolaemia. Management is aimed at treating the underlying causes. When sinus tachycardia is inappropriately fast, given the physiological state of the patient, slowing of the heart rate with β-blockade is helpful (Table 2), particularly if the patient has evidence of ongoing cardiac ischaemia.

## Atrial tachyarrhythmias

The incidence of atrial tachyarrhythmias during the peri-infarction period is estimated at 10–20%[40], with atrial fibrillation being the commonest atrial tachyarrhythmia (occurs in 10–15% of cases). Atrial flutter occurs in less than 5% of patients. These arrhythmias usually occur within 72 h of the index infarction with less than 3% arising in the very early phase (<3 h)[41].

Atrial fibrillation has been shown to be independently associated with in-hospital and long-term mortality, re-infarction rates, ventricular arrhythmias, advanced atrioventricular conduction disturbances, asystole, cardiogenic shock, and ischaemic strokes. It is also more likely to be associated with extensive coronary artery disease and poor reperfusion of the infarct related artery[42,43] and, therefore, the threshold for cardiac catheterisation should be low.

Factors associated with the development of peri-infarction atrial fibrillation include: atrial infarction/ischaemia, sinus node dysfunction, older age, metabolic abnormalities, pericarditis, pericardial effusion, right ventricular infarction, congestive heart failure, higher peak cardiac enzyme concentration, increased heart rate, diabetes mellitus, history of hypertension and inotropic drugs. The development of atrial fibrillation within 24 h is usually associated with inferior wall myocardial infarction from right coronary artery occlusion. In contrast, atrial fibrillation developing more than 24 h afterwards is associated with anterior wall myocardial infarction and left ventricular dysfunction.

### Treatment of atrial tachyarrhythmias

The early treatment of atrial tachyarrhythmias is important as increased ventricular rates and loss of atrial systole result in a significant reduction in cardiac output and an increase in cardiac ischaemia. When there is significant haemodynamic compromise, then DC cardioversion is indicated. If the patient is haemodynamically stable, early control of the ventricular rate with either a β-blocker, calcium antagonist or digoxin is satisfactory (Table 2). Alternatively, pharmacological cardioversion to sinus rhythm can be attempted with amiodarone or dofetilide[44,45]. Dofetilide has recently been shown to be effective in cardioverting atrial fibrillation in the post-infarction period in patients with left ventricular dysfunction without affecting all-cause, cardiac and arrhythmic mortality[45]. However, dofetilide is associated with an increased incidence of torsades de pointes and close ECG monitoring is mandatory when it is administered. Although newer class III agents such as ibutilide and azimilide have been successful in the treatment of atrial fibrillation, data concerning their efficacy and safety in the peri-infarction period are currently limited. Elective DC cardioversion should be considered if the patient remains in atrial fibrillation after the acute infarction period has passed. Atrial fibrillation is associated with an increased risk of thrombo-embolism, and provided there are no contra-indications, all patients should be heparinised and considered for oral anticoagulation if atrial fibrillation persists or is paroxysmal.

## Conduction disturbances

Myocardial ischaemia can produce a broad range of conduction disturbances, involving both the atrioventricular node and infranodal structures. Although early reperfusion with thrombolysis can shorten the duration of AV block and reduce the need for temporary pacing, it has not reduced the incidence of atrioventricular block, which has remained relatively constant[46].

First degree AV block is the most common conduction disturbance occurring in up to 14% of patients with acute myocardial infarction. It is usually associated with inferior myocardial infarction and may be a manifestation of hypervagotonia or functional damage of the AV node. First degree heart block that is below the His bundle is more commonly associated with anterior myocardial infarction and has a worse prognosis. Iatrogenic causes of first degree heart block include drugs such as β-blockers, calcium antagonists and digoxin. Mobitz type 1 heart block (Wenckebach) is present in 4–10% of patients with acute myocardial infarction and accounts for about 90% of patients with second degree heart block[47]. It is usually transient and is more common following inferior infarctions. Mobitz type 2 heart block is less common and is more associated with anterior infarction, indicating damage to the AV junction or His bundle[48]. The QRS complexes are usually wide implying bundle branch involvement and may herald the onset of complete heart block. Complete heart block (CHB) has an incidence of about 6% and is more common with inferior/posterior infarctions. CHB occurring in association with anterior myocardial infarctions implies extensive myocardial damage and has a worse prognosis. CHB complicating either inferior or anterior wall myocardial infarctions is independently associated with mortality and in-hospital complications[46].

Conduction disturbances involving the left and right bundle branches occur in 10–24% of patients with acute myocardial infarction. Persistent bundle branch block is an independent marker of mortality, whereas, transient blocks which recover normal conduction during hospitalisation have similar prognosis to patients who never develop this complication.

Left anterior hemiblock occurs in 3–5% of acute myocardial infarctions and mortality is slightly increased[49]. Left posterior hemiblock occurs in 1–2% of cases and, because of its large size, disturbances of this conduction pathway reflect significant myocardial damage, and it is associated with a higher mortality[46].

## Treatment of conduction disturbances

First degree heart block in the peri-infarction period does not require any specific treatment. Similarly, Mobitz type 1 (Wenckebach) heart block does not require specific treatment provided that the ventricular rate is adequate; if there is associated haemodynamic compromise, not responsive to atropine (Table 2), then temporary transvenous ventricular pacing is indicated. Where possible, it is recommended to ensure AV synchronisation by inserting an atrial sensing/pacing electrode. As Mobitz type 2 heart block is at risk of progressing to CHB, the insertion of a temporary pacing wire is recommended. CHB occurring in the context of inferior wall myocardial infarction and hypervagotonia may respond to atropine; otherwise the patient should be temporarily paced. Table 3 summarises the indications for transvenous pacing as recommended by the ACC/AHA.

Although atrioventricular block and/or bundle branch block carry an independent risk for mortality and in-hospital complications, the use of pacing during this period does not alter mortality[46]. However, temporary cardiac pacing does serve to protect against hypotension and subsequent ischaemia exacerbation, as well as the development of bradycardia-dependent ventricular tachyarrhythmias. In the setting of inferior myocardial infarction, CHB is self-limiting and usually resolves within the first week but can last up to 14–16 days[50]. Therefore, decisions regarding the placement of a permanent pacemaker in patients with inferior myocardial infarctions should be delayed for at least a week to allow recovery of normal conduction. In contrast, there is a significant risk of

**Table 3** Indications for temporary transvenous pacing and permanent pacing in the peri-infarction and post-infarction periods, respectively

TEMPORARY TRANSVENOUS PACING

*Established (evidence supporting and/or general agreement)*

- Asystole
- Symptomatic bradycardia including sinus bradycardia and type 1 second-degree AV block with haemodynamic compromise, which is medically refractory
- New or age-indeterminate alternating bundle branch block (including RBBB with alternating LAFB/LAPB)
- New or age-indeterminate trifasicular block (RBBB+LAFB+FDHB, RBBB+LPFB+FDHB, or LBBB+FDHB)
- Mobitz type II second-degree AV block

*Less established*

- New or age-indeterminate bifasicular block (RBBB+LAFB, RBBB+LPFB or RBBB+FDHB)
- New or age indeterminate LBBB
- Atrial or ventricular overdrive/underdrive pacing for recurrent VT
- Recurrent sinus pauses (greater than 3 s) refractory to atropine

PERMANENT PACING

*Established (evidence supporting and/or general agreement)*

Persistent second-degree AV block in the His-Purkinje system with bilateral bundle branch block or third degree AV block within or below the His-Purkinje system

Transient advanced (second or third degree) infranodal AV block and associated bundle branch block

Symptomatic AV block independent of location

*Less established*

Persistent advanced (second or third degree) block at the AV node level

Note: decisions regarding the placement of a permanent pacemaker in patients with inferior myocardial infarction should be delayed for at least 1 week as the majority of conduction disturbances resolve by this time

**Note:** AV, atrioventricular; RBBB, right bundle branch block; LAFB, left anterior fasicular block; LPFB, left posterior fasicular block; FDHB, first degree heart block. Adapted from Ryan et al[39].

asystole in patients with anterior infarction and CHB (even if transient); therefore, permanent pacing is recommended (Table 3).

# Conclusions

Cardiac ischaemia causes complex interactions between ionic, metabolic and neurohormonal factors with deleterious effects on cardiac cellular electrophysiology. The end result is the induction and maintenance of supraventricular and ventricular tachyarrhythmias, and conduction disturbances. Despite improvements in the management of myocardial infarction, the arrhythmias generated during myocardial ischaemia contribute significantly to the morbidity and mortality seen in the peri- and post-infarction periods. At present, supraventricular tachyarrhythmias which are often not life-threatening are reasonably controlled with pharmacological intervention. In contrast, ventricular tachyarrhythmias which are life-threatening are less restrained by pharmacological therapy, and some agents may precipitate arrhythmic death. ICDs remain an effective tool in selected patient groups in the post-infarction period both in terms of primary and secondary prevention. It is imperative to ensure that all patients with CAD are optimally treated for on-going cardiac ischaemia, and are appropriately prescribed some form of antiplatelet therapy, β-blockers, cholesterol lowering therapy and ACE inhibitors. As CAD continues to be prevalent in today's society, it is inevitable that cardiologists and physicians will continue to be challenged with the arrhythmias generated from cardiac ischaemia.

## References

1   Gandhi MM. Clinical epidemiology of coronary heart disease in the UK. *Br J Hosp Med* 1997; **58**: 23–7

2   Corr PB, Yamada KA. Selected metabolic alterations in the ischemic heart and their contributions to arrhythmogenesis. In: Zehender M, Meinertz T, Just H. (eds) *Myocardial Ischaemia and Arrhythmia*. New York: Steinkopff Darmstadt, 1994; 15–33

3   Schwartz PJ. The autonomic nervous system and sudden death. *Eur Heart J* 1998; **19** (**Suppl F**): F72–80

4   Karlsberg RP, Penkoske PA, Cryer PE, Corr PB, Roberts R. Rapid activation of the sympathetic nervous system following coronary artery occlusion: relationship to infarct size, site, and haemodynamic impact. *Cardiovasc Res* 1979; **13**: 523–31

5   La Rovere MT, Bigger Jr JT, Marcus FI, Mortara A, Schwartz PJ. Baroreflex sensitivity and heart-rate variability in prediction of total cardiac mortality after myocardial infarction. ATRAMI (Autonomic Tone and Reflexes After Myocardial Infarction) Investigators. *Lancet* 1998; **351**: 478–84

6   Janse MJ, Wit AL. Electrophysiological mechanisms of ventricular arrhythmias resulting from myocardial ischemia and infarction. *Physiol Rev* 1989; **69**: 1049–169

7   Bigger Jr JT, Dresdale FJ, Heissenbuttel RH, Weld FM, Wit AL. Ventricular arrhythmias in ischemic heart disease: mechanism, prevalence, significance, and management. *Prog Cardiovasc Dis* 1977; **19**: 255–300

8   O'Doherty M, Tayler DI, Quinn E, Vincent R, Chamberlain DA. Five hundred patients with myocardial infarction monitored within one hour of symptoms. *BMJ* 1983; **286**: 1405–8

9   Maggioni AP, Zuanetti G, Franzosi MG *et al.* Prevalence and prognostic significance of ventricular arrhythmias after acute myocardial infarction in the fibrinolytic era. GISSI-2 results. *Circulation* 1993; **87**: 312–22

10  Hine LK, Laird N, Hewitt P, Chalmers TC. Meta-analytic evidence against prophylactic use of lidocaine in acute myocardial infarction. *Arch Intern Med* 1989; **149**: 2694–8

11  Echt DS, Liebson PR, Mitchell LB *et al.* Mortality and morbidity in patients receiving encainide, flecainide, or placebo. The Cardiac Arrhythmia Suppression Trial. *N Engl J Med* 1991; **324**: 781–8

12  Teo KK, Yusuf S, Furberg CD. Effects of prophylactic antiarrhythmic drug therapy in acute myocardial infarction. An overview of results from randomized controlled trials. *JAMA* 1993; **270**: 1589–95

13  Cairns JA, Connolly SJ, Roberts R, Gent M. Randomised trial of outcome after myocardial infarction in patients with frequent or repetitive ventricular premature depolarisations: CAMIAT. Canadian Amiodarone Myocardial Infarction Arrhythmia Trial Investigators. *Lancet* 1997; **349**: 675–82

14  Julian DG, Camm AJ, Frangin G *et al.* Randomised trial of effect of amiodarone on mortality in patients with left-ventricular dysfunction after recent myocardial infarction: EMIAT. European Myocardial Infarct Amiodarone Trial. *Lancet* 1997; **349**: 667–74

15  Eldar M, Sievner Z, Goldbourt U, Reicher-Reiss H, Kaplinsky E, Behar S. Primary ventricular tachycardia in acute myocardial infarction: clinical characteristics and mortality. The SPRINT Study Group. *Ann Intern Med* 1992; **117**: 31–6

16  Heidbuchel H, Tack J, Vanneste L, Ballet A, Ector H, Van de Werf F. Significance of arrhythmias during the first 24 hours of acute myocardial infarction treated with alteplase and effect of early administration of a beta-blocker or a bradycardiac agent on their incidence. *Circulation* 1994; **89**: 1051–9

17  Soyza ND, Bissett JK, Kane JJ, Murphy ML, Doherty JE. Ectopic ventricular prematurity and its relationship to ventricular tachycardia in acute myocardial infarction in man. *Circulation* 1974; **50**: 529–33

18  Cheema AN, Sheu K, Parker M, Kadish AH, Goldberger JJ. Non-sustained ventricular tachycardia in the setting of acute myocardial infarction: tachycardia characteristics and their prognostic implications. *Circulation* 1998; **98**: 2030–6

19  Mukharji J, Rude RE, Poole WK *et al.* Risk factors for sudden death after acute myocardial infarction: two-year follow-up. *Am J Cardiol* 1984; **54**: 31–6

20  Bigger Jr JT, Fleiss JL, Rolnitzky LM. Prevalence, characteristics and significance of ventricular tachycardia detected by 24-hour continuous electrocardiographic recordings in the late hospital phase of acute myocardial infarction. *Am J Cardiol* 1986; **58**: 1151–60

21  Boutitie F, Boissel JP, Connolly SJ *et al.* Amiodarone interaction with beta-blockers: analysis of the merged EMIAT (European Myocardial Infarct Amiodarone Trial) and CAMIAT (Canadian Amiodarone Myocardial Infarction Trial) databases. The EMIAT and CAMIAT Investigators. *Circulation* 1999; **99**: 2268–75

22  Moss AJ, Hall WJ, Cannom DS *et al.* Improved survival with an implanted defibrillator in patients with coronary disease at high risk for ventricular arrhythmia. Multicenter Automatic Defibrillator Implantation Trial Investigators. *N Engl J Med* 1996; **335**: 1933–40

23  Buxton AE, Lee KL, Fisher JD, Josephson ME, Prystowsky EN, Hafley G. A randomized study of the prevention of sudden death in patients with coronary artery disease. Multicenter Unsustained Tachycardia Trial Investigators [see comments] [published erratum appears in *N Engl J Med* 2000; **342**: 1300]. *N Engl J Med* 1999; **341**: 1882–90

24  Mont L, Cinca J, Blanch P *et al.* Predisposing factors and prognostic value of sustained monomorphic ventricular tachycardia in the early phase of acute myocardial infarction. *J Am Coll Cardiol* 1996; **28**: 1670–6

25  Ryan TJ, Antman EM, Brooks NH *et al.* 1999 update: ACC/AHA guidelines for the management of patients with acute myocardial infarction: executive summary and recommendations: a report of the American College of Cardiology/American Heart Association Task Force on Practice Guidelines (Committee on Management of Acute Myocardial Infarction). *Circulation* 1999; **100**: 1016–30

26  Nasir Jr N, Taylor A, Doyle TK, Pacifico A. Evaluation of intravenous lidocaine for the termination of sustained monomorphic ventricular tachycardia in patients with coronary artery disease with or without healed myocardial infarction. *Am J Cardiol* 1994; **74**: 1183–6

27  Gorgels AP, van den Dool A, Hofs A *et al.* Comparison of procainamide and lidocaine in terminating sustained monomorphic ventricular tachycardia. *Am J Cardiol* 1996; **78**: 43–6

28  Ho DS, Zecchin RP, Richards DA, Uther JB, Ross DL. Double-blind trial of lignocaine versus sotalol for acute termination of spontaneous sustained ventricular tachycardia. *Lancet* 1994; **344**: 18–23

29  Kowey PR, Bharucha DB, Rials SJ, Marinchak RA. Intravenous antiarrhythmic therapy for high-risk patients. *Eur Heart J* 1999; **1 (Suppl C)**: C36–40

30  Anonymous. Guidelines 2000 for cardiopulmonary resuscitation and emergency cardiovascular care. Part 6: advanced cardiovascular life support: 7D: the tachycardia algorithms. The American Heart Association in collaboration with the International Liaison Committee on Resuscitation. *Circulation* 2000; **102**: I158–65

31  Wolfe CL, Nibley C, Bhandari A, Chatterjee K, Scheinman M. Polymorphous ventricular tachycardia associated with acute myocardial infarction. *Circulation* 1991; **84**: 1543–51

32  Campbell RW, Murray A, Julian DG. Ventricular arrhythmias in first 12 hours of acute myocardial infarction. Natural history study. *Br Heart J* 1981; **46**: 351–7

33  Kudenchuk PJ, Cobb LA, Copass MK *et al*. Amiodarone for resuscitation after out-of-hospital cardiac arrest due to ventricular fibrillation. *N Engl J Med* 1999; **341**: 871–8

34  Nademanee K, Taylor R, Bailey WE, Rieders DE, Kosar EM. Treating electrical storm : sympathetic blockade versus advanced cardiac life support-guided therapy. *Circulation* 2000; **102**: 742–7

35  Furniss S, Anil-Kumar R, Bourke JP, Behulova R, Simeonidou E. Radiofrequency ablation of haemodynamically unstable ventricular tachycardia after myocardial infarction. *Heart* 2000; **84**: 648–52

36  Connolly SJ, Hallstrom AP, Cappato R *et al*. Meta-analysis of the implantable cardioverter defibrillator secondary prevention trials. *Eur Heart J* 2000; **21**: 2071–8

37  Gregoratos G, Cheitlin MD, Conill A *et al*. ACC/AHA guidelines for implantation of cardiac pacemakers and antiarrhythmia devices: a report of the American College of Cardiology/American Heart Association Task Force on Practice Guidelines (Committee on Pacemaker Implantation). *J Am Coll Cardiol* 1998; **31**: 1175–209

38  Brugada J, Aguinaga L, Mont L, Betriu A, Mulet J, Sanz G. Coronary artery revascularisation in patients with sustained ventricular arrhythmias in the chronic phase of a myocardial infarction: effects on the electrophysiologic substrate and outcome. *J Am Coll Cardiol* 2001; **37**: 529–33

39  Kelly P, Ruskin JN, Vlahakes GJ, Buckley Jr MJ, Freeman CS, Garan H. Surgical coronary revascularization in survivors of prehospital cardiac arrest: its effect on inducible ventricular arrhythmias and long-term survival. *J Am Coll Cardiol* 1990; **15**: 267–73

40  Liberthson RR, Salisbury KW, Hutter Jr AM, DeSanctis RW. Atrial tachyarrhythmias in acute myocardial infarction. *Am J Med* 1976; **60**: 956–60

41  Hod H, Lew AS, Keltai M *et al*. Early atrial fibrillation during evolving myocardial infarction: a consequence of impaired left atrial perfusion. *Circulation* 1987; **75**: 146–50

42  Crenshaw BS, Ward SR, Granger CB, Stebbins AL, Topol EJ, Califf RM. Atrial fibrillation in the setting of acute myocardial infarction: the GUSTO-I experience. Global Utilization of Streptokinase and TPA for Occluded Coronary Arteries. *J Am Coll Cardiol* 1997; **30**: 406–13

43  Sakata K, Kurihara H, Iwamori K *et al*. Clinical and prognostic significance of atrial fibrillation in acute myocardial infarction. *Am J Cardiol* 1997; **80**: 1522–7

44  Vardas PE, Kochiadakis GE, Igoumenidis NE, Tsatsakis AM, Simantirakis EN, Chlouverakis GI. Amiodarone as a first-choice drug for restoring sinus rhythm in patients with atrial fibrillation: a randomized, controlled study. *Chest* 2000; **117**: 1538–45

45  Køber L, Thomsen PEB, Møller M *et al*. Effect of dofetilide in patients with recent myocardial infarction and left-ventricular dysfunction: a randomised trial. *Lancet* 2000; **356**: 2052–8

46  Simons GR, Sgarbossa E, Wagner G, Califf RM, Topol EJ, Natale A. Atrioventricular and intraventricular conduction disorders in acute myocardial infarction: a reappraisal in the thrombolytic era. *Pacing Clin Electrophysiol* 1998; **21**: 2651–63

47  Feigl D, Ashkenazy J, Kishon Y. Early and late atrioventricular block in acute inferior myocardial infarction. *J Am Coll Cardiol* 1984; **4**: 35–8

48  Antman EM, Braunwald E. Acute myocardial infarction. In: Braunwald E. (ed) *Heart Disease*, 5th edn. Philadelphia: WB Saunders, 1997; 1245–54

49  Klein RC, Vera Z, Mason DT. Intraventricular conduction defects in acute myocardial infarction: incidence, prognosis, and therapy. *Am Heart J* 1984; **108**: 1007–13

50  Barold SS. American College of Cardiology/American Heart Association guidelines for pacemaker implantation after acute myocardial infarction. What is persistent advanced block at the atrioventricular node? *Am J Cardiol* 1997; **80**: 770–4

# Angiogenesis, protein and gene delivery

**Michael Azrin**

*Cardiology Division, University of Connecticut Health Center, Farmington, Connecticut, USA*

Advances in our understanding of angiogenesis and blood vessel growth have given rise to efforts to develop novel therapeutic approaches for patients with ischaemia who are not adequately treated with presently available therapies. Among the growth factors that play a role in blood vessel growth and development, vascular endothelial growth factors and fibroblast growth factors have been the most extensively studied. Various methods of delivery have been utilized to enhance localization and persistence, including methods for delivery of proteins as well as gene transfer techniques. Initial clinical trials have now been undertaken. Preliminary information on efficacy is beginning to become available, raising hopes, as well as questions about the future direction and potential success of therapeutic angiogenesis as a clinical approach to the treatment of ischaemia.

In spite of significant advances in the treatment of coronary artery disease, a substantial number of patients remain inadequately treated with anti-anginal medications or with coronary revascularization thereby prompting great interest in alternative therapeutic approaches. One approach utilizes the knowledge that the collateral circulation can play an important role in patients with coronary artery disease. Advances in our understanding of the process of angiogenesis, and the recognition that collateral formation can be altered by growth factors have given rise to the concept of therapeutic angiogenesis. This refers to the therapeutic administration of agents such as growth factors or cytokines to enhance collateral development and reduce vascular insufficiency. Demonstrated efficacy in animal studies then led to initial human clinical trials of therapeutic angiogenesis using both protein delivery and gene transfer therapy. Clinical trials are currently being designed and performed, and the future of therapeutic angiogenesis is just beginning to unfold.

The importance of collateral vessels has long been recognized and is often evident in the clinical practice of cardiology. For example, one patient with an occluded left anterior descending (LAD) coronary artery and inadequate collaterals might present with an acute myocardial infarction and severe left ventricular dysfunction, while another patient, who also has an occluded LAD, but in whom the only evident difference

Correspondence to:
Michael Azrin MD,
Cardiology Division,
University of Connecticut
Health Center, 263
Farmington Ave,
Farmington,
CT 06030, USA

is the presence of abundant collaterals, may have only angina and preserved left ventricular function. The importance of the collateral circulation has been studied systematically, and the ability of collateral circulation to limit ischaemia has been demonstrated prospectively[1]. During acute coronary occlusion, a gradient develops between a patent vessel and the occluded coronary resulting in the recruitment or filling of dormant collateral vessels; this has been demonstrated in the setting of acute coronary occlusion such as occurs during coronary spasm or during balloon angioplasty[2]. Furthermore, the presence of collateral vessels has been demonstrated to modify the functional effects of coronary occlusion by reducing ST changes, metabolic effects and infarct size, and to improve ejection fraction and long-term outcomes[3]. Thus, it is evident that collaterals can play an important functional role.

In addition to recruitment of pre-existing collaterals, collateral flow may be enhanced by both enlargement of existing channels, as well as by the development of new collateral channels[4]. The former is arteriogenesis, which refers to the remodelling and structural enlargement of pre-existing arteriolar connections, and the latter is angiogenesis which refers to extension of the existing vasculature through the development of capillary sprouts (a process that also occurs in the setting of tumour neovascularization, wound healing and pathological diabetic retinopathy). Angiogenesis is a complex multistep process. In response to an angiogenic stimulus, the normally quiescent endothelial cells become activated. Local vasodilation, increased permeability and proteolytic disruption of the basement membrane then lead to migration of endothelial cells through the basement membrane into the surrounding matrix with proliferation and formation of capillary sprouts. Formation of a lumen and connection to other vascular structures with reformation of the basement membrane results in a functional vascular connection.

Several factors can influence collateral development. Ischaemia is felt to be a strong stimulant. For example, enhanced collaterals have been demonstrated in dogs subjected to long-term hypoxia or with chronic anaemia and in animal models of coronary or limb ischaemia. Similarly, humans with chronic anaemia or chronic obstructive pulmonary disease have more extensive collaterals, and extensive collateralization can be observed in the setting of chronic coronary disease or claudication. But, collateral development is also under the influence of factors other than ischaemia. For example, patients with distal lower extremity ischaemia will often develop extensive collaterals proximally, in the thigh, in an area that is not itself ischaemic. Increased shear forces develop due to the pressure differential caused by vessel occlusion. The stimuli for collateral development include these increased shear forces which result in endothelial activation, as well as an important contribution by monocytes. While both small vessel collaterals arising from capillaries and post-capillary venules, and larger visible collaterals arising from pre-existing interconnecting arterioles both may contribute to tissue perfusion in the setting of vessel occlusion, the larger collateral vessels are felt to contribute more to meaningful perfusion[5].

Regulation of angiogenesis and collateral formation has been demonstrated to be complex, involving stimulators, inhibitors and modulators. While a number of cytokines play important roles, two families of growth factors which play key roles (and that have been the most extensively investigated and utilized in clinical and preclinical studies) are the vascular endothelial growth factor (VEGF) and the fibroblast growth factor (FGF) protein families.

## Vascular endothelial growth factor (VEGF)

VEGF is a key factor in the process of angiogenesis[6]. It is secreted by a number of cell types and acts in a paracrine fashion. VEGF exists as a number of isoforms that are produced by alternative splicing resulting in isoforms of 121, 145, 165, 189 or 206 amino acids. VEGF also contains a typical signal sequence enabling secretion by intact cells. The 165 and 121 residue forms are the most abundantly expressed. The larger isoforms contain the binding sites for heparan sulphate and extracellular matrix; therefore, a significant portion of the larger isoforms remains bound to the cell surface or extracellular matrix. In contrast, $VEGF_{121}$ does not contain the heparin- or matrix-binding domains making it the most freely diffusible form.

VEGF is a highly specific mitogen for vascular endothelial cells. *In vitro*, VEGF induces endothelial cell proliferation and chemotaxis. VEGF also induces vascular hyperpermeability allowing small molecules to pass into the extravascular space. There are two well-described VEGF receptors: FLT-1 (VEGFR-1) and KDR (FLK-1, VEGFR-2) which are found almost exclusively on endothelial cells. FLT-1 (VEGFR-1) appears to be involved in vessel permeability, while KDR (VEGFR-2) mediates the angiogenic process.

The VEGF protein family includes VEGF (also called VEGF-A) as well as VEGF-B, VEGF-C (VEGF-2), VEGF-D and placental growth factor. While VEGF has been investigated the most extensively, both VEGF-2 and VEGF-D have also been studied for therapeutic angiogenesis, in part because, like VEGF, they too interact with the KDR (VEGFR-2) receptor involved in angiogenesis.

VEGF plays a key role in angiogenesis and has effects on all of the key steps in this process, including endothelial cell mitogenesis and chemotaxis, vascular permeability, and proteolysis. Both VEGF and its endothelial specific receptors are up-regulated in the setting of hypoxia

– potentially enabling localization of the effect to areas of hypoxia or ischaemia[7]. These key characteristics have made VEGF an appealing candidate for use in therapeutic angiogenesis.

# Fibroblast growth factor (FGF)

The fibroblast growth factor family includes more than 20 different structurally-related polypeptides characterized by high affinity binding to cellular heparan sulphates. The first two members of the fibroblast growth factor family identified, FGF-1 (acidic FGF) and FGF-2 (basic FGF), have been extensively studied and have significant effects on the processes involved in angiogenesis[8]. In spite of the historical name of 'fibroblast' growth factors, they are in fact potent mitogens for numerous cell types including endothelial cells, smooth muscle cells and cells of mesenchymal, neural and epithelial origin. FGFs regulate the key migratory and proliferative processes involved in angiogenesis. The prototypic fibroblast growth factors, FGF-1 and FGF-2, are chemotactic and mitogenic for endothelial cells, they induce matrix-resorbing activity and proteolytic systems that are necessary for matrix degradation involved in angiogenesis, and they are powerful angiogenic agents both *in vitro* and *in vivo*[9].

# Methods of delivery

Therapeutic angiogenesis represents an attempt to induce blood vessel growth in an area of ischaemia while avoiding unwanted angiogenesis elsewhere. While some degree of localization might be expected through the up-regulation of receptors for angiogenic growth factors in regions of ischaemia[10], there remains a need to localize the effects of therapy to avoid such potential side-effects as unwanted angiogenesis, mitogenesis or growth factor-mediated hypotension, as well as to deliver a sufficient quantity of therapy locally for a sufficient duration. Two different approaches have been taken to achieve localization and persistence. The first is to localize physically the protein (or the gene) to the region of interest; the second is to utilize gene therapy to achieve more prolonged local expression.

Techniques for localization of drug delivery have been developed, and several have been utilized in clinical or preclinical trials of therapeutic angiogenesis. The simplest delivery techniques have included intra-venous, intra-arterial, or peripheral intramuscular injection. Although the delivery techniques required are more involved, angiogenic growth factors have also been delivered directly to the myocardium, either as epicardial injections at the time of surgery or through catheter-based endomyocardial injection techniques. In addition, perivascular delivery has been employed either by peri-adventitial delivery using sustained-release polymers at the time of surgery or by intrapericardial delivery. All of these techniques have the same goal which is to enhance the local effect while avoiding systemic effects. Each of these techniques has apparent benefits and drawbacks[11]. The relative ease of delivery by methods such as intracoronary or intravenous delivery, may result in more systemic exposure, and will have to be compared in terms of safety, efficacy and clinical applicability to techniques designed to localize delivery.

# Gene therapy

Gene therapy for angiogenesis involves transfer of the gene encoding the angiogenic protein into a host cell to obtain over-expression of the protein. Several different means of gene transfer have been considered, including both viral and non-viral methods. Viral vectors have been employed because viruses have evolved highly efficient mechanisms to transfer their genetic material to target cells. Viral gene delivery involves the incorporation of the chosen DNA sequences into the genome of the parent virus, which then transfers the gene to the target cells.

## Viral-based gene therapy

Retroviral vectors have been used extensively for gene transfer. However, their use in clinical angiogenesis trials has several limitations. Retroviral (RNA) vectors integrate into the host genome, resulting in permanent expression of the therapeutic gene. This is in contrast to adenoviral (DNA) vectors which remain independent of the host genome and are gradually lost with cell division. Retroviral vectors are truly defective and none of the viral proteins are expressed in the target cell, thereby avoiding an immune response. However, retroviruses are small, limiting the size of genes that can be incorporated. In addition, transfer efficiency is low, and they are not infective in non-dividing cells, which is a major limitation for this application. Also, because retroviral vectors integrate into the host cell chromosome, insertional mutagenesis is possible.

Adenoviral vectors have become widely used for experimental gene transfer. They can infect non-dividing cells, do not integrate into the host genome and have a high efficiency of transfer. The production of 'replication-deficient' vectors results in a reduced host immune response, and is also important for patient safety, as well as to prevent transfer to other individuals. For adenoviral vectors, the approach taken was to remove critical viral genes necessary for viral propagation. The gene for the angiogenic growth factor is then inserted along with a promoter, such as the CMV promoter, which can then drive constitutive expression of the inserted protein gene. The duration of effect is limited to only a few weeks because cells derived from the modified cells will not express the transgene, and because genes expressed by adenoviral vectors elicit an immune response. Early non-specific inflammation may occur, and this is followed by a specific host immune response resulting in a shortened duration of transgene expression. While transient expression is a limitation of therapy for genetic disorders, it may actually be a beneficial safety attribute in the treatment of ischaemia where indefinite growth factor expression may not be required or desirable.

### Non-viral gene therapy

One of the simplest means of delivery of a gene to a target cell is through the use of 'naked' or plasmid DNA. Plasmid DNA expression vectors are comprised of DNA sequences in addition to the gene of interest. These include a transcriptional promoter, as well as sequences that impart stability and functionality to the mRNA.

When plasmid DNA is placed in contact with the cell membrane, a small amount will pass into the cell. This non-viral means of delivery of genes to target cells has a number of potential advantages. Several of the safety concerns associated with viral vectors, including an immune response, insertional mutagenesis or viral transmission, may be avoided. However, plasmid-based gene therapy must overcome several obstacles including penetration of the cell plasma membrane, passage through the cytoplasm, entry into the nucleus, transcription of DNA into functional mRNA, transport of the mRNA to the cytoplasm, and translation into a functional protein. While viruses have evolved to transfer efficiently their nucleic acid to mammalian cells, plasmid gene transfer remains inefficient. In spite of this, two factors may enable therapeutic angiogenesis using plasmid gene therapy. First, there is evidence that gene transfer is enhanced in ischaemic muscle[12]. Second, use of a secreted protein may have paracrine effects in spite of low transfection efficiency[13]. Furthermore, successful gene transfer for therapeutic angiogenesis has been achieved in animals as well as in preliminary clinical trials using plasmid VEGF[14].

## Clinical trials

A number of clinical trials have now been performed (Table 1). While most of these are small trials, they have provided preliminary information regarding safety, feasibility and dosing which is now leading to larger clinical trials to evaluate efficacy. A number of approaches have been undertaken. These include use of proteins, plasmids or viral-based gene transfer therapy, use of both VEGF and FGFs, as well as various delivery approaches including intravenous, intra-arterial, intramuscular, perivascular and therapy administered in concert with revascularization.

## VEGF protein therapy

A series of studies has been performed which ultimately led to the use of VEGF protein in clinical trials of therapeutic angiogenesis. First, it was recognized that VEGF plays a key role in a number of settings, ranging from vascular embryogenesis to pathological angiogenesis. Angiogenic properties were demonstrated in experimental angiogenesis models such as the chick chorio-allantoic membrane and the rabbit cornea, and then in ischaemic animal models including the rabbit hindlimb model and canine and porcine coronary ischaemia models. In addition, various routes of administration were utilized including intravenous, intra-arterial, peri-adventitial and intramyocardial routes in animal models. These studies, which have been reviewed elsewhere[6,15] provided the basis for initiating clinical trials of VEGF.

Phase I trials were performed to evaluate safety and tolerability of both intracoronary[16] and intravenous administration[17]. These studies were performed on patients with demonstrable myocardial ischaemia who were not candidates for revascularization by surgery or by percutaneous coronary intervention. $VEGF_{165}$ protein was administered to 15 patients by intracoronary infusion in escalating doses. Hypotension was found to be dose-limiting with a maximal tolerated dose of 50 ng/kg/min. While there was no placebo group, there was nevertheless a suggestion of improvement clinically and by functional testing. Of the 15 patients, 13 had a decrease in angina class; 7 of 14 patients had an improvement in myocardial perfusion imaging on the rest studies, though not in the stress studies, and each of those 7 patients had a corresponding increase in angiographic collateral density[16]. In a second phase I trial[17], VEGF was administered intravenously to 28 patients. The maximal tolerated dose was again 50 ng/kg/min, and there were again suggestions of improvement in rest myocardial perfusion (which improved in two or more segments in 54% of patients) and in collateral density in this small dose-finding study.

With these dose finding studies as background, the VIVA trial (VEGF in Ischemia for Vascular Angiogenesis) was then performed[18]. This was a phase II double-blind placebo-controlled trial of $VEGF_{165}$ by intra-coronary (17 or 50 ng/kg/min) followed by intravenous administration of the same dose on days 3, 6 and 9. VEGF was well tolerated with no

| | Growth factor | Study type | n | Method of administration | Dose |
|---|---|---|---|---|---|
| **Coronary disease** | | | | | |
| ***VEGF*** | | | | | |
| Hendel et al 2000[16] | VEGF 165 | Phase I | 15 | Intracoronary infusion | 5–167 ng/kg/min |
| Gibson et al 1999[17] | VEGF 165 | Phase I | 28 | Intravenous infusion | |
| Henry et al 1999[18,19] Henry et al 2000[15] | VEGF 165 | Phase II placebo-controlled | 178 (63 placebo) | Intracoronary and intravenous infusions | 17 or 50 ng/kg/min |
| Laitinen et al 2000[25] | Plasmid VEGF liposome | Phase I placebo-controlled | 15 (5 placebo) | Intracoronary infusion via perfusion catheter | 1000 mcg |
| Losordo et al 1998[29] Symes et al 1999[30] Vale et al 2000[31] Lathi et al 2001[32] | Plasmid VEGF 165 | Phase I | 30 | Intramyocardial injection via mini-thoracotomy | 125, 250 or 500 µg |
| Rosengart et al 1999[35] | Adenoviral vector VEGF121 | Phase I | 15 | Combined CABG and intramyocardial injection | $4 \times 10^8$ to $4 \times 10^{10}$ pu |
| Rosengart et al 1999[34] | Adenoviral vector VEGF122 | Phase I | 6 | Intramyocardial injection via mini-thoracotomy | $4 \times 10^9$ pu/patient |
| ***FGF*** | | | | | |
| Schumacher et al 1998[36] Pecher et al 2000[37] | FGF-1 | Phase II placebo-controlled | 40 (20 placebo) | Combined CABG and intramyocardial injection | 0.1 mg/kg |
| Selke et al 1998[38] | FGF-2 | Phase I | 8 | Epicardial heparin alginate | 1 or 10 µg |
| Laham et al 1999[39] | FGF-2 | Phase I placebo-controlled | 24 (8 placebo) | Combined CABG and peri-adventitial delivery | 10 or 100 µg in heparin-alginate microcapsules |
| Unger et al 2000[40] | FGF-2 | Phase I placebo-controlled | 25 (8 placebo) | Intracoronary | 3–100 µg/kg |
| Laham et al 2000[41] | FGF-2 | Phase I | 52 | Intracoronary | 0.33–48 µg/kg |
| Udelson et al 2000[42] | FGF-2 | Phase I | 59 | Intracoronary (n = 45) Intravenous (n = 14) | 0.33–48 µg/kg |
| Chronos 2000[43] | FGF-2 | Phase II placebo-controlled | 337 | Intracoronary | 0.3, 3.0 or 30 µg |
| **Peripheral vascular disease** | | | | | |
| ***VEGF*** | | | | | |
| Isner et al 1996[24] Isner 1998[23] | Plasmid VEGF 165 | Phase I | 8 | Intra-arterial local delivery catheter | 100–2000 µg |
| Baumgartner et al 1998[14] Isner et al 1998[27] Baumgartner 2000[26] | Plasmid VEGF 165 | Phase I | 50 | Intramuscular lower extremity | 100–4000 µg |
| ***FGF*** | | | | | |
| Lazarous et al 2000[44] | FGF-2 | Phase I placebo-controlled | 19 (6 placebo) | Intra-arterial | 10 or 30 µg/kg, or two daily 30 µg/kg doses |
| Lederman et al 2001[45] | FGF-2 | Phase II placebo-controlled | 190 (63 placebo) | Intra-arterial infusion | 30 µg/kg on day 1 ± on day 30 |

**Table 1** Clinical therapeutic angiogenesis trials

significant increase in adverse events. The primary end-point was exercise treadmill time at day 60. There was a notable improvement in all three groups, including the placebo group, at 60 days, in exercise time, angina class, as well as quality of life compared to baseline values. However, compared with the placebo group, there was no improvement in the primary end-point. While these early results were disappointing, subsequent findings suggest that the placebo effect, which was prominent at 60 days, subsequently diminished, whereas the improvements in the high dose group were maintained or increased[19,20]. At 120 days, there was improvement in angina class in the high dose group in comparison with the placebo group ($P = 0.04$), and a trend for improvement in exercise time ($P = 0.17$). While this trial was not a definitive phase 3 trial of efficacy, it was nevertheless important because of the larger number of patients enrolled and because it was double-blind, randomized and placebo-controlled. It demonstrated the critical importance of careful placebo controls in studies of angiogenesis The explanation for the absence of clear benefit may lie in methodological issues, the marked placebo effect, a more delayed time-course than could be identified in this short-term study, or simply may reflect an inadequate effect on angiogenesis and collateral development.

## VEGF plasmid DNA therapy

Clinical trials of VEGF using direct injection of plasmid VEGF DNA were stimulated by a series of illustrative animal studies. After demonstration of the angiogenic potential of VEGF protein in preclinical studies, similar studies were performed using plasmid DNA. An initial animal study utilized specialized catheters to achieve localized, intra-arterial delivery[21]. However, subsequent studies demonstrated that intramuscular injection, which is potentially simpler to achieve and does not require arterial cannulation, could also result in functional effects in spite of low efficiency of transduction[22].

Clinical trials were performed in patients with peripheral vascular disease using catheter-based direct intra-arterial delivery including a dose finding study in 8 patients using Plasmid VEGF$_{165}$ delivered with the hydrogel-coated balloon[23]. Although there were no placebo controls, there were improvements in symptoms and blood flow at the high dose, as well as a transient telangiectasia and peripheral oedema in one patient at the highest dose[24]. Similarly, in the coronary circulation catheter-based techniques for local gene delivery using a perfusion catheter were utilized to deliver plasmid VEGF/liposome which demonstrated feasibility and safety, although efficacy of therapeutic angiogenesis was not evaluated[25].

The demonstration of successful skeletal muscle VEGF gene transfer in animal studies suggested that intra-arterial delivery might not be required and led to clinical trials of intramuscular injection of plasmid $VEGF_{165}$ in patients with peripheral vascular disease in a total of 50 patients[26]. Preliminary reports describing 9 patients with critical limb ischaemia[14] and 6 patients with Buerger's disease[27] both demonstrated transgene expression. In addition, some patients in these studies, which did not include placebo controls, did have functional improvement including improved blood flow, healing of ulcers and improved symptoms, particularly in patients with Buerger's disease. These preliminary feasibility studies, as well as a promising preliminary report of 13 patients receiving plasmid VEGF-2 in a placebo-controlled trial[28], have given rise to the initiation of clinical trials with intramuscular plasmid DNA injection.

The demonstration of possible clinical benefits with intramuscular injection for peripheral vascular disease also led to trials of intra-myocardial VEGF gene transfer. Initially, intramyocardial injection could only be achieved intra-operatively either at the time of bypass surgery or through direct injection through a thoracotomy. A series of 30 patients were treated with intramyocardial plasmid $VEGF_{165}$ as sole therapy (*i.e.* without concomitant CABG) in a dose escalation trial[29–32]. Serum VEGF levels increased, confirming successful gene transfer. There were also improvements in angina, exercise time, and nuclear perfusion studies compared to baseline.

Studies involving surgical intramyocardial injections are limited by the morbidity of concomitant surgery, the inability to enroll patients in a placebo arm of a trial of surgical therapy, and the confounding effects of concomitant bypass grafting in combination trials. The development of percutaneous techniques for intramyocardial injection has enabled the initiation of placebo-controlled trials for coronary ischaemia and also may enable repeat dosing[31].

## VEGF adenoviral vector gene therapy

In addition to trials of VEGF protein, plasmid $VEGF_{165}$ or VEGF-2[33], trials of gene transfer using an adenoviral vector are also underway. An adenoviral $VEGF_{121}$ vector was utilized in a dose escalation trial in 21 patients (15 patients underwent concomitant coronary bypass grafting, and 6 patients received sole therapy with adenoviral $VEGF_{121}$ through a mini-thoracotomy or thorocoscopy), further demonstrating the feasibility of intramyocardial angiogenic therapy[34,35]. There was no evident cardiac or systemic toxicity. In the sole therapy arm, all patients had improved angina, and there were trends for improvement in angiographic collaterals, stress wall motion, reversible ischaemia and exercise parameters. A randomized, double-blind, placebo-controlled phase 2 trial of intramuscular adenoviral VEGF$_{121}$ is now underway in patients with claudication.

## FGF protein therapy for myocardial ischaemia

FGF-2 and to a lesser extent FGF-1 have been extensively studied in animal models of both peripheral and myocardial ischaemia. Several different routes of administration including intra-arterial, intravenous, intramuscular, perivascular and subcutaneous routes have been utilized. Reviews of the preclinical data have been published[9] and, based on promising preclinical data in animal models of ischaemia, clinical trials of both protein and gene therapy with FGFs have been undertaken.

Schumacher and colleagues[36,37] published the first placebo-controlled therapeutic angiogenesis trial. They administered FGF-1 protein at the time of bypass surgery as an intramyocardial injection distal to the site of the LAD anastomosis in 40 patients undergoing LIMA grafting of the LAD where an additional stenosis was present in the distal LAD or one of the diagonals. Initial evaluation by digital subtraction angiography at 3 months demonstrated a significant increase in capillary density, as well as collateral filling of non-bypassed vessels in the treated patients, but not in the control patients. While the initial report did not evaluate the functional benefit of this therapy, subsequent follow-up at 3 years in 31 of the original 40 patients demonstrated an improvement in ejection fraction and NYHA functional class.

FGF-2 has also been utilized as an adjunct to bypass surgery. Sellke and colleagues[38] performed a small study in 8 patients in whom FGF-2 was administered epicardially in a slow-release formulation within heparin alginate beads placed epicardially at the time of CABG in areas of incomplete revascularization. In this study, as well as in an expanded series[39] of 24 patients (which included 8 controls) there was evidence of improved perfusion by magnetic resonance imaging as well as by nuclear perfusion imaging, particularly at the highest dose. These studies are nevertheless limited by the confounding effect of the concomitant bypass surgery as well as the small number of patients enrolled.

FGF-2 protein has also been delivered as an intracoronary infusion. Unger and colleagues[40] performed a phase 1 study of intracoronary FGF-2 infusion in 25 patients with stable angina which included 8 placebo-treated patients. Hypotension, bradycardia, and transient mild thrombocytopenia and proteinuria were noted in this dose ranging study. A larger phase I dose-finding study by Laham and colleagues[41], in 52 patients with ischaemia who were not amenable to revascularization, demonstrated that intracoronary FGF-2 was safe and well-tolerated up to a dose of 36 µg/kg. While this was a patient population at high risk for cardiac and other adverse events, there was also dose-related hypotension and proteinuria in 4 patients. Follow-up evaluation demonstrated improvements in angina, measures of quality of life, exercise tolerance and ejection fraction, as well as a reduction in the extent of ischaemia by magnetic resonance imaging. Nuclear perfusion studies also suggested improvement after FGF-2 in some measures including a reduction in segmental reversible ischaemia at 29, 57 and 180 days, and improved rest perfusion in patients that had areas of mild or moderate (but not severe) resting hypoperfusion[42]. While the dose ranging nature of these trials, the small size and the lack of a blinded placebo group limited the strength of any conclusions about efficacy, they nevertheless provided the groundwork for a subsequent larger trial.

Preliminary results of a phase II randomized, double-blind, placebo-controlled trial of intracoronary FGF-2 (the FIRST study) have recently been presented[43]. In this trial, 337 patients with angina, who were ineligible for angioplasty or CABG were randomized to receive either placebo or one of three doses of FGF-2 (0.3, 3.0 or 30 mcg/kg) by a single intracoronary infusion. The primary end-point was exercise capacity evaluated at 90 days. There was a 65 s improvement in patients receiving one of the FGF doses; however, there was a 45 s improvement in the placebo group and this difference was not significant. In subgroups, including older patients and patients with more baseline angina, there were significant differences in exercise time as well as in angina class Nevertheless, in spite of promising preclinical and preliminary clinical data, the FIRST trial, like the VIVA trial of VEGF which also utilized recombinant protein, demonstrated a significant placebo effect and no significant difference in the primary endpoint.

## FGF protein therapy for peripheral vascular disease

FGF-2 has also been administered to patients with peripheral vascular disease. Lazarous and colleagues[44] performed a phase 1 double-blind, placebo-controlled trial in 19 patients with claudication in which FGF-2 was administered as an intra-arterial infusion. They reported significantly increased blood flow assessed by plethysmography, compared with baseline blood flow, as well as a decrease in claudication at the highest dose of 30 µg/kg.

Preliminary results of a larger double-blind, placebo-controlled trial in patients with claudication have recently been presented[45]. In the TRAFFIC trial (therapeutic angiogenesis with FGF-2 for intermittent claudication), 190 patients with claudication were randomized to receive either one or two doses of intra-arterial FGF-2 protein (30 µg/kg) given 30 days apart. The primary end-point was the change in peak walking time at day 90. There was an acceptable safety profile including a low incidence of hypotension and proteinuria. At 90 days, there was a 14% increase in the peak walking time in the placebo group, while there was a 34% increase in the peak walking time in the single dose group, ($P = 0.026$) and a 20% increase in the double-dose group ($P = $ NS). This clinical improvement in the single-dose group was supported by measurement of ankle-brachial index, and by improvement in claudication severity. Although not a definitive phase 3 trial, this trial of intra-arterial protein therapy for claudication is the first phase 2 therapeutic angiogenesis trial to demonstrate a positive result in the primary endpoint.

## Conclusions

The identification of potent angiogenic proteins, the promising preclinical data and the development of methods of delivery suggested that therapeutic angiogenesis might be achievable. Approaches that were tested in preclinical studies have now been evaluated in small and often uncontrolled human feasibility studies. The limited clinical data now available contain evidence suggesting that functional benefit may be obtained in patients with symptomatic ischaemia. While the two phase 2 trials, the VIVA trial and the FIRST trial, did not demonstrate significant improvement in their primary end-points, a third, the TRAFFIC, trial has demonstrated improvement with one of two dosing regimens. In addition, suggestive, albeit not universally significant, benefits were seen in all three, and the safety data have been reassuring. Nevertheless, the number of questions that remain is substantial. Which patients should be treated? Which of the ever increasing number of angiogenic growth factors should be used? Or, will it require combinations of growth factors? Which method of delivery and which dosing regimen is best? Will functional collaterals be formed, or merely non-functioning capillary networks? Can exogenously administered growth factors or even gene transfer therapies succeed in a complex clinical setting where the adaptive responses to ischaemia have failed? There is certainly reason for optimism given the encouraging preliminary data, but there is also ample room for scepticism. The ideal angiogenic agent will be simple to administer, will be effective, and will have limited side effects. However, clinical trials that convincingly demonstrate the efficacy of any single approach are needed, before the differing approaches can be compared.

## References

1   Charney R, Cohen M. The role of the coronary collateral circulation in limiting myocardial ischemia and infarct size. *Am Heart J* 1993; **126**: 937–45
2   Rentrop KP, Cohen M, Blanke H, Phillips RA. Changes in collateral channel filling immediately after controlled coronary artery occlusion by an angioplasty balloon in human subjects. *J Am Coll Cardiol* 1985; **5**: 587

3    Goncalves LM. Angiogenic growth factors: potential new treatment for acute myocardial infarction. *Cardiovasc Res* 2000; **45**: 294–302

4    Schaper W, Ito WD. Molecular mechanisms of coronary collateral vessel growth. *Circ Res* 1996; **79**: 911–9

5    Schaper W, Schaper J. *Collateral Circulation*. Norwell, MA: Kluwer, 1993

6    Ferrara N. Vascular endothelial growth factor: molecular and biological aspects. *Curr Top Microbiol Immunol* 1999; **237**: 1–30

7    Shweiki D, Itin A, Soffer D, Keshet E. Vascular endothelial growth factor induced by hypoxia may mediate hypoxia-initiated angiogenesis. *Nature* 1992; **359**: 843–5

8    Slavin J. Fibroblast growth factors: at the heart of angiogenesis. *Cell Biol Int* 1995; **19**: 431–44

9    Simons M, Laham RJ. Therapeutic angiogenesis in myocardial ischemia. In: Ware JA, Simons M. (eds) *Angiogenesis and Cardiovascular Disease*. New York: Oxford University Press, 1999

10   Sellke FW, Wang SY, Stamler A *et al*. Enhanced microvascular relaxations to VEGF and bFGF in chronically ischemic porcine myocardium. *Am J Physiol* 1996; **271**: H713–20

11   Kornowski R, Fuchs S, Leon MB, Epstein SE. Delivery strategies to achieve therapeutic myocardial angiogenesis. *Circulation* 2000; **101**: 454–8

12   Takeshita S, Ishiki T, Sato T. Increased expression of direct gene transfer into skeletal muscles observed after acute ischemic injury in rats. *Lab Invest* 1996; **74**: 1061–5

13   Losordo DW, Pickering JG, Takeshita S *et al*. Use of the rabbit ear artery to serially assess foreign protein secretion after site specific arterial gene transfer *in vivo*: evidence that anatomic identification of successful gene transfer may underestimate the potential magnitude of transgene expression. *Circulation* 1994; **89**: 785–92

14   Baumgartner I, Pieczek A, Manor O *et al* Constitutive expression of phVEGF165 after intramuscular gene transfer promotes collateral vessel development in patients with critical limb ischemia. *Circulation* 1998; **97**: 1114–23

15   Henry TD, Abraham JA. Review of preclinical and clinical results with vascular endothelial growth factors for therapeutic angiogenesis. *Curr Intervent Cardiol* 2000; **2**: 228–41

16   Hendel RC, Henry TD, Rocha-Singh K *et al*. Effect of intracoronary recombinant human vascular endothelial growth factor (rhVEGF) on myocardial perfusion: evidence for a dose-dependent effect. *Circulation* 2000; **101**: 118–21

17   Gibson CM, Laham R, Giordano FJ *et al*. Magnitude and location of new angiographically apparent coronary collaterals following intravenous VEGF administration. *J Am Coll Cardiol* 1999; **33**: 384A

18   Henry T, Annex B, Azrin M *et al*. Double blind placebo controlled trial of recombinant human vascular endothelial growth factor – the VIVA trial. *J Am Coll Cardiol* 1999; **33**: 384A

19   Henry TD, Annex BH, Azrin MA *et al*. Final results of the VIVA trial of rhVEGF for human therapeutic angiogenesis. *Circulation* 1999; **100**: I-476

20   Henry T, McKendall GR, Azrin MA *et al*. Viva trial: one year follow up. *Circulation* 2000; **102**: II-129

21   Riessen R, Rahimizadeh H, Blessing B *et al*. Arterial gene transfer using pure DNA applied directly to a hydrogel-coated angioplasty balloon. *Hum Gene Ther* 1993; **4**: 749–58

22   Takeshita S, Weir L, Chen D *et al*. Therapeutic angiogenesis following arterial gene transfer of vascular endothelial growth factor in a rabbit model of hindlimb ischemia. *Biochem Biophys Res Commun* 1996; **227**: 628–35

23   Isner JM. Arterial gene transfer of naked DNA for therapeutic angiogenesis: early clinical results. *Adv Drug Delivery Rev* 1998; **30**: 185–97

24   Isner JM, Pieczek A, Schainfeld R *et al*. Clinical evidence of angiogenesis following arterial gene transfer of phVEGF165 in patient with ischemic limb. *Lancet* 1998; **348**: 370–4

25   Laitinen M, Hartikainen J, Hiltunen MO *et al*. Catheter-mediated vascular endothelial growth factor gene transfer to human coronary arteries after angioplasty. *Hum Gene Ther* 2000; **11**: 263–70

26   Baumgartner I, Rauh G, Pieczek A *et al*. Lower-extremity edema associated with gene transfer of naked DNA encoding vascular endothelial growth factor. *Ann Intern Med* 2000; **132**: 880–4

27   Isner JM, Baumgartner I, Rauh G *et al*. Treatment of thromboangitis obliterans (Buerger's disease) by intramuscular gene transfer of vascular endothelial growth factor: preliminary clinical results. *J Vasc Surg* 1998; **28**: 964–73

28  Rauh G, Gravereaux E, Pieczek A *et al.* Assessment of safety and efficiency of intramuscular gene therapy VEGF-2 in patients with critical limb ischemia. *Circulation* 1999; **100**: I-770

29  Losordo DW, Vale PR, Symes JF *et al.* Gene therapy for myocardial angiogenesis: initial clinical results with direct myocardial injection of phVEGF165 as sole therapy for myocardial ischemia. *Circulation* 1998; **98**: 2800–4

30  Symes JF, Losordo DW, Vale PR *et al.* Gene therapy with vascular endothelial growth factor for inoperable coronary artery disease. *Ann Thorac Surg* 1999; **68**: 830–7

31  Vale PR, Losordo DW, Milliken CE *et al.* Left ventricular electromechanical mapping to assess efficacy of phVEGF165 gene transfer for therapeutic angiogenesis in chronic myocardial ischemia. *Circulation* 2000; **102**: 965–74

32  Lathi KG, Vale PR, Losordo DW *et al.* Gene therapy with vascular endothelial growth factor for inoperable coronary artery disease: anesthetic management and results. *Anesth Analg* 2001; **92**: 19–25

33  Hendel RC, Vale PR, Losordo DW *et al.* The effects of VEGF-2 gene therapy on rest and stress myocardial perfusion: results of serial SPECT imaging. *Circulation* 2000; **102**: II-769

34  Rosengart TK. Six-month assessment of a phase I trial of angiogenic gene therapy for the treatment of coronary artery disease using direct intramyocardial administration of an adenovirus vector expressing the $VEGF_{121}$ cDNA. *Ann Surg* 1999; **230**: 466–70

35  Rosengart TK, Lee LY, Patel SR *et al.* Angiogenesis gene therapy: phase I assessment of direct intramyocardial administration of an adenovirus vector expressing $VEGF_{121}$ cDNA to individuals with clinically significant severe coronary artery disease. *Circulation* 1999; **100**: 468–74

36  Schumacher B, Pecher P, von Specht BU *et al.* Induction of neoangiogenesis in ischemic myocardium by human growth factors. *Circulation* 1998; **97**: 645–50

37  Pecher P, Schumacher BA. Angiogenesis in ischemic human myocardium: clinical results after 3 years. *Ann Thorac Surg* 2000; **69**: 1414–9

38  Selke FW, Laham RJ, Edelman ER *et al.* Therapeutic angiogenesis with basic fibroblast growth factor. *Ann Thorac Surg* 1998; **65**: 1540–4

39  Laham RJ, Selke FW, Edelman ER *et al.* Local perivascular delivery of basic fibroblast growth factor in patients undergoing coronary bypass surgery. *Circulation* 1999; **100**: 1865–71

40  Unger EF, Goncalves L, Epstein SE *et al.* Effects of a single intracoronary injection of basic fibroblast growth factor in stable angina pectoris. *Am J Cardiol* 2000; **85**: 1414–9

41  Laham RJ, Chronos NA, Pike M *et al.* Intracoronary basic fibroblast growth factor (FGF-2) in patients with severe ischemic heart disease: results of a phase I open-label dose escalation study. *J Am Coll Cardiol* 2000; **36**: 2132–9

42  Udelson JE, Dilsizian V, Laham RJ *et al.* Therapeutic angiogenesis with recombinant fibroblast growth factor-2 improves stress and rest myocardial perfusion abnormalities in patients with severe symptomatic chronic coronary artery disease. *Circulation* 2000; **102**: 1605–10

43  Chronos N. *FIRST, FGF-2 Initiating Revascularization Support Trial.* Meeting of the American College of Cardiology, Anaheim, CA, USA, March 2000

44  Lazarous DF, Unger EF, Epstein SE *et al.* Basic fibroblast growth factor in patients with intermittent claudication: results of a phase I trial. *J Am Coll Cardiol* 2000; **36**: 1239–44

45  Lederman R. American Heart Association Scientific Conference on *Therapeutic Angiogenesis and Myocardial Laser Revascularization*, Santa Fe, NM, USA, January 2001

# Stent development and local drug delivery

**E Regar, G Sianos** and **P W Serruys**

*Department of Cardiology, Thoraxcentre, Erasmus Medical Centre Rotterdam, The Netherlands*

Stent implantation has become the new standard angioplasty procedure. In-stent re-stenosis remains the major limitation of coronary stenting. Re-stenosis is related to patient-, lesion- and procedure-specific factors.

Patient-specific factors can not be influenced to any extent. Procedure-specific factors are affected by implantation technique and stent characteristics. Design and material influence vascular injury and humoral and cellular response. Radiation has been shown to have inhibitory effects on smooth muscle cell growth and neo-intima formation, but in clinical trials the outcome has been hampered by re-stenosis at the edges of the radioactive stent ('candy wrapper').

New approaches target pharmacological modulation of local vascular biology by local administration of drugs. This allows for drug application at the precise site and time of vessel injury. Systemic release is minimal and this may reduce the risk of toxicity. The drug and the delivery vehicle must fulfil pharmacological, pharmacokinetic and mechanical requirements and the application of eluting degradable matrices seems to be a possible solution. Numerous pharmacological agents with antiproliferative properties are currently under clinical investigation, *e.g.* actinomycin D, rapamycin or paclitaxel. Another approach is for stents to be made of biodegradable materials as an alternative to metallic stents. Their potential long-term complications, such as in-stent re-stenosis and the inaccessibility of the lesion site for surgical revascularization, needs to be assessed.

Current investigational devices and the line of (pre)clinical investigation are discussed in detail. Currently, there is little experimental, and only preliminary clinical, understanding of the acute and long-term effects of drug-eluting or biodegradable stents in coronary arteries. The clinical benefit of these approaches still has to be proven.

Correspondence to:
Prof. P W Serruys,
Thoraxcentre (Bd 406),
Erasmus Medical Centre
Rotterdam,
Dr Molewaterplein 40,
3015 GD Rotterdam,
The Netherlands

Over the last decade, coronary stents have revolutionized the field of interventional cardiology. Stent implantation has become the new standard angioplasty procedure[1-3]. This popularity is mainly for two reasons: (i) the unique capability to master a major complication of balloon angioplasty – (sub)acute vessel closure; and (ii) a superior long-term outcome in comparison to balloon angioplasty[4-8]. The high reliability of the acute angioplasty result after stenting allowed for a dramatic expansion in the indication for catheter-based intervention (ostial lesions[9], bifurcation lesions[10,11], left main lesions[12,13], multiple lesions[14]).

In the early phase, device technology was directed toward improving the accessibility of lesions, *e.g.* in tortuous, small and/or calcified vessels. The advances included premounted stents, reduced crossing profile and improved flexibility. Modifications in stent design such as 'rotating' and 'locking' mechanisms afforded them high flexibility when unexpanded and remarkable radial strength when expanded. Further development included specifically configured stents for distinct indications, such as bifurcation lesions, lesions with side branch take-off, aneurysms and vessel rupture.

## The problem: re-stenosis

As most acute aspects of stenting are resolved, the long-term outcome becomes more and more the focus of attention. In-stent re-stenosis remains for several reasons the major limitation of coronary stenting. The absolute number of in-stent re-stenotic lesions is increasing in parallel with the steadily increasing number of stenting procedures and with the complexity of culprit lesions. The treatment of in-stent re-stenosis is, despite progresses in radiation therapy, technically challenging and costly. In subsets of lesions (such as small vessel size and diffuse disease), an anticipated high risk for re-stenosis may prevent the use of stents.

Re-stenosis is considered as a local vascular manifestation of the general biological response to injury. Catheter-induced injury consists of denudation of the intima and stretching of the media. The wound-healing reaction consists in an inflammatory phase, a granulation phase and a remodelling phase. The inflammatory phase is characterized by platelets and growth factor activation, the granulation phase by smooth muscle cell and fibroblast migration and proliferation into the injured area, the remodelling phase by proteoglycan and collagen synthesis, which replaces early fibronectin as major component of extracellular matrix[15]. Current concepts describe three mechanisms of the re-stenotic process: early elastic recoil, late vessel remodelling and neo-intimal growth[16,17]. Coronary stents provide mechanical scaffolding that virtually eliminates recoil and remodelling[18]. However, neo-intimal growth continues to be a major problem.

Neo-intimal proliferation occurs principally, but not exclusively, at the site of the primary lesion within the first 6 months after stent implantation. Neo-intima is basically an accumulation of smooth muscle cells within a proteoglycan matrix that narrows the previously enlarged lumen. Neo-intima formation is triggered by a cascade of cellular and molecular events including platelet activation, leukocyte infiltration, smooth muscle cell expansion, extracellular matrix elaboration and re-endothelialization.

In the clinical setting, neo-intimal formation and in-stent re-stenosis are related to patient-specific factors such as genetic predisposition or diabetes mellitus[19], to lesion-specific factors such as vessel calibre[20], lesion length or plaque burden [21] and to procedure-specific factors such as extent of vessel damage, residual dissections[22], number of stents, minimal stent diameter or minimal stent area[23].

Patient-specific factors can not be influenced to any extent. Attempts to modulate lesion-specific factors by pharmacological therapy have not been not successful so far[24,25]. Procedure-specific factors may be favourably affected by the stent implantation technique and stent characteristics[26].

## The solution: the ideal stent?

From the interventionist's technical point of view, the ideal stent should have at least the following features:
- Reach any location within the coronary artery system
- Have a low profile, high trackability and flexibility
- Allow for precise placement with good visibility
- Guarantee predictable expansion with minimal foreshortening
- Provide equally distributed radial strength, be rigid and have many, thick struts
- Prevent plaque protrusion having many struts with small spaces between struts
- Allow for side-branch access having few struts with large spaces between struts
- Reduce acute thrombotic and inflammatory vessel response, *i.e.* have few, thin struts
- Allow wound healing but inhibit exaggerated neo-intimal growth. It should be thromboresistant and have high hydrodynamic compatibility
- Guarantee vessel accessibility for further intervention (PCR, bypass grafting) and thus possibly disappear after 6 months.

Unfortunately, all these requirements on stent characteristics are mutually incompatible.

## The ideal stent: small steps towards a big goal

The focus of stent development in the first decade of stenting was on optimization of stent characteristics. Systematic investigations were performed to gain insights into mechanisms of stent action and vessel biology. This resulted in a huge variety of stents, differing in design, material, surface, radioactivity and coatings[27].

## Design

Stent design varies in the geometry (number of intersections and interstrut area), in the strut configuration and the metal-to-artery ratio. These are the major determinants of stent profile, flexibility, radial strength and (elastic) expansion characteristics.

Presently, more than 55 stents are available (12 with FDA-approval) which are manufactured by more than 30 companies. They use two different expansion principles (balloon-expansion and self-expansion) and can be categorized in five basic design types: tubular, ring, multi-design, coil, and mesh.

The physical properties affect vascular injury and response. The different stent designs show a considerable range of the elastic moduli[28] which affect stent expansion properties as late as 8 weeks after deployment[29]. Reduction of strut–strut intersections can reduce the vascular injury score, thrombosis and neo-intimal hyperplasia[30]. Non-uniform stent expansion increases vascular injury and in-stent re-stenosis[31].

## Material and surface (texture)

Stent materials and surface are relevant to in-stent re-stenosis. Surface characteristics can be modulated by (electromechanical) polishing, ion implantation or coating. Suitable stent materials are metals, metal-alloys or polymers. Chemistry, charge, and texture[32] modulate humoral and

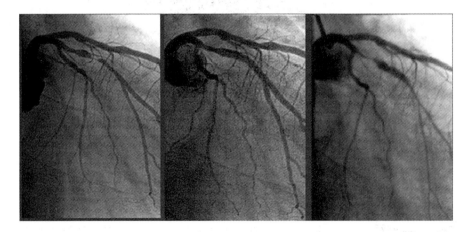

**Fig. 1** Coronary angiogram of a the left coronary artery, showing a lesion of the circumflex artery pre-intervention (left), immediately after radioactive stent implantation (mid) and at 6-months' follow-up (right). At 6 months, there is significant narrowing at the proximal and at the distal edge of the radioactive stent ('candy wrapper' effect), while the lumen within the stent shows only minimal neo-intimal growths.

**Table 1** Results of [$^{32}$P]-radioactive stents at 6-month follow-up

| Study | Patients (n) | Stent activity (μCi) | Lesion length (mm) | Restenosis rate | TLR |
|---|---|---|---|---|---|
| IRIS 1A | 32 | 0.5–1.0 | <15 | 31 | 21 |
| IRIS 1B | 25 | 0.75–1.5 | <15 | 50 | 32 |
| IRIS Heidelberg | 11 | 1.5–3.0 | <15 | 54 | N/A |
| IRIS Rotterdam | 26 | 0.75–1.5 | <28 | 17 | 12 |
| [$^{32}$P]-Dose response Rotterdam | 40 | 6.0–12 | <28 | 44 | 25 |
| [$^{32}$P]-Dose Response Milan | 23 | 0.75–3.0 | <28 | 52 | 52 |
| | 29 | 3.0–6.0 | | 41 | 41 |
| | 30 | 6.0–12 | | 50 | 50 |
| | 40 | 12–21 | | 30 | 30 |

N/A, not available; TLR, target lesion revascularization.

cellular vessel response (plasma proteins, inflammatory and proliferative mediators, platelet and leukocyte activation). Copper is more frequently associated with subacute thrombosis than steel[33].

## Radioactivity

Another possible way to modify the physical properties is the introduction of radioactivity[34,35]. Radiation has proven inhibitory effects on smooth muscle cell growth and neo-intima formation[36]. However, clinical trials utilizing radioactive stents have been disappointing. Despite effective prevention of neo-intimal growth with the stent, clinical and angiographic outcomes have been hampered by re-stenosis at the edges of the radioactive stent; termed the 'candy wrapper' effect (Fig. 1)[37]. This unfavourable phenomenon occurred irrespective of the stent design (cold end, hot end) or the dose rate (high activity *versus* low activity; Table 1).

## Coating

Coating categories are various (Table 2). Stent coatings can dramatically reduce protein deposition and platelet adhesion in experimental settings (Fig. 2)[38]. However, polymers have shown conflicting results in the experimental setting[39–41] with some provoking a severe tissue response[42].

**Table 2** Stent coating categories

| | |
|---|---|
| Inorganic/ceramic materials | *Gold, si-carbide, diamond-like carbon, biogold* |
| Synthetic and biological polymers | *Phosphorylcholine, polyurethane, polyester, polylactic acid, cellulose* |
| Human polymers | *Chondroitin sulphate, hyaluronic acid, fibrin* |
| Immobilized drugs | *Heparin, paclitaxel, abciximab, P-15 (peptide)* |
| Membrane-covered | *PTFE, autologous vein and artery* |
| Eluting, degradable matrices | |

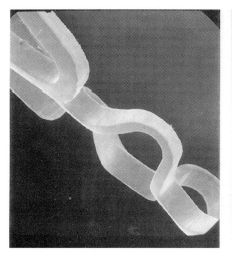
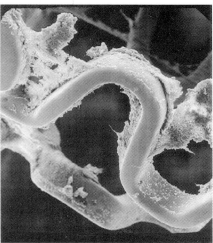

**Fig. 2** SEM of a heparin coated (left) and a non-coated stent.

A number of other coatings like inert polymer[30], phosphorylcholine[43,44] or heparin[45-47], demonstrated a reduction in (sub)acute stent thrombosis rate and possible effects on neo-intimal hyperplasia[48].

In clinical practice, however, the acute beneficial effect on stent thrombosis is of minor relevance as already modern uncoated stents show a very low (sub)acute thrombosis rate. Furthermore, the acute beneficial effect did not result in a substantial decrease in in-stent re-stenosis[49]. In response to this, the interest in coatings has shifted towards considering coatings as vehicles for local drug delivery. So far, phosphorylcholine is the only clinically-available, polymer coated stent (Fig. 3)[50].

## A big step: local drug delivery?

New approaches target not only the stent characteristics but also the pharmacological modulation of the local vascular biology. A proposed

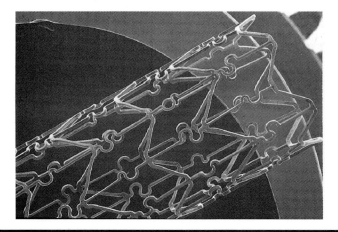

**Fig. 3** Phosphoryl-choline-coated stent (BiodivYsioTMTM SV stent; Biocompatibles Ltd, Surrey, UK).

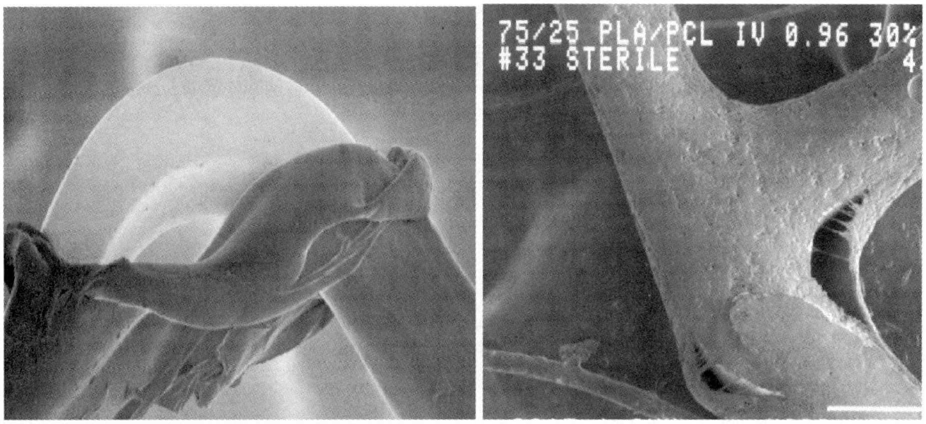

**Fig. 4** SEM of a coated stent, showing the effect of stent expansion (left) and the effect of sterilization (right) on the coating.

explanation for the repeated failure of clinical drug studies has been that agents given systemically cannot reach sufficient levels in injured arteries to impact significantly on the re-stenotic process. Local administration of drugs offers advantages. The active drug is applied to the vessel at the precise site and at the time of vessel injury. Local drug delivery might be able to achieve higher tissue concentrations of the drug. No additional materials or procedures are required. Systemic release is minimal and may reduce the risk of remote or systemic toxicity.

## Candidate delivery vehicles

The delivery vehicle must fulfil pharmacological, pharmacokinetic and mechanical requirements. The release of the drug into the vessel must take place in a manner that is consistent with the drug's mode of action. Drug-release must be in predictable and controllable concentrations and within a known time span. The delivery vehicle must be suitable for sterilisation. It must follow the stent changes of configuration during stent expansion and resist mechanical injury caused by the implantation balloon. An example of possible deleterious effects of stent expansion and sterilisation on the coating is given in Figure 4. Currently, these problems are controlled, guaranteeing intact coating during clinical application (Fig. 5). The application of eluting, degradable matrices seems to be a possible solution. An overview of delivery vehicles for drug eluting systems is given in Table 3.

## Candidate drugs

The drug should be able to inhibit the multiple components of the complex re-stenosis process. Uncontrolled neo-intima tissue accumulations shows

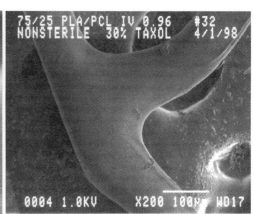

**Fig. 5** SEM of a contemporary coated and drug loaded stent. The integrity of the coating is not affected by stent expansion or sterilization.

**Table 3** Overview of drug delivery vehicles

| | |
|---|---|
| * | Polyvinyl pyrolidone/cellulose esters |
| * | Polyvinyl pyrolidone/polyurethane |
| * | Polymethylidene maloleate |
| * | Polylactide/glycoloide co-polymers |
| * | Polyethylene glycol co-polymers |
| * | Polyethylene vinyl alcohol |
| * | Polydimethylsiloxane (silicone rubber) |

some parallels to tumour growths; thus, the use of anti-tumour strategies seems to be a logical choice. Numerous pharmacological agents with antiproliferative properties have been tested for their potential to inhibit re-stenosis with mostly disappointing results[51]. Antimitotic compounds (like methotrexate and colchicine) have failed to inhibit smooth muscle cell proliferation and intimal thickening[52,53]. In contrast, other agents such as angiopeptin[54], GP IIb/IIIa inhibitors or steroids[55] [56] have shown a promising inhibitory effect on neo-intimal proliferation. Potential candidates for local drug delivery are given in Table 4. The following drugs are now being tested in randomized clinical trials.

**Table 4** Potential candidates for drug elution

| | |
|---|---|
| Antineoplastic | Dexamethasone |
| Paclitaxel (Taxol™) | Tacrolimus (FK506) |
| Taxol derivative (QP-2) | |
| Actinomycin D | Collagen synthetase inhibitor |
| Vincristine | Halofuginone |
| | Propyl hydroxylase |
| Antithrombins | C-proteinase inhibitor |
| Hirudin and iloprost | Metalloproteinase inhibitor |
| Heparin | |
| | AngiopeptinV |
| Immunosuppressants | |
| Sirolimus (Rapamycin™) | VEGF |
| Tranilast | |

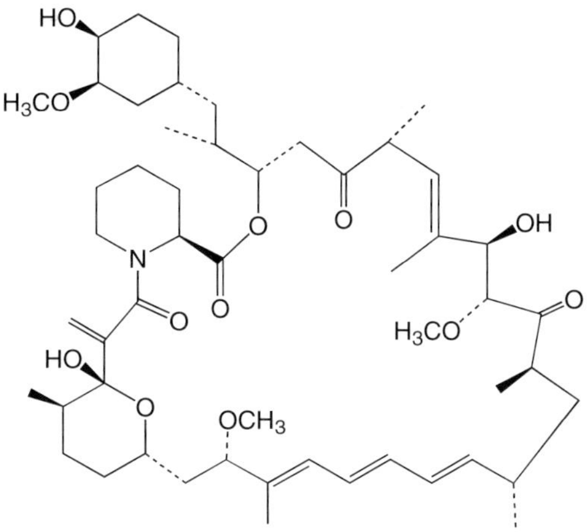

Fig. 6 Chemical structure of rapamycin (Sirolimus).

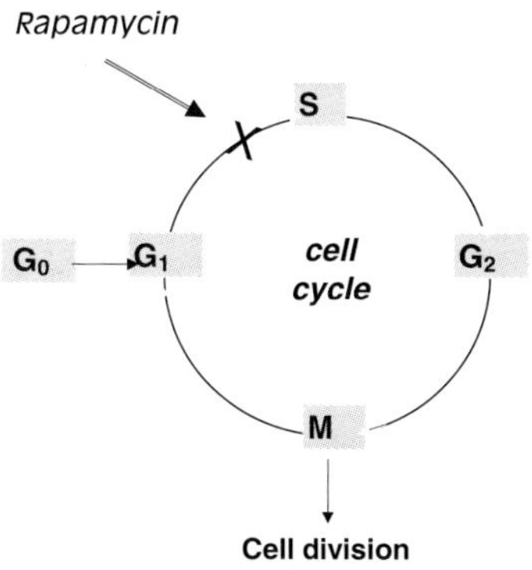

Fig. 7 Schematic of the mechanism of action of rapamycin within the cell cycle.

## Actinomycin D (Cosmegen®)

Actinomycin D has been marketed world-wide since the 1960s. It is an antibiotic used for its antiproliferative properties in the treatment of various malignant neoplasmas (*e.g.* Wilms tumour, sarcomas, carcinoma of testis and uterus). It inhibits the proliferation of cells. Actinomycin D ($C_{62}H_{86}N_{12}O_{16}$) forms, via deoxyguanosine residues, a stable complex with double-stranded DNA and inhibits DNA-primed RNA synthesis.

## Rapamycin (Sirolimus; Rapamune®)

Rapamune® is an FDA approved drug for the prophylaxis of renal transplant rejection in use since 1999. It is a naturally occurring macrocyclic lactone (Fig. 6) which is highly effective in preventing the onset and severity of disease in several animal models of autoimmune disease, such as insulin-dependent diabetes mellitus, systemic lupus erythematosus and arthritis.

The class of macrocyclic immunosuppressive agents (rapamycin, cyclosporin A, tacrolimus) bind to specific cytosolic proteins called immunophilins to gain their immunosuppressive activity. Rapamycin blocks G1 to S cell cycle progression (Fig. 7) by interacting with a specific target protein (mTOR, mammalian target of rapamycin) and inhibiting its activation. The inhibition of mTOR suppresses cytokine-driven (IL-2, IL-4, IL-7 and IL-15) T-cell proliferation.

mTOR is a key regulatory kinase and its inhibition has several important effects including: (i) inhibition of translation of a family of mRNAs that code for proteins essential for cell cycle progression; (ii) inhibition of IL-2-induced transcription of proliferating cell nuclear antigen (PCNA) that is essential for DNA replication; (ii) blocking CD28-mediated sustained up-regulation of IL-2 transcription in T cells; and (iv) inhibition of the kinase activity of the cdk4/cyclin D and cdk2/cyclin E complexes, essential for cell

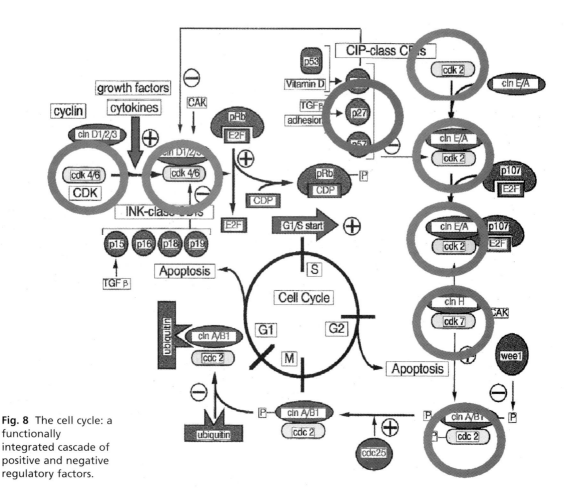

**Fig. 8** The cell cycle: a functionally integrated cascade of positive and negative regulatory factors.

cycle progression. On overview of rapamycin effects within the cell cycle is given in Figure 8.

The mechanism of action is distinct from other immunosuppressive drugs that act solely by inhibiting DNA synthesis, such as mycophenolate mofetil (CellCept) and azathioprine (Imuran). Rapamycin is synergistic with cyclosporin A and has much lower toxicity than other immunosuppressive agents.

In *in vitro* and *in vivo* studies, rapamycin prevents proliferation of T cells but also proliferation[57,58] and migration[59] of smooth muscle cells. Furthermore, rapamycin has been shown to diminish smooth muscle cell hyperproliferation in several animal models of arteriopathy[60–62].

### Paclitaxel (Taxol®)
Paclitaxel was originally isolated from the bark of the Pacific Yew. It is an antineoplastic agent that is currently used to treat several types of cancer, most commonly breast and ovarian cancer.

It is a diterpenoid with a characteristic taxane-skeleton of 20 carbon atoms and has a molecular weight of 853.9 Da. Paclitaxel exerts its pharmacological effects through formation of numerous decentralized and unorganized microtubules. This enhances the assembly of extraordinarily stable microtubules, interrupting proliferation, migration and signal transduction[63,64] Unlike other antiproliferative agents of the colchicine type, which inhibit microtubuli assembly, paclitaxel shifts the microtubule equilibrium towards microtubule assembly. It is highly lipophylic, which promotes a rapid cellular uptake, and has a long-lasting effect in the cell due to the structural alteration of the cytoskeleton.

*In vitro* and *in vivo* studies have shown that paclitaxel may prevent or attenuate re-stenosis. Paclitaxel inhibits proliferation and migration of cultured smooth muscle cells in a dose-dependent manner[65]. In a rat balloon injury model, intraperitoneal administration of paclitaxel reduced neo-intimal area. In a rabbit atherosclerotic model where plaque burden was increased by electrical injury, local administration of paclitaxel reduced neo-intimal thickness[66,67].

## Investigational devices

### Actinomycin D: Multi-Link Tetra™-D stent (Guidant, Santa Clara, CA, USA)

The stent is fabricated from medical 316L stainless steel tubing and is composed of a series of cylindrically oriented rings aligned along a common longitudinal axis. Each ring consists of 3 connecting bars and 6 expanding elements. The stent is premounted on a delivery catheter.

The antiproliferative drug is actinomycin D. The finished Multi-Link Tetra stent is coated with a polymer matrix (semicrystalline ethylene-vinyl alcohol co-polymer: EVAL) containing a maximal dose of 150 µg actinomycin D. This is equivalent to 20–200 times less than the recommended total human adult dose of 500 µg/day given intravenously for 5 days.

The delivery catheter is a rapid exchange design (0.014 inch guidewire). It is equipped with two radiopaque markers located underneath the balloon to mark the ends of the stent and has a 'stepped' balloon design to optimize stent and balloon shoulder configuration.

### NIRx™ – paclitaxel-coated conformer coronary stent (Boston Scientific, USA)

The stent is fabricated from medical 316LS stainless steel. The geometry is a continuous, uniform, multicellular design with adaptive cells capable of differential lengthening. This enables the stent to be flexible in the unexpanded configuration. Stent length is 15 mm. The stent is premounted on a delivery catheter (Fig. 9).

The antiproliferative drug is paclitaxel. Paclitaxel is incorporated into a fast-release triblock co-polymer carrier system on the stent. There are two drug concentration. The 'low dose' concentration is 1.0 µg/mm$^2$

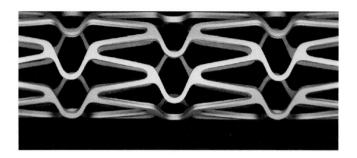

**Fig. 9** NIRx™-Paclitaxel-coated conformer coronary stent (Boston Scientific, USA.

(loaded drug/stent surface area; total dose 85 µg per stent) and gives sustained release over ~28 days. The 'moderate dose' is 2.0 µg/mm² (loaded drug/stent surface area).and provides a rapid release in the first 24 h, followed by a slower release over the following 28 days.

The delivery catheter is a monorail design (0.014 inch guidewire/7F guiding catheter). It is equipped with two radiopaque markers located underneath the balloon to mark the ends of the stent. The delivery balloon will be 3.0 mm and 3.5 mm in diameter.

**Rapamycin-coated BX™ VELOCITY stent (Cordis, Warren, USA)**
The stent is fabricated from medical 316LS stainless steel. It is available in 2 configurations: a 6-cell configuration (expanded diameter 2.5–3.25 mm) and a 7-cell design (expanded diameter 3.5–3.75 mm). Stent length is 18 mm. The stent is premounted on a delivery balloon with diameters of 2.5 mm, 3.0 mm and 3.5 mm (Fig. 10).

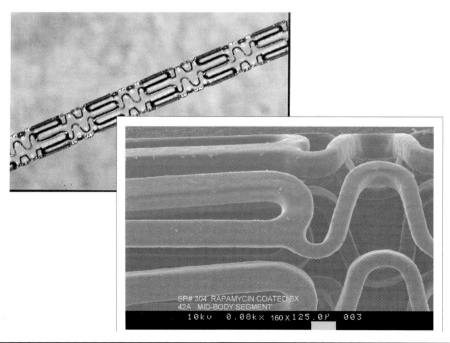

**Fig. 10** Rapamycin coated BX™ VELOCITY stent (Cordis, Warren, USA).

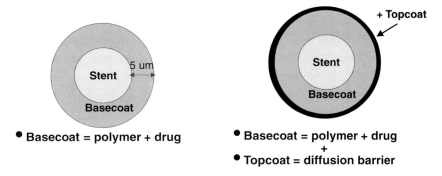

**Fig. 11** Coating structure for fast drug release (left) and slow drug release (right).

# Fast drug release    Slow drug release

The antiproliferative drug is rapamycin. The stent contains 140 µg/cm$^2$ which gives a total rapamycin content of 153 µg on the 6-cell stent and 180 µg on the 7-cell stent. The coating formulation consists of 30% rapamycin by weight in a 50:50 mixture of the polymers polyethylenevinylacetate (PEVA) and polybutylmethacrylate (PBMA; Fig. 11).

The delivery catheter utilizes a rapid exchange design (0.014 inch guidewire/7F guiding catheter). It is equipped with two radiopaque markers located underneath the balloon to mark the ends of the stent. The delivery balloon will be 3.0 mm and 3.5 mm in diameter.

## Clinical studies

### Actinomycin D

There is no published research to date documenting the use of actinomycin D for treatment of coronary artery disease and/or re-stenosis. A phase 1, randomized clinical trial ACTION (ACTinomycin eluting stent Improves Outcomes by reducing Neointimal Hyperplasia) started in June 2001 to evaluate the safety and performance of the Multi-Link Tetra™-D stent system: 360 patients will be randomized to receive an actinomycin D coated stent or a non-coated stent for treatment of *de novo* lesions in native coronary arteries with a vessel calibre of 3.0–4.0 mm. Six month angiographic follow-up is expected to be completed in February 2002, 12-month clinical follow-up up is expected to be completed in August 2002.

### Rapamycin (Sirolimus)

A first clinical application of the rapamycin-coated stents was performed in Sao Paulo and Rotterdam. Thirty patients with angina pectoris were electively treated with 2 different formulations of rapamycin-coated BX™ VELOCITY stents (Cordis) (slow release [SR], $n$ = 15, and fast release [FR], $n$ = 15). All stents (18 mm) were successfully delivered, (3.0–3.5 mm vessel calibre) and patients were discharged without clinical complications. At 4 months angiographic and IVUS follow-up, there was minimal neo-intimal hyperplasia in both groups (11.0 ± 3.0% in the SR group and 10.4 ± 3.0% in the FR group, $P$ = NS) by ultrasound and quantitative coronary angiography (in-stent late loss, 0.09 ± 0.3 mm [SR] and –0.02 ± 0.3 mm [FR]. No in-stent or edge re-stenosis was observed. No major clinical events (stent thrombosis, repeat revascularization, myocardial infarction, death) had occurred by 8 months[68]. At 1 year follow-up, IVUS volumetric analysis and angiography indicated minimal amounts of neo-intimal hyperplasia that were scarcely different from the 4 month data in both groups, with some patients showing no evidence of hyperplasia whatsoever. There were no MACE and no re-stenosis in either of the groups. One late acute MI occurred in the fast-release group at 14 months[69].

The randomized RAVEL study with the rapamycin-coated BX™ VELOCITY balloon-expandable stent in the treatment of patients with *de novo* lesions in native coronary arteries is a multicenter, prospective, randomized double-blind clinical trial comparing bare metal and the drug-coated stents. A total of 220 patients were randomized for treatment with either a single rapamycin-coated (140 µg.cm$^{-2}$) or a bare metal BX™ VELOCITY stent. At 6-month follow-up, the restenosis rate of the treated group was zero, the loss in minimal lumen diameter was zero, there was no target lesion reintervention and the event-free survival was 96.5%[74].

The SIRIUS study is a multicentre, prospective, randomized double-blind trial that is being conducted in 55 centres in the USA. Eleven hundred patients with focal *de novo* native coronary arterial lesions (2.5 to 3.5 mm diameter, 15 to 30 mm long) will be randomized for treatment with either rapamycin-coated (109 mg.cm$^{-2}$) or bare metal BX™ VELOCITY balloon expandable stents. The primary endpoints of the SIRIUS trial are target vessel failure (death, myocardial infarction, target lesion revascularization) at 9 months. In addition, secondary endpoints are core laboratory analysis of angiographic and intravascular ultrsound data to determine treatment effects on neointimal hyperplasia and in-stent restenosis. Clinical follow-up will continue for 3 years in order to assess late events. In addition to the pivotal RAVEL and SIRIUS trials, feasibility studies are ongoing to assess efficacy of rapamycin-coated stents in more complex lesion subsets, such as in-stent restenosis.

### Paclitaxel

There are several ongoing clinical trials of paclitaxel-coated stents. In the TAXUS I trial 61 patients were randomized to receive a paclitaxel-coated (1.0 µg/mm$^2$) or a bare NIR stent. At 6-month follow-up, no restenosis was seen in the paclitaxel-coated stent group, while the restenosis rate in the bare stent group was 11%. The late lumen loss of 0.35±0.47 mm was significantly lower in the paclitaxel-coated stent group (0.71±0.88 mm). The Asian ASPECT trial showed a clear dose response. Patients ($n = 177$) were randomized to receive a high dose (3.1 $\mu$g.mm$^{-2}$) paclitaxel-coated, a low dose (1.3 $\mu$g.mm$^{-2}$) paclitaxel-coated, or a bare stent. The restenosis rate at 6 months was 4%, 12%, and 27%, respectively[75]. The ongoing ELUTES trial randomises 180 patients into 5 groups – 4 different dose levels and a bare stent control group.

In other clinical trials, the taxol derivate QP2 was used. The QP2 pilot study included 32 patients with *de novo* or restenosis lesions who underwent QuaDS-QP2 stent implantation. The stainless steel, slotted tube stent was 13 or 17 mm in length and coated with multiple ploymer sleeves that slowly release QP2 (up to 4000 $\mu$g). A 2-year follow-up of 25 patients recorded that they were all asymptomatic[76]. Another group reported on the 8 month IVUS follow-up. IVUS revealed only moderate neointima formation with a neointima burden of 13.6±14.9%[77]. Another multicenter, trial randomized 266 patients to receive a QuaDS-QP2 stent (4000 mg with an elution over 180d) or a bare stent. Follow-up angiography at 6 months showed a significant reduction in restenosis in the QuaDS-QP2 stent group (6.9% v. 36%). However, this trial has been stopped by the safety committee because of an excessive adverse event rate in the QuaDS-QP2 stent group of 10.2% – periprocedural myocardial infarction and subacute stent thrombosis[78].

# Another step: biodegradable stents

Coronary stents exert their beneficial clinical effect within a relatively narrow time frame. Stent scaffolding is needed from the acute procedural phase (in case of threatened or actual vessel closure) until the first 6 months after the procedure to overcome late negative vessel remodelling. In the long-term perspective, metallic stents have potential complications such as in-stent re-stenosis and the inaccessibility of the lesion site for surgical revascularization. Thus stents made of bio-degradable materials may be an ideal alternative.

## Experimental data

The first requirement for polymeric materials in intracoronary stents is biocompatibility. In animal studies, the biocompatibility of polymer stents has been controversial suggesting that tissue incompatibility may be a major obstacle.

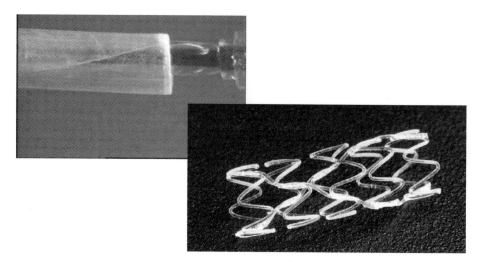

**Fig. 12** Poly-l-lactic monopolymer Igaki-Tamai biodegradable stent (Igaki Medical Planning Co, Ltd.

Marked inflammatory response after the implantation of 5 different polymer-loaded stents (polyglycolic acid/polylactic acid, polycaprolactone, polyhydroxybutyrate valerate, polyorthoester, and polyethyleneoxide/polybutylene terephthalate) has been reported in a porcine coronary model[42]. Thrombotic occlusion of polymeric stents was seen in other experiments[70].

In contrast, Zidar *et al* reported only a minimal inflammatory reaction and minimal neo-intimal hyperplasia with the use of poly-l-lactic acid (PLLA) stents in canine femoral arteries. *In vitro* data revealed a reduced platelet adherence and thrombogenicity of the PLLA stent as compared with slotted-tube stainless steel metallic stents[70].

### Investigational device: poly-l-lactic monopolymer Igaki-Tamai biodegradable stent (Igaki Medical Planning Co, Ltd)

The Igaki-Tamai stent is a coil stent made of a poly-l-lactic (PLLA) monofilament (molecular mass, 183 kDa). PLLA has been used for orthopaedic applications in humans and has generally been found to be biocompatible. The stent is self-expanding with a zigzag helical design. The stent length is 12 mm. The thickness of the stent strut is 0.17 mm. In its expanded state, the stent covers 24% of the vessel area. The stent has a radiopaque gold marker at both ends of the prosthesis. Stents are mounted on standard angioplasty balloon catheters that are the same size as the stent with diameters of 3.0, 3.5, and 4.0 mm (Figure 12). It takes the stent 18–24 months to biodegrade fully.

Deployment of the stent is currently done with a balloon-expandable covered sheath system through an 8 French guiding catheter. The stent delivery balloon inflation is performed with a heated dye at 80°C using a 30 s inflation at 6–14 atm. This temperature ensures adequate stent expansion within 30 s and may minimize vessel injury caused by a heated balloon. The stent continues to expand gradually to its original size after deployment *in vivo*.

### Clinical data

The first clinical data are available in 15 patients who underwent elective coronary PLLA Igaki-Tamai stent implantation: 25 stents were successfully implanted in 19 lesions. Angiographic success was achieved in all procedures. No stent thrombosis and no major cardiac event occurred within 30 days. Angiographically, both the re-stenosis rate and target lesion revascularization rate were 10.5% at 6 months. Intravascular ultrasound revealed no significant stent recoil at 1 day and stent expansion at follow-up. No major cardiac event, except for repeat angioplasty, developed within 6 months[71].

Long-term data (12 months) of 63 lesions in 50 patients have been previously presented. Angiographic analysis showed a good procedural result with was a 12 ± 8% final diameter stenosis post-stent implantation. At 6 months, diameter stenosis was 38 ± 23% and decreased slightly to 33 ± 23% at 12 months. Subacute thrombosis occurred in one patient at day 5, but no other MI, urgent CABG, or death occurred over the 12 months[72].

## Limitations

Although the principle of stent implantation is well established and although (most of) the applied drugs and polymers have been used in clinical practice for many years, there is little experimental and only preliminary clinical knowledge of the acute and long-term effects of drug-eluting or biodegradable stents in coronary arteries. Thus, a number of concerns and open questions have to be investigated in the future.

The concerns include drug toxicity as well as acute and late vascular effects. A number of toxic effects are known for all drugs applied in cancer therapy such haematological toxicity (neutropenia), neurotoxicity (peripheral neuropathy), hypersensitivity reactions, or cardiac disturbances. However, these side-effects are described in patients undergoing high-dose chemotherapy for a malignant disease with plasma levels 100–1000 times higher (and over longer time periods) than plasma levels that result from a local delivery. Another concern is possible delayed wound healing and endothelialization. This would increase thrombogenicity and the danger of (late) stent thrombosis.

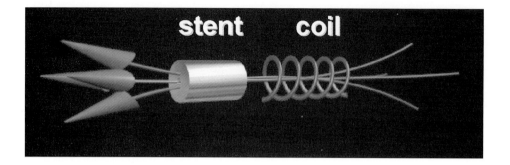

**Fig. 13** Potential prevention of stent re-stenosis by non-invasively heating the stent, using alternating magnetic fields. High frequency alternating magnetic fields cause hysteresis phenomenon on the metallic stent, generating energy loss that appears as heat.

Further potential side-effects could be late positive remodelling and aneurysmal formation. Thus the most suitable antithrombotic regimen following drug-eluting and/or biodegradable stent implantation still has to be evaluated.

A series of open questions exists on the mechanism of action and also the design of local drug delivery systems and drug-eluting stents. Little is known of specific pharmacokinetic issues. There is a paucity of data on the most appropriate tissue concentration and the rate and duration of drug-release over time. The tissue concentration is dependent on close mechanical contact of the stent to the vascular tissue and on physiological transport forces into the tissue. Hydrophobic drugs, like paclitaxel, have greater variability in terms of drug delivery, while hydrophilic drugs, like heparin, have less variability and achieve higher local concentrations. Local concentrations and concentration gradients, however, are crucial parameters for biological effects. The relationship between vascular effects and physicochemical properties of the drug-loaded stent is poorly understood. Drug distribution within the vessel wall seems to be significantly affected by the stent expansion pattern (uniform versus non-uniform)[73].

## Conclusions and future perspectives

Drug-eluting and biodegradable stents represent one of the fastest growing fields in interventional cardiology today. However, many unanswered questions still have to be resolved before determining the potential of these techniques. Hopefully, after the completion of planned and on-going trials many of these issues will be answered. Furthermore, these new technologies will have to prove effective in the daily routine of treating patients presenting with long lesions, small vessels, chronic occlusion, bifurcation, multi-vessel and/or left main stem disease or acute myocardial infarction.

Stent development will investigate a variety of possibilities to resolve the re-stenosis problem. Possibilities range from the further exploitation of different classes of drugs which are potential candidates for the inhibition of re-stenosis to the combination of biodegradability with drug delivery, local gene therapy (*e.g.* local expression of proliferation regulatory genes; transfer of cytotoxic genes, VEGF) or external heating of stents (Fig. 13).

# Acknowledgement

ER was supported by a grant from the Deutsche Forschungsgemeinschaft.

## References

1 Ruygrok PN, Ormiston JA, O'Shaughnessy B. Coronary angioplasty in New Zealand 1995–1998: a report from the National Coronary Angioplasty Registry. *N Z Med J* 2000; **113**: 381–4

2 Ikeda S, Bosch J, Banz K, Schneller P. Economic outcomes analysis of stenting versus percutaneous transluminal coronary angioplasty for patients with coronary artery disease in Japan. *J Invasive Cardiol* 2000; **12**: 194–9

3 Al Suwaidi J, Berger PB, Holmes DR. Coronary artery stents. *JAMA* 2000; **284**: 1828–36

4 Serruys PW, de Jaegere P, Kiemeneij F *et al*. A comparison of balloon-expandable-stent implantation with balloon angioplasty in patients with coronary artery disease. Benestent Study Group [see comments]. *N Engl J Med* 1994; **331**: 489–95

5 Fischman DL, Leon MB, Baim DS *et al*. A randomized comparison of coronary-stent placement and balloon angioplasty in the treatment of coronary artery disease. Stent Restenosis Study Investigators [see comments]. *N Engl J Med* 1994; **331**: 496–501

6 Kimmel SE, Localio AR, Brensinger C *et al*. Effects of coronary stents on cardiovascular outcomes in broad-based clinical practice. *Arch Intern Med* 2000; **160**: 2593–9

7 Angelini P, Vaughn WK, Zaqqa M, Wilson JM, Fish RD. Impact of the 'stent-when-feasible' policy on in-hospital and 6-month success and complication rates after coronary angioplasty: single-center experience with 17,956 revascularization procedures (1993–1997). *Tex Heart Inst J* 2000; **27**: 337–45

8 Heuser R, Houser F, Culler SD *et al*. A retrospective study of 6,671 patients comparing coronary stenting and balloon angioplasty. *J Invasive Cardiol* 2000; **12**: 354–62

9 Rocha-Singh K, Morris N, Wong SC, Schatz RA, Teirstein PS. Coronary stenting for treatment of ostial stenoses of native coronary arteries or aortocoronary saphenous venous grafts. *Am J Cardiol* 1995; **75**: 26–9

10 Popma JJ, Lansky AJ, Ito S, Mintz GS, Leon MB. Contemporary stent designs: technical considerations, complications, role of intravascular ultrasound, and anticoagulation therapy. *Prog Cardiovasc Dis* 1996; **39**: 111–28

11 Carlier SG, van der Giessen WJ, Foley DP *et al*. Stenting with a true bifurcated stent: acute and mid-term follow-up results. *Cathet Cardiovasc Diagn* 1999; **47**: 361–96

12 Laham RJ, Carrozza JP, Baim DS. Treatment of unprotected left main stenoses with Palmaz-Schatz stenting. *Cathet Cardiovasc Diagn* 1996; **37**: 77–80

13 Lopez JJ, Ho KK, Stoler RC *et al*. Percutaneous treatment of protected and unprotected left main coronary stenoses with new devices: immediate angiographic results and intermediate-term follow-up. *J Am Coll Cardiol* 1997; **29**: 345–52

14  Moussa I, Reimers B, Moses J *et al.* Long-term angiographic and clinical outcome of patients undergoing multivessel coronary stenting. *Circulation* 1997; **96**: 3873–9

15  Forrester JS, Fishbein M, Helfant R, Fagin J. A paradigm for restenosis based on cell biology: clues for the development of new preventive therapies. *J Am Coll Cardiol* 1991; **17**: 758–69

16  Lafont A, Guzman LA, Whitlow PL, Goormastic M, Cornhill JF, Chisolm GM. Restenosis after experimental angioplasty. Intimal, medial, and adventitial changes associated with constrictive remodeling. *Circ Res* 1995; **76**: 996–1002

17  Schwartz RS, Topol EJ, Serruys PW, Sangiorgi G, Holmes Jr DR. Artery size, neointima, and remodeling: time for some standards. *J Am Coll Cardiol* 1998; **32**: 2087–94

18  Mudra H, Regar E, Klauss V *et al.* Serial follow-up after optimized ultrasound-guided deployment of Palmaz- Schatz stents. In-stent neointimal proliferation without significant reference segment response. *Circulation* 1997; **95**: 363–70

19  Sobel BE. Acceleration of restenosis by diabetes: pathogenetic implications. *Circulation* 2001; **103**: 1185–7

20  Mintz GS, Popma JJ, Pichard AD *et al.* Intravascular ultrasound predictors of restenosis after percutaneous transcatheter coronary revascularization. *J Am Coll Cardiol* 1996; **27**: 1678–87

21  Prati F, Di Mario C, Moussa I *et al.* In-stent neointimal proliferation correlates with the amount of residual plaque burden outside the stent: an intravascular ultrasound study. *Circulation* 1999; **99**: 1011–4

22  Kornowski R, Hong MK, Tio FO, Bramwell O, Wu H, Leon MB. In-stent restenosis: contributions of inflammatory responses and arterial injury to neointimal hyperplasia. *J Am Coll Cardiol* 1998; **31**: 224–30

23  de Feyter PJ, Kay P, Disco C, Serruys PW. Reference chart derived from post-stent-implantation intravascular ultrasound predictors of 6-month expected restenosis on quantitative coronary angiography. *Circulation* 1999; **100**: 1777–83

24  Lefkovits J, Topol EJ. Pharmacological approaches for the prevention of restenosis after percutaneous coronary intervention. *Prog Cardiovasc Dis* 1997; **40**: 141–58

25  Rosanio S, Tocchi M, Patterson C, Runge MS. Prevention of restenosis after percutaneous coronary interventions: the medical approach. *Thromb Haemost* 1999; **82** (**Suppl 1**): 164–70

26  de Feyter PJ, Vos J, Rensing BJ. Anti-restenosis trials. *Curr Interv Cardiol Rep* 2000; **2**: 326–31

27  Gunn J, Cumberland D. Does stent design influence restenosis? *Eur Heart J* 1999; **20**: 1009–13

28  Lossef SV, Lutz RJ, Mundorf J, Barth KH. Comparison of mechanical deformation properties of metallic stents with use of stress-strain analysis. *J Vasc Interv Radiol* 1994; **5**: 341–9

29  Hofma SH, Whelan DM, van Beusekom HM, Verdouw PD, van der Giessen WJ. Increasing arterial wall injury after long-term implantation of two types of stent in a porcine coronary model. *Eur Heart J* 1998; **19**: 601–9

30  Rogers C, Edelman ER. Endovascular stent design dictates experimental restenosis and thrombosis. *Circulation* 1995; **91**: 2995–3001

31  Carter AJ, Scott D, Rahdert D et al. Stent design favorably influences the vascular response in normal porcine coronary arteries. *J Invasive Cardiol* 1999; **11**: 127–34

32  Edelman ER, Seifert P, Groothuis A, Morss A, Bornstein D, Rogers C. Gold-coated NIR stents in porcine coronary arteries. *Circulation* 2001; **103**: 429–34

33  Wilczek KL, De Scheerder I, Wang K. Implantation of balloon expandable copper stents in porcine coronary arteries. A model for testing the efficacy of stent coating in decreasing stent thrombogenicity. *Circulation* 1995; **92** (**Suppl**): 455

34  Fischell TA, Hehrlein C. The radioisotope stent for the prevention of restenosis. *Herz* 1998; **23**: 373–9

35  Carter AJ, Fischell TA. Current status of radioactive stents for the prevention of in-stent restenosis. *Int J Radiat Oncol Biol Phys* 1998; **41**: 127–33

36  Rubin P, Williams JP, Riggs PN *et al.* Cellular and molecular mechanisms of radiation inhibition of restenosis. Part I: role of the macrophage and platelet-derived growth factor [see comments]. *Int J Radiat Oncol Biol Phys* 1998; **40**: 929–41

37  Albiero R, Nishida T, Adamian M *et al.* Edge restenosis after implantation of high activity (32)P radioactive beta-emitting stents. *Circulation* 2000; **101**: 2454–7

38  Simon C, Palmaz JC, Sprague EA. Protein interactions with endovascular prosthetic surfaces. *J Long Term Eff Med Implants* 2000; **10**: 127–41

39  van Beusekom HM, Serruys PW, van der Giessen WJ. Coronary stent coatings. *Coron Artery Dis* 1994; **5**: 590–6

40  van Beusekom HM, Schwartz RS, van der Giessen WJ. Synthetic polymers. *Semin Interv Cardiol* 1998; **3**: 145–8

41  van der Giessen WJ, Schwartz RS. Coated and active stents: an introduction. *Semin Interv Cardiol* 1998; **3**: 125–6

42  van der Giessen WJ, Lincoff AM *et al*. Marked inflammatory sequelae to implantation of biodegradable and nonbiodegradable polymers in porcine coronary arteries. *Circulation* 1996; **94**: 1690–7

43  Malik N, Gunn J, Shepherd L, Crossman DC, Cumberland DC, Holt CM. Phosphorylcholine-coated stents in porcine coronary arteries: *in vivo* assessment of biocompatibility. *J Invasive Cardiol* 2001; **13**: 193–201

44  Whelan DM, van der Giessen WJ, Krabbendam SC *et al*. Biocompatibility of phosphorylcholine coated stents in normal porcine coronary arteries. *Heart* 2000; **83**: 338–45

45  Serruys PW, Emanuelsson H, van der Giessen W *et al*. Heparin-coated Palmaz-Schatz stents in human coronary arteries. Early outcome of the Benestent-II Pilot Study. *Circulation* 1996; **93**: 412–22

46  Ahn YK, Jeong MH, Kim JW *et al*. Preventive effects of the heparin-coated stent on restenosis in the porcine model. *Cathet Cardiovasc Interv* 1999; **48**: 324–30

47  van der Giessen WJ, van Beusekom HM, Eijgelshoven MH, Morel MA, Serruys PW. Heparin-coating of coronary stents. *Semin Interv Cardiol* 1998; **3**: 173–6

48  Holmes DR, Camrud AR, Jorgenson MA, Edwards WD, Schwartz RS. Polymeric stenting in the porcine coronary artery model: differential outcome of exogenous fibrin sleeves versus polyurethane-coated stents. *J Am Coll Cardiol* 1994; **24**: 525–31

49  Serruys PW, van Hout B, Bonnier H *et al*. Randomised comparison of implantation of heparin-coated stents with balloon angioplasty in selected patients with coronary artery disease (Benestent II) [published erratum appears in *Lancet* 1998; 352: 1478]. *Lancet* 1998; **352**: 673–81

50  Galli M, Bartorelli A, Bedogni F *et al*. Italian BiodivYsio open registry (BiodivYsio PC-coated stent): study of clinical outcomes of the implant of a PC-coated coronary stent. *J Invasive Cardiol* 2000; **12**: 452–8

51  Mak KH, Topol EJ. Clinical trials to prevent restenosis after percutaneous coronary revascularization. *Ann N Y Acad Sci* 1997; **811**: 255–84; discussion 284–8

52  O'Keefe JH, McCallister BD, Bateman TM, Kuhnlein DL, Ligon RW, Hartzler GO. Ineffectiveness of colchicine for the prevention of restenosis after coronary angioplasty. *J Am Coll Cardiol* 1992; **19**: 1597–600

53  Muller DW, Topol EJ, Abrams GD, Gallagher KP, Ellis SG. Intramural methotrexate therapy for the prevention of neointimal thickening after balloon angioplasty. *J Am Coll Cardiol* 1992; **20**: 460–6

54  De Scheerder I, Wilczek K, Van Dorpe J *et al*. Local angiopeptin delivery using coated stents reduces neointimal proliferation in overstretched porcine coronary arteries. *J Invasive Cardiol* 1996; **8**: 215–22

55  de Scheerder I, Wang K, Wilczek K *et al*. Local methylprednisolone inhibition of foreign body response to coated intracoronary stents. *Coron Artery Dis* 1996; **7**: 161–6

56  Lincoff AM, Furst JG, Ellis SG, Tuch RJ, Topol EJ. Sustained local delivery of dexamethasone by a novel intravascular eluting stent to prevent restenosis in the porcine coronary injury model. *J Am Coll Cardiol* 1997; **29**: 808–16

57  Marx SO, Jayaraman T, Go LO, Marks AR. Rapamycin-FKBP inhibits cell cycle regulators of proliferation in vascular smooth muscle cells. *Circ Res* 1995; **76**: 412–7

58  Mohacsi PJ, Tuller D, Hulliger B, Wijngaard PL. Different inhibitory effects of immunosuppressive drugs on human and rat aortic smooth muscle and endothelial cell proliferation stimulated by platelet-derived growth factor or endothelial cell growth factor. *J Heart Lung Transplant* 1997; **16**: 484–92

59  Poon M, Marx SO, Gallo R, Badimon JJ, Taubman MB, Marks AR. Rapamycin inhibits vascular smooth muscle cell migration. *J Clin Invest* 1996; **98**: 2277–83

60  Gregory CR, Huie P, Billingham ME, Morris RE. Rapamycin inhibits arterial intimal thickening caused by both alloimmune and mechanical injury. Its effect on cellular, growth factor, and cytokine response in injured vessels. *Transplantation* 1993; **55**: 1409–18

61  Gregory CR, Huang X, Pratt RE *et al*. Treatment with rapamycin and mycophenolic acid reduces arterial intimal thickening produced by mechanical injury and allows endothelial replacement. *Transplantation* 1995; **59**: 655–61

62  Poston RS, Billingham M, Hoyt EG *et al*. Rapamycin reverses chronic graft vascular disease in a novel cardiac allograft model. *Circulation* 1999; **100**: 67–74

63  Schiff PB, Fant J, Horwitz SB. Promotion of microtubule assembly *in vitro* by taxol. *Nature* 1979; **277**: 665–7

64  Rowinsky EK, Donehower RC. Paclitaxel (taxol). *N Engl J Med* 1995; **332**: 1004–14

65  Sollott SJ, Cheng L, Pauly RR *et al*. Taxol inhibits neointimal smooth muscle cell accumulation after angioplasty in the rat. *J Clin Invest* 1995; **95**: 1869–76

66  Axel DI, Kunert W, Goggelmann C *et al*. Paclitaxel inhibits arterial smooth muscle cell proliferation and migration *in vitro* and *in vivo* using local drug delivery. *Circulation* 1997; **96**: 636–45

67  Herdeg C, Oberhoff M, Baumbach A *et al*. Local paclitaxel delivery for the prevention of restenosis: biological effects and efficacy *in vivo*. *J Am Coll Cardiol* 2000; **35**: 1969–76

68  Sousa JE, Costa MA, Abizaid A *et al*. Lack of neointimal proliferation after implantation of Sirolimus-coated stents in human coronary arteries: a quantitative coronary angiography and three-dimensional intravascular ultrasound study. *Circulation* 2001; **103**: 192–5

69  Sousa JEMR, Costa MA, Abizaid A *et al*. Mid- (4 months)and long-term (1 year) QCA and three-dimensional IVUS follow-up after implantation of Sirolimus-coated stent in human coronary arteries. *J Am Coll Cardiol* 2001; **37**: 8A

70  Zidar J, Lincoff AM, Stack R. Biodegradable stents. In: Topol EJ. (ed) *Textbook of Interventional Cardiology*. Philadelphia, PA: WB Saunders, 1994; 787–802

71  Tamai H, Igaki K, Kyo E *et al*. Initial and 6-month results of biodegradable poly-l-lactic acid coronary stents in humans. *Circulation* 2000; **102**: 399–404

72  Tsuji T, Tamai H, Igaki K *et al*. One year follow-up of biodegradable self-expanding stent implantation in humans. *J Am Coll Cardiol* 2001; **37**: 47A

73  Hwang CW, Wu D, Edelman ER. Stent-based delivery is associated with marked spatial variations in drug distribution. *J Am Coll Cardiol* 2001; **37**: 1A

74  Morice M, Serruys P, Sousa J, Fajadet J, Perin M, Ben Hayashi E *et al*. The RAVEL study: a randomized study with the sirolimus-coated BX™ VELOCITY balloon-expandable stent in the treatment of patients with de novo native coronary artery lesions. *Eur Heart J* 2001: (Abstract)

75  The Asian paclitaxel eluting stent clinical trial. *TCT*. 2001; http://www.tetmd.com/clinical-trials/breaking/one.html?presentation_id=261&start_idx=1

76  de la Fuente LM, Miano J, Mrad J, Penazola E, Yeung AC, Eury R *et al*. Initial results of the Quanam drug eluting stent (QuaDS-QP2) registry (BARDDS) in human subjects. *Cathet Cardiovasc Intervent* 2001; **53**: 480–8

77  Honda Y, Grube E, de la Fuente LM, Yock PG, Stertzer SH, Fitzgerald PJ. Novel drug-delivery stent: intravascular ultrasound observations from the first human experience with the QP2-eluting polymer stent system. *Circulation* 2001; **104**: 380–3

78  Liistro F, A C. Late acute thrombosis after paclitaxel eluting stent implantation. *Heart* 2001; **86**: 262–4

# Laser revascularisation

**S C Clarke** and **P M Schofield**

*Department of Cardiology, Papworth Hospital, Cambridge, UK*

Patients who present with angina pectoris due to underlying coronary artery disease which is not controlled by medical therapy, and who have disease which is not amenable to conventional forms of revascularisation, present an increasing clinical problem. Laser techniques have been introduced to improve myocardial perfusion in this group of patients. The surgical technique of transmyocardial laser revascularisation has been evaluated in this patient population. Generally, there has been a good symptomatic response in terms of improvement in angina, and in some studies an increase in exercise capacity. The technique, however, does carry significant morbidity and mortality. More recently, a catheter-based technique has been introduced – percutaneous myocardial laser revascularisation. This technique seems to improve symptoms of angina, produce an increase in exercise capacity, with a much more favourable procedural risk profile.

Effective treatment is available for the vast majority of patients with angina pectoris due to underlying coronary artery disease. The majority of patients respond adequately to medical therapy. The remaining patients usually have disease which is amenable to coronary angioplasty/stenting or coronary artery bypass surgery. There is, however, a group of patients who have severe angina despite medication, and who have coronary artery disease which is not amenable to either coronary angioplasty/stenting or coronary artery surgery. This cohort of patients is increasing in number, and they have usually had several revascularisation procedures in the past. Typically, they have diffuse disease within their coronary circulation, which particularly affects the distal part of the vessel.

The use of thoracic artery implantation many years ago[1] was an attempt to provide direct myocardial perfusion. This was based on the description of a sinusoidal network in the human heart. Sen *et al*[2] proposed the creation of transmural channels in the left ventricular wall to permit direct perfusion of ischaemic myocardium with oxygenated left ventricular blood. This concept was based on the model of the reptilian heart, in which the left ventricle is directly perfused from endothelium lined channels that radiate out from the left ventricular cavity. Mirhoseni and colleagues[3] advanced the concept by using laser energy rather than mechanical energy to create the transmural channels. There has been a series of clinical trials which have evaluated transmyocardial laser revas-

*Correspondence to: Dr P M Schofield, Consultant Cardiologist, Papworth Hospital, Papworth Everard, Cambridge CB3 8RE, UK*

cularisation (TMR) in patients with advanced coronary artery disease. More recently, a catheter-based technique has been introduced and evaluated.

# Transmyocardial laser revascularisation

The rationale for introducing TMR into clinical practice was based on the knowledge of a rich sinusoidal network within the left ventricular myocardium. It was hoped that the creation of laser channels would enable direct perfusion of the myocardium from within the left ventricular cavity. Although studies have demonstrated an improvement in angina in patients following TMR, the mechanism of action remains uncertain. From histological evidence, it appears that the channels close following the procedure, and it is unlikely that direct perfusion of the myocardium plays a significant role. Currently, angiogenesis seems to be the most likely explanation for the symptomatic improvement noted in this patient population. Other possible explanations include a degree of denervation as well as a placebo effect. The placebo effect, in this group of patients with 'end stage disease' should not be underestimated.

## The procedure

TMR is usually carried out under general anaesthesia using a left anterolateral thoracotomy. It is also possible to carry out the procedure less invasively using thoracoscopic techniques. The patient is investigated prior to the procedure using angiographic techniques, as well as an assessment of myocardial perfusion using either nuclear cardiology or positron emission tomography (PET). The area, or areas, to be treated by TMR are, therefore, determined beforehand using a combination of the findings from angiography and myocardial perfusion assessment. The laser probe is placed on the surface of the left ventricle, and is activated when the ventricle is maximally distended with blood. The density of the channels within each of the ischaemic zones to be treated, is usually about one every 1.0 cm$^2$. The initial trials of TMR utilised a high energy carbon dioxide laser (The Heart Laser, PLC Medical Systems, USA), and more recently a Holmium:YAG laser system has been used (Eclipse Surgical Technologies, USA). A transoesophageal echocardiogram was used initially to demonstrate the transmural nature of the laser channel. There was a characteristic appearance within the left ventricular cavity as the laser channel penetrated the myocardium. A transoesophageal echocardiogram, however, is not now used routinely – it is clear that a transmyocardial channel has been created since bleeding occurs at the epicardial surface. This bleeding from the channels usually stops spontaneously. Sometimes, digital pressure is required to stop the bleeding, and occasionally a suture is necessary.

## Clinical trials

One of the early trials of TMR was reported by Horvath et al[4]. This was an uncontrolled study of patients with angina which was not adequately controlled by medical therapy. The patients had evidence of reversible myocardial ischaemia, and they had coronary artery disease which was not amenable to treatment by either coronary angioplasty/stenting or coronary artery bypass grafting. The majority of patients experienced a significant improvement in terms of angina. Some 75% of patients experienced a reduction of at least two Canadian cardiovascular scores (CCS) classes in terms of their angina. The procedure, however, was not without significant risk. There was a peri-operative mortality of some 9%. The results from a registry of TMR, using a high energy $CO_2$ laser, has been reported[5]. The registry included sites within Europe and Asia. In the registry report, 50% of patients demonstrated an improvement of at least two CCS angina classes, and there was an operative mortality of almost 10%.

Following on from these initial uncontrolled trials, there have been several trials of TMR, some of which have used the $CO_2$ laser, and some the Holmium:YAG laser equipment. There have been prospective randomised trials carried out in the US[6] and also in the UK[7] using the high energy $CO_2$ laser. These trials were similar in design. Following assessment, suitable patients were randomised to either continued medical therapy, or TMR plus their standard medical treatment. In both trials, there was an improvement in angina. In the US trial[6], 72% of patients in the TMR group experienced an improvement in angina of at least two classes. In the control group (medication only), only 13% of patients experienced an improvement in angina of at least two classes. The symptomatic benefit noted in the UK trial[7] was less impressive. In the TMR group, at 12 months only 25% of patients had an improvement of at least two angina classes, as compared with 4% of the control group. The US trial was also criticised because of a high cross-over rate from the control group (medical therapy) to the TMR group. Clearly, this made interpretation of results much more difficult. A further problem was the fact that the 12 month follow-up data were incomplete. The UK trial also assessed exercise capacity, using both treadmill exercise times as well as the 12 min walking distance. Both of these measures of exercise capacity improved slightly in the TMR group, although the difference between the TMR group and the control group was not statistically significant. In the UK trial, the peri-operative mortality was 5%. The periprocedural morbidity was significant. One-third of patients developed either a wound infection or respiratory infection which required treatment with antibiotic. Transient arrhythmia, which was usually atrial fibrillation, occurred in the peri-operative phase in some 15% of patients, and 12% of patients developed symptoms from left ventricular failure which required a transient increase in their diuretic therapy. These trials, therefore, demonstrate that whilst TMR may improve angina, and result in some increase in exercise capacity, it does carry significant morbidity and mortality.

There have also been two large studies of TMR using the Holmium:YAG laser. The ATLANTIC study[8] randomised a total of 182 patients to either continued medical therapy or TMR with continued medication. In the TMR group, there was a reduction of at least two angina classes at 12 months of 61% of patients, as compared with 11% of patients in the control group. The ATLANTIC study also demonstrated an improvement in exercise capacity at 12 months follow-up. There was an improvement in exercise capacity in the TMR group of a mean of 65 s, whereas in the control group there was a mean decrease of 46 s – this difference was statistically significant. A further study of TMR using a Holmium:YAG laser was reported by Allen et al[9]. This randomised, prospective study involved 275 patients in 18 centres. Following assessment, 143 patients were randomised to medical therapy alone, and 132 were randomised to TMR plus continued medication. At 12 month follow-up, there was a decrease in at least two angina classes noted in 76% of the patients treated with TMR, whereas a reduction in two angina classes in the control group occurred in 32% of patients. The operative mortality in this study was 5%, and in the ATLANTIC study[8] the operative mortality was 1%.

Therefore, in both the initial uncontrolled trials, as well as in the subsequent prospective randomised trials, TMR seems to produce symptomatic benefit. Usually, at least half of patients with angina and disease not suitable for conventional revascularisation techniques, experience a reduction in at least two angina classes at 12 months of follow-up. Secondly, exercise capacity has usually increased following TMR, although this has not always been a statistically significant improvement. It is clear, however, that the technique of TMR is associated with significant morbidity, as well as a peri-operative mortality of 5–10%. These results are summarised in Table 1.

## Percutaneous myocardial laser revascularisation

In view of the morbidity and mortality associated with the surgical approach of TMR, catheter-based laser techniques have been developed. It is now possible to deliver laser energy percutaneously, using a Holmium:YAG laser introduced using a femoral artery approach. Using

**Table 1** Summary of clinical trials of transmyocardial laser revascularisation

| | Type of laser | Peri-operative mortality | Improvement of at least 2 angina classes at 12 months | | Improvement in exercise time at 12 months | |
| --- | --- | --- | --- | --- | --- | --- |
| | | | TMR group | Control group | TMR group | Control |
| Horvath[4] | $CO_2$ | 9% | 75% | – | – | – |
| Burns[5] | $CO_2$ | 9.7% | 50% | – | +110 s | |
| March[6] | $CO_2$ | 8% | 72% | 13% | – | – |
| Schofield[7] | $CO_2$ | 5% | 25% | 4% | +70 s | +12 s |
| Burkhoff[8] | Ho:YAG | 1% | 61% | 11% | +64 s | –46 s |
| Allen[9] | Ho:YAG | 5% | 76% | 32% | – | – |

Ho:YAG, Holmium:YAG.

this technology, the laser energy is delivered to the endocardial surface of the ventricle, rather than the epicardial surface utilised with TMR. The percutaneous approach is carried out under local anaesthetic. Since there is no requirement for general anaesthesia, and since there is no requirement for a thoracotomy, the technique is much more attractive from the patient's view-point. Following TMR, patients often need to stay in hospital for up to 10 days, whereas patients can usually be discharged the following day after a percutaneous procedure.

## The procedure

Currently, there are two systems available to deliver Holmium:YAG laser energy to the endocardial surface of the left ventricle. The first technique, percutaneous myocardial laser revascularisation (PMR, Eclipse Surgical Technologies, USA) involves a standard radiographic technique. The second approach of direct myocardial revascularisation (DMR, Biosense, Johnson & Johnson, USA) uses an electromechanical mapping system and catheter location technology.

The Eclipse PMR system was originally developed by CardioGenesis, USA. Access to the left ventricle is gained using a 9 French sheath which is introduced into the femoral artery. There are essentially three parts to the equipment. The first is an 'aligning catheter', which is advanced and positioned in the left ventricular cavity. This is available in a variety of curves. The shape selected depends on the configuration of the left ventricle, as well as the area to be treated. The second part of the equipment is the 'laser catheter'. This has a right-angled bend just before the tip. The laser catheter is advanced though the aligning catheter and rotation of the laser catheter facilitates access to the various parts of the left ventricle. The third part of the equipment is the 'laser fibre'. This is advanced through the laser catheter, in order to make contact with the endocardial surface of the left ventricle. The manipulation and positioning of the equipment is carried out using radiographic screening. It is standard practice to use the 40° right anterior oblique projection, together with the 50° left anterior oblique projection, usually with 10° of cranial angulation. Once the views have been selected, it is important that the patient does not move during the laser procedure.

The aligning catheter is advanced into the left ventricular cavity at the start of the procedure. Following this, two left ventricular angiograms are performed – one in the right anterior oblique, and one in the left anterior oblique projections. The outline of the left ventricular angiogram is then traced onto the acetate sheets which have been fixed over the viewing screens. During the procedure, these traced outlines act as 'maps' of the left ventricular cavity. The patient is assessed prior to the PMR procedure by angiography, as well as an evaluation of myocardial perfusion. This may be carried out using nuclear cardiology, or alternatively PET. The findings from the angiogram and the perfusion scan indicate which area of the left ventricle requires laser therapy. By manipulating the aligning catheter, and/or the laser catheter, it is possible to access most parts of the left ventricle. The region selected for treatment may be the anterior wall, the inferior wall, the lateral wall or the septum. Once the laser catheter is orientated towards the region to be treated, the laser fibre is advanced in order to make contact with the left ventricular endocardium. This can be 'felt' by the operator, and can also be seen radiographically since the laser catheter is 'pushed back' from the endocardial surface of the left ventricle. Contact with the anterior or inferior wall of the left ventricle is best seen using the right anterior oblique projection. Contact with the lateral wall or septum of the left ventricle is usually best seen in the left anterior oblique projection.

The laser is activated once an appropriate site has been selected, and contact has been made. Activation of the laser produces a channel which is approximately 3 mm deep into the left ventricular myocardium. The laser fibre is then usually advanced slightly, and a further burst of laser energy is delivered. This results in a channel which is around 6 mm in depth. The laser fibre is then withdrawn into the laser catheter. A different site is then selected by further manipulation of the guiding catheter and/or laser catheter. Prior to the PMR procedure, the patient undergoes transthoracic echocardiography. It is important to ensure that the area to be treated is at least 8 mm in thickness – this reduces the risk of left ventricular perforation. The apex of the left ventricle is usually the thinnest part of the left ventricular wall. When treating the apex, typically only one burst of laser energy is delivered. Once the laser energy has been delivered, the site is marked in the two views on the acetate sheet. The channels are created about 1 cm apart. The map of the channels is usually best seen in the left anterior oblique projection when treating the anterior wall or the inferior wall. The right anterior oblique projection is best for mapping the channels created when treating the lateral wall or septum. Usually, 10–15 channels are created in each of the regions which have been shown to have evidence of reversible myocardial ischaemia.

Patients are anticoagulated during the PMR procedure. A bolus of 10,000 units of heparin is usually given at the start of the procedure, and the ACT is monitored throughout. During manipulation of the guiding catheter and laser catheter, ventricular arrhythmias occur commonly – this is usually ventricular premature beats, although non-sustained ventricular tachycardia can be induced. During manipulation, it is also possible to induce left bundle branch block. This does not usually have any sequelae, although it is important to position a temporary pacing wire prior to PMR if the patient has pre-existing right bundle branch block. If the patient has a thin left ventricular wall in the region to be treated, then it may be feasible to proceed with the treatment, although only one burst of laser energy being used, thereby minimising the risk of perforation. If the patient has definite evidence of left ventricular thrombus on the transthoracic echocardiogram, then PMR should not be undertaken. Access to the left ventricle may also be precluded by the presence of advanced peripheral vascular disease, or significant aortic stenosis.

The equipment used for DMR enables both electromechanical mapping of the left ventricle, as well as the delivery of laser treatment, without the need for radiographic screening. The sophisticated mapping system with DMR uses a very low energy source, together with catheter electrodes which have sensors at their tip, in order to locate the exact position of the catheter in three dimensional space. The mapping catheter is positioned at many sites on the endocardial surface of the left ventricle. The electrical and mechanical information received is then integrated. This technology is useful in determining whether the left ventricle at that site is normal, scar tissue, or ischaemic tissue. The electromechanical maps which are generated are, therefore, useful in identifying the target regions of the left ventricle to be treated by laser energy. Using the location sensors, the laser catheter can be guided towards the region to be treated. An additional application of this technology is for the delivery of other intramyocardial treatments, such as growth factors.

A triangular location pad generates an electromagnetic field, and this interfaces with a catheter which has a deflectable tip, and which contains a miniature location system. Therefore, a 'real time' electrical and anatomical map of the endocardial surface of the left ventricle can be created. The system also requires a stationary reference catheter, which is usually placed externally on the body surface. The information received from the mapping catheter is processed by a workstation (the NOGA unit) in order to construct the three dimensional left ventricular image.

The position of the mapping catheter is gated to the end of diastole. Its position is recorded relative to the location of the fixed reference catheter on the body surface. This compensates for both patient or cardiac motion. The mapping catheter tip is positioned at multiple sites on the endocardial surface of the left ventricle. This facilitates the three-dimensional reconstruction of the left ventricle anatomically. In addition to the mechanical activity, electrical signals are acquired from the mapping catheter , and these can be superimposed on the three-dimensional anatomical map. Regions of the left ventricle which have low electrical activity and impaired mechanical activity usually represent areas of previous myocardial infarction. A region with high electrical and mechanical activity usually represents normal myocardium. In sites where there is normal electrical activity, but impaired mechanical activity, there is typically severe ischaemia/hibernating myocardium.

The Biosense system, therefore, has many potential applications. First, the electromechanical maps which are acquired help to identify the ischaemic parts of the left ventricular myocardium, which may be targets for DMR laser treatment. Second, the navigation system may also be useful for guiding the laser catheter during the DMR procedure. The channels which have been created during laser treatment can be indicated on the electromechanical map in real time. Third, the technology may prove to be useful for the intramyocardial delivery of growth factors, or other agents.

## Clinical trials

The results of a randomised prospective trial of PMR were published in November 2000[10]. A total of 221 patients were recruited and randomised from 13 centres – 12 in the US and 1 UK site. All of the patients who were randomised had angina which persisted despite medical treatment, and they had angiographically proven coronary artery disease which was not suitable for conventional forms of revascularisation. In the trial, 111 patients were randomised to medical treatment alone, and 110 to PMR and continued medical treatment. In the PMR group, at 6 months there was a mean reduction of 1.4 CCS angina classes, compared with 0.13 in the control group ($P = 0.001$). In terms of treadmill exercise time at 6 months, there was a 30% increase in exercise time in the PMR group, as compared to 5% in the control group. This was statistically significant, and the baseline values were around 400 s in both of the groups. At 12 months, exercise tolerance increased by a mean of 89 s in the PMR group, compared with 12.5 s in the control group ($P = 0.008$; Fig. 1). Angina status was evaluated using a masked assessment. At 12 months, angina class fell by two or more classes in 34% of the PMR patients, compared

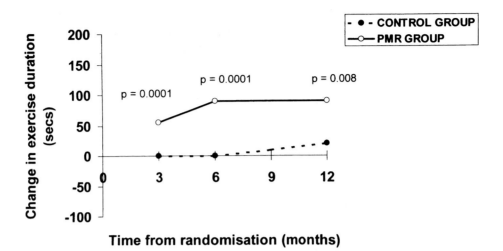

**Fig. 1** The change in exercise duration during the 12 months' following randomisation in the control group and the active treatment group.

with 13% of the medically treated group. There were no peri-operative deaths in the PMR group. The morbidity associated with the PMR procedure was low. Of the 110 patients who underwent PMR, one developed cardiac tamponade requiring percutaneous drainage and one patient developed atrio-ventricular block which required permanent pacing. It is clear, therefore, that the morbidity and mortality associated with PMR is vastly different to that encountered with TMR.

The criticism of the PACIFIC trial is that it was not a 'double blind trial'. A trial has been performed where the patients randomised to the control group underwent a 'sham' procedure. The laser equipment was positioned in the left ventricular cavity, but no laser energy was delivered. The results of this trial are not yet available, but are clearly awaited with interest.

In terms of clinical trials with the DMR laser system, preliminary results of a trial have been presented, but have not yet been published. The DIRECT trial involved a total of 298 patients who had angina despite medication, and who were not suitable for conventional forms of revascularisation. These patients were randomised to one of three groups. The first group, the 'placebo' group, received a mapping procedure only using the Biosense equipment, the second group underwent 'low dose laser therapy' (10–15 laser channels per treatment zone) and the third group had 'high dose laser therapy' (20–25 laser channels per treatment zone). In the DIRECT trial, the patient was blinded to their treatment group. At 6 months' follow-up, there was an increase in treadmill exercise time of 7–10%, but there was no significant difference between the three groups. The baseline exercise time was 360–390 s. At 6 months, there was also an improvement in angina class in all three groups, but again there was no significant difference between the groups. It was suggested by the presenters of the preliminary results from the DIRECT trial that the changes demonstrated in symptoms and exercise capacity were due to the placebo effect. It is interesting to note that the improvement in exercise duration on treadmill testing in the DIRECT trial ($\leq 10\%$) was much lower than that found in the PACIFIC trial (30%). As outlined above, there are substantial differences in the techniques utilised for PMR and DMR, and these may account for some of the differences in the findings from clinical trials. First, the technique for selecting the region to treat is quite different with PMR and DMR. With PMR, the angiogram and perfusion scan are used, whereas with DMR there is an influence from the electromechanical map which is generated at the start of the procedure. Second, the amount of energy delivered is different between PMR and DMR, and this affects the depth of the channels created – there is greater penetration with the PMR technique than with DMR. Finally, with the PMR technique it is extremely clear when contact has been made with the endocardial surface of the left ventricle. With the DMR technology, contact with the endocardial surface prior to laser therapy delivery, is less certain.

## Conclusions

We look forwards to reviewing the results of the DIRECT trial when published. The findings of the PMR trial in which the control group underwent a 'sham' procedure are also awaited with interest. If the future trials of catheter-based laser therapy confirm a beneficial effect, then it is likely that the percutaneous approach will be preferred. It is clear from the results of clinical trials to date that PMR carries a much lower morbidity and mortality than TMR. This may not necessarily, however, be 'the end of the road' for TMR treatment. It may still have a role as an adjunct to coronary artery bypass surgery. There are many patients undergoing coronary artery bypass surgery who have some vessels suitable for grafting, and other vessels which are not. In this patient group, a hybrid approach has been used. The vessels suitable for surgery are grafted, whereas the regions supplied by vessels which are not suitable for surgery are treated by TMR. Several centres continue to carry out these combined procedures.

If the future trials confirm the benefits demonstrated in the PACIFIC study, then it is likely that PMR will continue to be used in patients with angina and coronary artery disease which is not suitable for conventional forms of revascularisation. Indeed, its use would continue to increase. There may also be a role for hybrid procedures using percutaneous coronary intervention. Patients would undergo angioplasty/stenting to lesions that were amenable to this form of treatment. The areas of myocardium supplied by vessels which were diffusely diseased, and not suitable for conventional revascularisation may be amenable to treatment by PMR.

## References

1   Vineberg A. Clinical and experimental studies in the treatment of coronary artery insufficiency by internal mammary artery implant. *J Int Coll Surg* 1954; **22**: 503–18

2   Sen PK, Udwadia TE, Kinare SG *et al*. Transmyocardial acupuncture: a new approach to myocardial revascularisation. *J Thorac Cardiovasc Surg* 1965; **50**: 181–9

3   Mirhoseini M, Muckerheidi M, Cayton M. Transventricular revascularisation by laser. *Lasers Surg Med* 1982; **2**: 187–98

4   Horvath KA, Cohn LH, Cooley DA. Transmyocardial laser revascularisation: results of a multicentre trial with transmyocardial laser revascularisation used as sole therapy for end-stage coronary artery disease. *J Thorac Cardiovasc Surg* 1997; **113**: 645–54

5   Burns SM, Sharples LD, Tait S *et al*. The transmyocardial laser revascularisation international registry report. *Eur Heart J* 1999; **20**: 31–7

6   March RJ. Transmyocardial laser revascularisation with the $CO_2$ laser: one year results of a randomised controlled trial. *Semin Thorac Cardiovasc Surg* 1999; **11**: 12–8

7   Schofield PM, Sharples LD, Caine N *et al*. Transmyocardial laser revascularisation in patients with refractory angina: a randomised controlled trial. *Lancet* 1999; **353**: 519–24

8   Burkhoff D, Schmidt S, Shulman S *et al*. Transmyocardial revascularisation compared with continued medical therapy for treatment of refractory angina pectoris: a prospective randomised trial. *Lancet* 1999; **354**: 885–90

9   Allen K, Dowling R, Fudge T *et al*. Comparison of transmyocardial revascularisation with medical therapy in patients with refractory angina. *N Engl J Med* 1999; **341**: 1029–36

10  Oesterle SN, Sanborn TA, Ali N *et al*. Percutaneous transmyocardial laser revascularisation for severe angina: the PACIFIC randomised trial. *Lancet* 2000; **356**: 1705–10

# Minimally invasive therapy and robotics

**T J Spyt\*** and **A C De Souza†**

*\*Glenfield Hospital, University Hospitals of Leicester NHS Trust, Leicester, UK and †Royal Brompton Hospital, London, UK*

Considerable progress in the surgical management of coronary artery disease over the last several years has undoubtedly been influenced by developments in the technology of extracorporeal circulation and refinements in myocardial protection during surgery[1]. This was associated with improvements in surgical technique, the introduction of quality suturing material, recognition of the importance of the choice of conduit and more appropriate selection of patients for intervention.

The introduction of safe cardioplegic arrest enabled immobilisation of the heart for a period of time necessary for the construction of multiple bypasses. The majority of cardiac surgeons adopted this strategy as safe for the patient and comfortable for the operator.

However, effective bypass grafting can be performed without the use of cardiopulmonary bypass. A small group of surgeons continued to follow the pioneering work of Kolesow who, in 1964, bypassed the anterior descending artery on the beating heart[2,3]. Between 1995 and 1997, considerable interest was raised by Benetti, who postulated that bypass grafting can be performed satisfactorily through a limited left thoracotomy and without cardiopulmonary bypass[4-8]. Benetti named this intervention MIDCAB (minimally invasive direct coronary artery bypass).

In parallel with the emergence of new surgical approaches, a number of reports claimed non-physiological impact of extracorporeal circulation. It has now been documented that cardiopulmonary bypass reduces quantity and quality of blood flow to vital organs, micro-embolisation, impairment of immunological response leading to increased rate of infections, renal dysfunction and the most important of all, neurological complications[9-13]. As early as 1991, Benetti published the first comparison of costs of surgery with and without cardiopulmonary bypass, claiming considerable savings in the latter[4]. The trend of limiting trauma caused by the access of surgery has not been unique to cardiac surgery. There is a considerable belief that, in some patients, trauma of the traditional access may be greater than the actual benefit of the surgical procedure. In fact, cardiac surgeons were late to join the trend seen in many other surgical specialties.

There are many reasons why cardiac surgeons started to look for new ways of performing myocardial revascularisation. Frequently, failures of cardiac surgical intervention are not caused by inadequate technique or errors, but by complications related to extracorporeal circulation and

*Correspondence to: T J Spyt, Consultant Cardiothoracic Surgeon, Glenfield Hospital, University Hospitals of Leicester NHS Trust, Groby Road, Leicester LE3 9QP, UK*

myocardial reperfusion. Generalised inflammatory reaction and activation of complement results in increased permeability of blood vessels, leading to fluid overload producing pulmonary and renal impairment. The release of complement C3A and endothelin 1 leads to spasm of coronary arteries; cytokinins, TNF-$\alpha$, IL-6 and IL-8 contribute to negative influence on myocardial contractility and lead to a reduction in vascular resistance in patients undergoing surgery with cardiopulmonary bypass. Macro- and micro-embolisation seen following open heart surgery frequently originates from oxygenators, filters and atherosclerotic arteries. It is now documented that surgery without cardiopulmonary bypass does not lead to complement activation and embolisation is incidental. Cardiopulmonary bypass and sternotomy leads to a significant blood loss, hence the need for blood transfusion and clotting factors. In operations without cardiopulmonary support and through a small access, this problem does not exist. Limited surgical access makes the operation more difficult for the surgeon but a smaller wound, as in the case of the left limited thoracotomy, avoids injury to the sternum, producing a better cosmetic result and more effective postoperative analgesia. The hospital stay and convalescence in patients undergoing bypass grafting through a small thoracotomy is reduced in comparison with patients subjected to median sternotomy[14,15]. Not surprisingly, this procedure has generated considerable interest amongst patients and hospital managers.

## Minimally invasive direct coronary artery bypass

Patients suitable for MIDCAB procedures are those with obstruction in the proximal left anterior descending artery (LAD). Patients who benefit the most are those with: (i) severe impairment of left ventricular function; (ii) important co-existing co-morbidities; (iii) failed bypass grafting to left anterior descending coronary artery with venous conduit; and (iv) re-stenosis following angioplasty.

The anterior descending artery should be at least 2 mm diameter and it is essential that the course of the artery is superficial. Intramyocardial position of the LAD could put construction of the anastomosis at risk. It is essential that the artery is not calcified. In ideal circumstances, the anterior descending artery would be occluded with a good collateral filling. In some patients, it is possible to combine the left internal thoracic artery bypass to LAD with angioplasty to the circumflex and right coronary arteries (hybrid procedures). Measurable benefits of the operation are minimalisation of surgical trauma, reduction in hospital stay and cost of treatment, elimination of complications specific to cardiopulmonary bypass, and the ability to accept patients with particularly high risks. The cosmetic results are excellent[6–8].

Bypass grafting through limited access is performed on the beating heart without the support of cardiopulmonary bypass. It is desirable that the heart rate is reduced to 60 beats/min using pharmacological preparation with β-blockers and calcium channel blockers. The patient receives standard premedication. Either endotracheal intubation or laryngeal mask is used and thoracic epidural anaesthesia is essential. Left anterolateral thoracotomy is carried out through the fourth intercostal space. The length of the incision is usually 7–10 cm. Occasionally it is necessary to remove part of the fourth cartilage. The left internal thoracic artery is dissected using either direct visual control or thoracoscopy. It is necessary to detach the left internal thoracic artery from the chest wall to obtain a segment of artery approximately 10 cm long. The pericardium is opened next and the anterior descending artery identified. The artery needs to be occluded above and below the site of planned arteriotomy. Alternatively, an intravascular shunt may be used. A segment of the anterior left ventricular wall containing the anterior descending artery is immobilised using a commercially available instrument (Cardiothoracic System® or Medtronic Octopus® device). Heparin is administered in a dose of 1 mg/kg body weight. The anastomosis of the left internal thoracic artery to the anterior descending artery is carried out using a conventional technique of continuous either 7/0 or 8/0 Prolene. During the anastomosis, the ECG is closely monitored. It is desirable to monitor the function of the left ventricle using transoesophageal echocardiography. Once the anastomosis is completed, the chest wall is closed in layers over a single intercostal chest drain. Reversal of heparin is not necessary.

An alternative to the small left anterior thoracotomy is partial sternotomy. The sternum is incised from the xiphoid to the level of the third intercostal space where it is transected. The left internal thoracic artery is dissected and the rest of the operation is carried out as described above. The partial sternotomy does not disrupt the integrity of the sternum to the same extent as the standard approach. The advantage of performing the operation through a partial sternotomy is simplicity of dealing with potential complications which may require the institution of cardiopulmonary bypass. No new incision is required except extension of the existing one.

Operations using limited access are technically difficult. This is mainly because the majority of cardiac surgeons are used to larger access. Movement of the heart has been eliminated by recently developed instruments. Limited access creates concern that incomplete dissection of the internal thoracic artery may lead to a 'steal syndrome'. This concern has led to the introduction of video-assisted thoracoscopic techniques for harvesting of the internal thoracic artery. An increasing number of surgeons are capable of performing procedures using endoscopic instruments. As this experience increases, it creates potential that in the future the vascular anastomosis itself could be carried out endoscopically.

Results of coronary artery bypass grafting through limited access are not different from those performed using classical approaches. Early patency rates are as high as 98–99%. Mortality of the procedure is less than 1% and only very few patients need to be converted to bypass grafting with the use of extracorporeal circulation[16–18]. If the long-term results remain as good as early outcomes, the operation may become a useful choice, even for patients with multivessel disease. This is because, even now, it can be successfully complimented by angioplasty. A large multicentre trial is currently being carried out in Britain to compare the outcome of angioplasty and stenting to the anterior descending artery with bypass grafting through a limited anterior thoracotomy (Angioplasty versus Minimally Invasive Surgery trial – AMIST trial).

# Off pump CABG (OPCAB)

Multivessel coronary artery disease can also be treated surgically without the use of extracorporeal circulation. Easy access to the coronary arteries, which are on the surface of the heart, and introduction of instrumentation enabling immobilisation of the left ventricle have made the procedures possible[19]. However, complete modification of the anaesthetic and surgical techniques had to follow. It is desirable to perform the operation with the use of arterial conduits only, which avoids manipulation of the ascending aorta, frequently affected by atherosclerosis. The third bypass can be constructed using the radial artery which in its proximal part is anastomosed to the side of the left or right internal thoracic artery. The most severely affected coronary artery should be dealt with first. This strategy allows protection of the most vulnerable part of the myocardium. Bypasses to the remaining arteries are carried next. The most treacherous part of the procedure is the bypass grafting to the dominant right coronary artery. This is frequently associated with episodes of hypotension and arrhythmia varying from atrial fibrillation to a complete standstill. Insertion of intravascular stent may prevent these unwelcome occurrences. In practice, the anterior descending artery is bypassed first. This offers protection not only to the anterior wall of the left ventricle, but also to the intraventricular septum. Exposure of the heart is facilitated by placement of traction sutures at the back of the pericardium, mainly above the left upper pulmonary vein or between the left upper pulmonary vein and the diaphragm, or between the left upper pulmonary vein and the inferior vena cava. Manipulation of the heart and stabilisation of the part of the left ventricular wall may lead to sudden hypotension. Reduction of the preload caused by lifting the heart should be corrected by changing the position of the patient and by administration of intravenous fluids. Occasionally it is necessary to administer catecholamines. Intra-operative tachycardia can be treated with an infusion of short acting β-blockers and profound bradycardia will require temporary pacing. Patients need careful monitoring which includes ECG, pulse oximetry and measurement of peripheral arterial and central venous pressures. Intra-operative transoesophageal echocardiography and Swan Ganz catheterisation are desirable. Heparin is given in a dose of 1 mg/kg body weight to achieve activated clotting time of 250–300 s. Maintenance of normothermia is essential and this is achieved by relatively high temperature in theatre (22°C or more), preheating of the patient during induction of anaesthesia, active warming during surgery using air blankets (Bear Hugger®) and also by administration of warmed intravenous fluids. Early results of the more complex revascularisation procedures off pump are good, although no large randomised trials exist to encourage further dissemination of the technique. Early psychoneurological assessments of the patients, however, indicate better outcomes amongst patients who underwent surgery without cardiopulmonary bypass.

## Coronary artery bypass grafting through limited access with the use of extracorporeal circulation (port access CABG)

This method of coronary artery bypass grafting involves cardio-pulmonary bypass and cardioplegic arrest. Surgical access is obtained through several smaller incisions; in some cases, a limited left anterior thoracotomy is performed. The patient is intubated with a double lumen tube. Arterial pressure is monitored in both radial arteries. Debrillator pads are attached to the chest. One or both internal thoracic arteries are dissected using video-assisted thoracoscopy. After heparinisation, the femoral artery and vein are cannulated in the groin. It is also possible to cannulate the ascending aorta through a separate incision in the first intercostal space[20]. The venous cannula is advanced to the level of the ostium of the superior vena cava. The internal thoracic artery is divided distally and the pericardium is opened vertically through a mini-thoracotomy. Cardiopulmonary bypass is supported usually with a centrifugal pump. If venous conduits are used, the proximal anastomosis on the aorta is carried out using a small side-biting clamp. The ascending aorta is clamped and cardioplegia administered. The heart is decompressed through a separate cannula which also serves to occlude the aorta from inside by expanding a balloon (endoclamp) positioned above the aortic valve under echocardiographic control. The same cannula is also used for the delivery of cardioplegic solution once the ascending aorta has been occluded. Misplacement of endoclamp will be noticed by a difference in arterial pressure monitored from both radial arteries. Observation of arterial pressure is important, as misplacement of the balloon may occlude branches of the aorta, thus jeopardising cerebral blood supply. Bypass grafting is performed once the heart is stopped. Some surgeons prefer mini-thoracotomy, others use multiple small incisions employing small ports for access for which specially designed instruments are essential. Once all distal anastomoses are completed, the endoclamp is deflated and removed. Cardiopulmonary bypass is discontinued and heparin reversed. The femoral vessels are decannulated and all incisions closed.

Port-access surgery is usually performed in selected patients with a low risk of peri-operative mortality[21], in centres with a large surgical experience. To date, published data describe no more than 2000 patients who have undergone this form of surgery. The time of cardiopulmonary bypass and ischaemic cardiac arrest is considerably longer and the operation takes 4–5 h[22,23]. The number of patients requiring conversion to a standard sternotomy is minimal. Peri-operative mortality is also less than 1%. Neurological complications, however, are seen in approximately 2% of cases[24-26]. The important complication of this approach is the possibility of dissection of the aorta observed in 1% of patients[27]. This is considerably higher than during standard procedures. Re-exploration for bleeding is more frequent. Some patients develop healing problems in the groin. Hospital stay is short and early angiographic results of surgery indicate 97–100% graft patency. As this form of surgery has been carried out only since 1996, there are no published reports describing long-term outcome.

The idea of endoscopic cardiac surgery, supported by cardiopulmonary bypass, was initiated as early as 1991 in Stamford Surgical Technologies. This development was kept secret until 1995, when the company changed its name to Heartport Inc. An undoubted advantage of port-access is the ability to perform full revascularisation on the still heart through surgically small incisions, which gives an excellent cosmetic result. However, this is achieved by increased cardiopulmonary bypass and ischaemic time, and increased risk of serious vascular complications. The technique requires a long training, the operations take considerable time and the equipment is expensive[28,29]. In comparison with the MIDCAB and OPCAB procedures, port-access is unlikely to become common place. In wealthy societies, where small incisions may be attractive to the patients for cosmetic reasons, port-access may be an alternative to the traditional approach as long as there are no major systemic risk factors, no peripheral vascular disease and the function of the left ventricle is good enough to withstand 2–5 h of extracorporeal circulation. To our knowledge, no British centre at present carries out a regular programme of port access coronary artery bypass grafting.

# References

1. Aris A. One hundred years of cardiac surgery. *Ann Thorac Surg* 1996; **62**: 636–7

2. Kolessov VI. Mammary artery – coronary artery anastomosis as method of treatment for angina pectoris. *J Thorac Cardiovasc Surg* 1967; **54**: 535–44

3. Trapp WG, Bisarya R. Placement of coronary artery bypass graft without pump oxygenator. *Ann Thorac Surg* 1975; **19**: 1–9

4. Benetti FJ. Coronary artery bypass without extracorporeal circulation versus percutaneous transluminal coronary angioplasty: comparison of costs. *J Thorac Cardiovasc Surg* 1991; **102**: 802–3

5. Benetti F, Ballester C. Use of thoracoscopy and a minimal thoracotomy, in mammary coronary bypass to left anterior descending artery, without extracorporeal circulation. *J Cardiovasc Surg* 1995; **36**: 159–61

6. Bufollo E, Andrade JCS, Branco JNR, Aguiar LF, Ribeiro EE, Jatene AD. Myocardial revascularisation without extracorporeal circulation, seven-year experience in 593 cases. *Eur J Cardiovasc Thorac Surg* 1990; **4**: 504–8

7. Calafiore AM, Angelini GD, Bergsland J, Salerno TA. Minimally invasive coronary artery bypass grafting. *Ann Thorac Surg* 1996; **62**: 1545–8

8. Calafiore AM, Teodori G, Giammaraco G et al. Minimally invasive coronary artery bypass grafting on a beating heart. *Ann Thorac Surg* 1997; **63**: S72–5

9. Ascione R, Lloyd C, Underwood M, Gomes W, Angelini G. On-pump versus off-pump coronary revascularization: evaluation of renal function. *Ann Thorac Surg* 1999; **68**: 493–8

10. Ascione R, Lloyd C, Underwood M, Lotto AA, Pitsis A, Angelini GD. Economic outcome of off-pump coronary artery bypass surgery: a prospective randomized study. *Ann Thorac Surg* 1999; **68**: 2237–42

11. Baufreton C, Intrator L, Jansen PG et al. Inflammatory response to cardiopulmonary bypass using roller or centrifugal pumps. *Ann Thorac Surg* 1999; **67**: 972–7

12. Clark RE. Microemboli during coronary artery bypass grafting. *Thorac Cardiovasc Surg* 1995; **109**: 249–58

13. Gaudino M, Glieca F, Alessandrini F et al. The unclampable ascending aorta in coronary artery bypass patients. *Circulation* 2000; **102**: 1497

14. King RC, Reece TB, Hurst JL et al. Minimally invasive coronary artery bypass grafting decreases hospital stay and costs. *Ann Surg* 1997; **225**: 805–11

15. Glower DD, Clements FM, Debruijin NP et al. Comparison of direct aortic and femoral cannulation for port-access cardiac operations. *Ann Thorac Surg* 1999; **68**: 1529–31

16. Biglioli P, Antona C, Alamanni F et al. Minimally invasive direct coronary artery bypass grafting: midterm results and quality of life. *Ann Thorac Surg* 2000; **70**: 456–60

17. Doty JR, Fonger JD, Salazar JD, Walinsky PL, Salomon NW. Early experience with minimally invasive direct coronary artery bypass grafting with the internal thoracic artery. *J Thorac Cardiovasc Surg* 1999; **117**: 873–80

18. Gill IS, Higginson LA, Maharajh GS, Keon WJ. Early and follow-up angiography in minimally invasive coronary bypass without mechanical stabilization. *Ann Thorac Surg* 2000; **69**: 56–60

19. Jansen EW, Borst C, Lahpor J. CABG without cardiopulmonary bypass using the 'Octopus' method: results in the first 100 patients. *J Thorac Cardiovasc Surg* 1998; **116**: 60–7

20. Glower DD, Clements FM, Debruijin NP et al. Comparison of direct aortic and femoral cannulation for port-access cardiac operations. *Ann Thorac Surg* 1999; **68**: 1529–31

21. Wimmer-Greinecker G, Matheis G, Dogan S et al. Patient selection for port-access multi vessel revascularization. *Eur J Cardiothorac Surg* 1999; **16 (Suppl 2)**: S43–7

22. Reichenspurner H, Boehm DH, Welz A et al. Minimally invasive coronary artery bypass grafting: port-access approach versus off-pump techniques. *Ann Thorac Surg* 1998; **66**: 1036–40

23. Falk V, Diegeler A, Walther T et al. Total endoscopic computer enhanced coronary artery bypass grafting. *Eur J Cardiothorac Surg* 2000; **17**: 38–45

24. Ribakove GH, Miller JS, Anderson RV et al. Minimally invasive port-access coronary artery bypass grafting with early angiographic follow-up: initial clinical experience. *J Thorac Cardiovasc Surg* 1998; **115**: 1101–10

25  Groh MA, Sutherland SE, Burton 3rd HG, Johnson AM, Ely SW. Port-access coronary artery bypass grafting: technique and comparative results. *Ann Thorac Surg* 1999; **68**: 1506–8

26  Grossi EA, Groh MA, Lefrak EA *et al*. Results of a prospective multicenter study on port-access coronary bypass grafting. *Ann Thorac Surg* 1999; **68**: 1475–7

27  Reichenspurner H, Gulielmos V, Wunderlick J *et al*. Port-access coronary artery bypass grafting with the use of cardiopulmonary bypass and cardioplegic arrest. *Ann Thorac Surg* 1998; **65**: 413–9

28  Watson DR, Duff SB. The clinical and financial impact of port-access coronary revascularization. *Eur J Cardiothorac Surg* 1999; **16** (**Suppl 1**): S103–6

29  Reichenspurner H, Boehm D, Detter C, Schiller W, Reichart B. Economic evaluation of different minimally invasive procedures for the treatment of coronary artery disease. *Eur J Cardiothorac Surg* 1999; **16** (**Suppl 2**): S76–9

# Neuromodulation for chronic refractory angina

**Roger Moore** and **Michael Chester**

*National Refractory Angina Centre, Mersey Regional Cardiothoracic Centre, Liverpool, UK*

Neuromodulation is the use of therapies which alter the relationship between the heart, its autonomic innervation and the central nervous system with the objective of reducing the ischaemic burden and diminishing the perception of angina.

Despite rapid innovations in percutaneous and surgical revascularisation techniques, increasing numbers of refractory angina patients are presenting to cardiologists with advanced coronary disease, which is unsuitable for further revascularisation. Such patients are often severely disabled by chronic angina pectoris, which often correlates poorly with the degree of observable ischaemia. It is with the background of this burgeoning group of patients, 'refractory' to revascularisation, that has led to increasing interest in the alternative strategies of neuromodulation.

Neuromodulation owes its origins to Melzack and Wall's gate theory of pain[1] that predicted that stimulation of vibratory afferent nerves would reduce or gate the transmission of pain traffic relaying through the cord at the same point. Transcutaneous electrical nerve stimulation (TENS)[2] was specifically designed to make use of this predicted effect and was used to treat a variety of pain conditions, before it was shown to be effective in angina. Spinal cord stimulation (SCS) was also used to good effect in non-cardiac pain conditions before being found to be effective in relieving angina in a patient implanted for cancer pain control.

The UK Pain Society Angina Special Interest Group and the Angina Special Interest Group of the International Association for the Study of Pain and the British Cardiovascular Interventional Society have endorsed the recommend-ation of the UK National Refractory Angina Group that neuromodulation should be offered as part of a multidisciplinary angina management pro-gramme based on the current guidelines (see <www.angina.org> for details).

Correspondence to:
Dr M R Chester, Director,
National Refractory
Angina Centre, Mersey
Regional Cardiothoracic
Centre, Thomas Drive,
Liverpool L14 3PE, UK

## Trancutaneous electrical nerve stimulation

### Clinical evidence for TENS treatment in angina

Early studies conducted on limbs compromised by peripheral vascular disease demonstrated improved microcirculatory blood flow as well as a direct analgesic effect[3]. These anti-ischaemic properties provoked interest in the possibility of treating coronary artery insufficiency, which led to Mannhiemer *et al*[4] producing the first reports of successful application of TENS for chronic angina pectoris in 1982. Several similar small randomised controlled studies[5–8] followed this publication, demonstrating that TENS could improve symptom control, reduce nitrate usage, increase exercise tolerance and extend walking times to ischaemia in chronic angina patients. In common with routine revascularisation strategies, none of the TENS trials attempted to evaluate the placebo effect of the treatment. There have been major difficulties in designing placebo studies because the treatment appears to require paraesthesia for efficacy and so blinding the patient is impossible.

TENS has also been shown to reduce the number of ischaemic episodes in patients presenting to the coronary care ward with unstable angina[9] {Borjesson 1999 5 /id}.

There have been no studies published looking at long-term effects of TENS on prolonged symptom improvement or impact on quality of life in the treatment of chronic angina. Although our own experience of a large series of 150 chronic refractory angina patients indicates significant and sustained improvement is possible in some patients and a randomised controlled study is underway.

## TENS application

The electrodes are placed on the chest either side of the maximal area of perceived pain. The electrodes are then connected to the generator and output set at a frequency of 70 Hz and a pulse width of 0.2 ms. The intensity is then increased from zero until the perceived sensation is just less prominent than the patient's typical angina episode[5].

Patients are advised to activate the TENS device for 1 h, three times per day for background control and also to use it prophylactically during acute angina attacks like GTN. A higher intensity level is required for prophylactic treatment during an acute angina episode with output increased to until the discomfort is relieved. In many patients, the analgesic effect is almost immediate with conversion of the pain to a less noxious sensation, which then gradually subsides. If the pain does not improve within 15 min, or sooner if associated with nausea, vomiting or sweating, patients are advised to attend hospital to exclude an acute coronary event.

## Complications

There are few complications in TENS therapy apart from interactions with pacemaker technology. Contact dermatitis is occasionally troublesome and can be avoided by rotating the electrode positions. If it does recur, varying the type of electrode and contact jelly can resolve the problem. In extreme cases a 'holiday' with local steroid treatment is helpful.

## Safety

TENS therapy is safe in the majority of patients. Permanent cardiac pacemakers are not a contra-indication and problems of abnormal sensing are rare[10]. Any misinterpretation can be avoided by reprogramming the device to a bipolar sensing configuration or altering sensing thresholds[11].

The TENS electrodes should not be placed directly over the pacemaker can.

There is a single case report of an implanted ventricular defibrillator misconstruing a TENS output as ventricular fibrillation resulting in an inappropriate shock. Care, therefore, must be taken when using TENS therapy in this situation.

# Spinal cord stimulation

## Clinical evidence

The first stimulator was implanted for intractable angina in Australia in 1987[12]. Subsequently, there has been extensive scrutiny of SCS in 'refractory' patients, with over 70 publications to date. SCS has been shown to diminish angina, reduce the frequency of hospital admissions and improve patients' quality of life[13–16]. These improvements appear to be persistent without generating additional risks for the patients.

Spinal cord stimulation was compared to high-risk non-prognostic coronary artery bypass surgery in the ESBY[17] randomized trial. Both groups displayed a significant reduction in angina frequency and short-acting nitrate requirements, whilst only the surgical group showed significant improvement of exercise induced ischaemia at 6 months. However, the surgical arm had a high procedural mortality rate which compared to no deaths in the SCS group.

## SCS implantation

Prior to implantation, it is essential that there is a clear understanding between the patient and carer and the medical team about the aims and objectives of therapy. Fear and anxiety are major problems in chronic refractory angina and SCS is not an anxiolytic nor is it implantable psychotherapy.

The device consists of three different components: the implanted pulse generator (IPG), the epidural electrode and a connecting lead. With the awake-patient placed in the prone or sitting position, a Touhy needle is placed in the epidural space using a paramedian approach at the T3–T5 level. Once in position, the electrode is advance to the appropriate level under fluoroscopy guidance (tip at C6–T1). The electrode is connected to an external generator and the final electrode level adjusted with reference to the patient's pattern of stimulatory anaesthesia. Once satisfied that the paraesthesia is pleasant and covers the area of referred pain, the patient is anaesthetized and the IPG is implanted subcutaneously on the anterior abdominal wall. The two units are then connected by a tunnelled lead.

The majority of implanters prefer to complete the entire procedure at one sitting to reduce cost and infection risk (1-stage procedure). If the initial on-table trial is unconvincing, then it is reasonable to externalise the trial lead and implant a few days later if appropriate (2-stage procedure).

## Complications

The main risk for patients is infection, which usually requires explantation of the entire system (viz. permanent pacemakers). All procedures are undertaken with sterile technique and covered with prophylactic anti-biotics. Because with the percutaneous approach the lead is free within the epidural space, lead displacement is relatively common and requires re-exploration of the epidural electrode. Lead fracture is relatively uncommon.

The most serious potential complication is epidural haemorrhage but is rare (approximately 1:2000), whilst an inadvertent dural tap though usually self-limiting can be quite distressing to the patient and occasionally requires a dural patch.

## Safety

Clinicians are naturally concerned over the potential risks of masking myocardial ischaemia. Cardiologists have been apprehensive, fearing that SCS might lead to an increase in the extent of silent ischaemic episodes and also affect the patient's ability to detect an acute coronary event[20].

Research, however, has established that with SCS the overall ischaemic burden is diminished, myocardial infarction is not disguised[21] and that mortality rates are similar to matched cohorts within the general population of coronary artery disease patients[19].

# General mechanisms of action

The precise method by which neuromodulation alleviates symptoms and reduces ischaemia has not yet been defined. Several possible mechanisms have been proposed.

## Placebo effect

Attempts to explain the clear clinical benefits of neuromodulation in terms of 'placebo' versus 'physiological' is impossible as both TENS and SCS produce a clearly perceived sensation when activated[22]. Any credible sham device would, therefore, be required to produce a discernible stimulus, which could then be criticized for providing neuro-stimulation. This creates an irresolvable dilemma.

The placebo effect relates to the psychological influence of a therapeutic agent based on the subject's own belief of the efficacy of the treatment rather than any direct physiological impact of the therapy. The reality is that placebo is a good thing and will influence the outcome from any therapy including angioplasty and bypass surgery. Although its influence is purely psychological, it has also been shown to be capable of eliciting a physiological response. The placebo response has been thought of as a transient phenomenon, but landmark trials in angina have demonstrated that the benefit of placebo can be long lasting[23,24]

## Gating theory

Melzack and Wall[1] proposed that the stimulation of large diameter type A (proprioceptive) fibres leads to attenuation of transmission from activated small unmyelinated type C fibres from the periphery to the central pain receptors via inhibitory interneurones, at the level of the dorsal horn of the spinal cord. Therefore, theoretically, either stimulation of peripheral nerves with TENS or stimulation at the level of the dorsal horn with SCS could lead to attenuation of incoming angina signals travelling along sympathetic efferent pathways. Investigation with SCS has revealed a generalized 'field effect' with reduced neural activity mediated by alteration in the balance of inhibitory and excitatory neurotransmitters. Linderoth et al[25] assayed dorsal horn neurotransmitter levels, demonstrating rises in the inhibitor γ-aminobutyric acid (GABA) and reduced level of excitatory amino acids (aspartate and glutamate) after SCS in rats. In addition, intrathecal administration of GABA antagonists and adenosine agonists have been shown to increase the effectiveness of SCS in the rat model[26]. This suggests that SCS may act, in part, by up-regulating the natural spinal GABAergic inhibitory interneurones. The GABA system is likely, however, merely to be an example, with the complete pattern of action liable to include the contribution of other messengers and involve their subtle and complex interactions.

## Endogenous opioids

It has been proposed that part of the effect of neurostimulation is mediated through heightening of endogenous endorphin activity both at the spinal and cardiac level. Administration of opiates has been shown to be clinically effective in this patient group and SCS has been demonstrated to increase spinal endorphin levels. Mannheimer et al[27] investigated the impact of SCS on cardiac β-endorphin levels using coronary sinus sampling in patients undergoing right atrial pacing. He established that SCS results in elevated cardiac β-endorphin levels, but interestingly also showed that the addition of the endorphin antagonist, nalaxone, failed to diminish the benefit of SCS. It is, therefore, not clear as to whether endorphins play a central role in the mechanism of neurostimulation or is just a peripheral phenomenon.

## Sympathetic nervous system

Increasing intrinsic cardiac sympathetic activity results in increased myocardial workload and, therefore, elevated oxygen demand. The epicardial and arteriolar coronary vessels are innervated by the sympathetic system, which has a pivotal role in vasomotor control through α-adrenergic receptors[28]. There are no consistent data on whether the sympathetic system exerts a resting vasoconstrictor tone on the resting coronary circulation, but clear evidence of sympathetic influence during exercise. It is, therefore, evident that any therapy that acts to minimize sympathetic activity will reduce the circumstances likely to potentiate ischaemia in patients with significant coronary artery disease.

In addition to its role in exacerbation of ischaemia, it is also becoming clear that the sympathetic system is also the main conduit in the transmission of angina, from ischaemic myocardium to the central nervous system[29].

### Sympathetic pathways
The heart has wide-spread sympathetic nerve endings, which coalesce to form the cardiac sympathetic plexus and collateral ganglia. Cardiac nerves link these structures to adjacent swellings within the cervical region of the paravertebral sympathetic ganglion chain[30]. These structures

are termed the stellate and middle cervical sympathetic ganglia. The sympathetic pathways connect with the intermediolateral grey column of the upper thoracic spinal cord (T1–T4) through the white and grey rami communicantes. The sympathetic pathway extends upward in the posterolateral brainstem terminating in the hypothalamus.

Studies have revealed that angina reaches consciousness not solely via the hypothalamus but by excitation of the upper thoracic spinothalamic tract, which relay through the ventroposterolateral thalamus and continue upward to the higher brain centres[31], although no anatomical relationship between the sympathetic pathway and the STT has been demonstrated.

The sympathetic/parasympathetic balance has been investigated by Hautvast *et al*[32] who failed to show any alteration in heart rate variability with SCS. However, Meglio *et al*[33] did find a decrease in resting heart rate and features suggestive of a functional sympathectomy in 25 patients with stimulators, and several investigators have demonstrated a small fall in systolic blood pressure during neurostimulation with both TENS and SCS[34]. Recent work by Foreman *et al*[35] has cast some light on the mechanism by which neurostimulation may alter cardiac sympathetic drive. They observed that spinal cord stimulation in dogs undergoing coronary artery ligature had a suppressive effect on intrinsic cardiac sympathetic activity. Furthermore, they also discovered that this effect could be neutralised by interrupting the afferent and efferent sympathetic tract in the subclavian ansea. This provides evidence that SCS may act through the influence of spinal cord neurons communicating with the intrinsic cardiac nervous system via intrathoracic cardiac nerves.

### Coronary blood flow and myocardial perfusion

Chauhan *et al*[35] used intracoronary Doppler wires to analyse the effect of TENS on coronary blood flow in CAD, Syndrome X and cardiac transplant patients. There was an increase in coronary flow at rest in all but the transplanted patients, which implied a sympathetic mediated mechanism. However, Sanderson[37] and Jessurun[38] were unable to verify these results in follow-up studies with Syndrome X and CAD patients, respectively. Likewise, Norsell *et al*[39] did not see an increase in coronary flow velocity in patients undergoing pacing stress with spinal cord stimulation. The coronary resistance vessels are, however, thought to consist of two resistance compartments in series. The first section consists of α-adrenergically constrained arterioles and the second section consisting of smaller vessels autoregulated by local metabolic factors. It is, therefore, possible that, whilst sympathectomy may reduce resistance in the first compartment, it may simultaneously, by reducing overall myocardial oxygen demand, increase resistance in the second. As a consequence, there may be no overall alteration in vasomotor tone and, therefore, no increase in coronary blood flow.

The effect of neuromodulation on myocardial perfusion during exercise has been investigated using positron emission tomography (PET)[40] in patients with ischaemic heart disease. The investigators found that although SCS failed to alter the overall blood flow, there was a redistribution of blood to previously ischaemic area producing a more homogeneous pattern.

## Algorithm

It is important to realize that, for the majority of patients, neuromodulation will lessen the intensity of their chest pain and reduce the frequency of attacks rather than completely eradicate symptoms. We have, therefore, found it necessary in our own department to provide the patient with education, counselling, help with relaxation and cognitive behaviour therapy as part of an integrated care algorithm[41]. This pathway is commenced prior to neurostimulation in order for the patients to gain maximum benefit from TENS and SCS. It provides an opportunity to reassure, change life-style patterns, such as minimal physical activity, and gain agreement with patients to realistic treatment goals.

## Conclusions

Neuromodulation has been shown to improve anginal symptoms and reduce ischaemia without placing the patient at significant risk. The exact mechanism of action remains unclear, but is likely to be a complex interaction involving placebo effect, nociceptive gating and cardiac sympathetic modulation.

### References

1   Melzack R, Wall PD. Pain mechanisms. *Science* 1965; **150**: 971–9
2   Hammond C, Murray S, Leach A, Chester R. Transcutaneous electrical nerve stimulation for the treatment of patients with chronic refractory angina. *Br J Cardiol* 2000; **7**: 293–5
3   Kaada B *et al*. Vasodilatation induced by of transcutaneous electrical nerve stimulation in peripheral ischaemia. *Eur Heart J* 1982; **3**: 303
4   Mannheimer C, Carlsson C-A, Emanuelsson H *et al*. TENS in severe angina pectoralis. *Eur Heart J* 1982; **3**: 297–302
5   Mannheimer C, Carlsson C-A, Emanuelsson H *et al*. The effects of transcutaneous electrical nerve stimulation in patients with severe angina pectoralis. *Circulation* 1985; **71**: 308–16
6   Mannheimer C, Carlsson C-A, Vedin A *et al*. Transcutaneous electrical nerve stimulation in angina pectoris. *Pain* 1986; **26**: 291–300
7   Kaada B *et al*. TENS in patients with coronary artery disease *Eur Heart J* 1990; **2**: 447–53
8   Nitz *et al*. Transcutaneous electrical nerve stimulation in chronic intractable angina pectoralis. *Aust J Physio* 1993; **39**: 109–13

9 Borjesson M, Ericsson P, Dellborg M *et al*. Transcutaneous electrical nerve stimulation in unstable angina pectoris. *Coron Artery Dis* 1997; **8**: 543–50

10 Rasmussen M, Hayes D, Vliesra R *et al*. Can transcutaneous electrical nerve stimulation be used safely in patients with permanent cardiac pacemakers? *Mayo Clin Proc* 1998; **63**: 443–5

11 Chen D, Philip M, Philip P *et al*. Cardiac pacemaker inhibition by transcutaneous electrical nerve stimulation. *Arch Phys Med Rehabil* 1990; **71**: 27–30{Rasmussen, Hayes *et al*. 1988 48 /id}

12 Murphy DF, Giles KE *et al*. Dorsal column stimulation for pain relief from intractable angina pectoris. *Pain* 1987; **28**: 365-8

13 Sanderson JE, Ibrahim B, Waterhouse D *et al*. Spinal electrical stimulation for intractable angina – long term clinical outcome and safety. *Eur Heart J* 1994; **15**: 810–4

14 Sanderson JE, Brooksby P, Waterhouse D *et al*. Epidural spinal electrical stimulation for severe angina: a study of its effect on symptoms, exercise tolerance and degree of ischaemia. *Eur Heart J* 1992; **13**: 628–33

15 Mannheimer C, Augustinsson LE, Carlsson C-A *et al*. Epidural spinal electrical stimulation in severe angina pectoris. *Br Heart J* 1988; **59**: 56–61

16 Dejonste M, Hautvast R, Hillege J *et al* on behalf of the Working Group on Neurocardiology. Efficacy of spinal cord stimulation as adjuvant treatment for intractable angina pectoris. *J Am Coll Cardiol* 1994; **23**: 1529–7

17 Mannheimer C, Eliasson T, Augustinsson L-E *et al*. Electrical stimulation versus coronary artery bypass surgery in severe angina pectoris. The ESBY study. *Circulation* 1998; **97**: 1157–63

18 Anderson C, Hole P, Oxhøj H. Does pain relief with spinal cord stimulation for angina conceal myocardial infarction? *Br Heart J* 1994; **71**: 419–21

19 Sanderson JE, Ibrahim B, Waterhouse D, Palmer RBG. Spinal electrical stimulation for intractable angina – long term clinical outcome and safety. *Eur Heart J* 1994; **15**: 810–4

20 Chandler M, Brennan T, Garrison D *et al*. A mechanism for of cardiac pain suppression by spinal cord stimulation.: implications for patients with angina pectoris. *Eur Heart J* 1993; **14**: 96–105

21 Dejonste M, Hautvast R, Hillege J *et al*. Effects of spinal cord stimulation on myocardial ischaemia during daily life in patients with severe coronary artery disease. A prospective ambulatory electrocardiographic study. *Br Heart J* 1994; **71**: 413–8

22 Melzack R, Wall PD. (eds) *Textbook of Pain*. Edinburgh: Churchill Livingstone, 1994: chapter 71

23 Cobb *et al*. An evaluation of internal mammary artery ligation by a double blind technique. *N Engl J Med* 1959; **20**: 1115–8

24 Dimond *et al*. Evaluation of internal mammary ligation and sham procedure in angina pectoris. *Circulation* 1958; **18**: 712–3

25 Stiller C, O'Connor W, Brodin E *et al*. Release of gamma-aminobutyric acid levels in the dorsal horn and suppression of tactile allodynia by spinal cord stimulation. *Neurosurgery* 1996; **39**: 367–74

26 Meyerson B, Linderoth B *et al*. Mechanisms of spinal cord stimulation in neuropathic pain. *Neurol Res* 2000; **22**: 285–92

27 Eliasson T, Mannheimer C, Waagstein F *et al*. Myocardial turnover of endogenous opioids and CGRP in the human heart and the effects of spinal cord stimulation on pacing induced angina pectoris. *Cardiology* 1998; **89**: 170–7

28 Young M, Vatner S. Regulation of large coronary arteries. *Circ Res* 1986; **59**: 579–96

29 Foreman R. Mechanisms of cardiac pain. *Annu Rev Physiol* 1999; **61**: 143–67

30 Janes RD, Brandys C, Hopkins DA, Johnstone DE, Murphy DA, Armour JA. Anatomy of extrinsic cardiac nerves and ganglia. *Am J Cardiol* 1986; **57**: 299–309

31 Chandler M, Zhang J, Foreman R *et al*. Cardiopulmonary sympathetic input excites primate cuneothalamic neurons: comparison with spinothalamic tract neurons. *J Neurophysiol* 1998; **80**: 628–37

32 Hauvast R, Brouwer J, Dejonste M *et al*. Effects of spinal cord stimulation on heart rate variability and myocardial ischaemia in patients with chronic intractable angina pectoris – a prospective ambulatory electrocardiographic study. *Clin Cardiol* 1998; **21**: 33–8

33 Meglio M, Cioni B, Rossi G *et al.* Spinal cord stimulation affects the central mechanisms of regulation of heart rate. *Appl Neurophysiol* 1986; **49**: 139–49

34 Emanuelsson H, Mannheimer C, Waagstein F *et al.* Catecholamine metabolism during pacing induced angina pectoris and the effect of transcutaneous electrical nerve stimulation. *Am Heart J* 1987; **114**: 1360–6

35 Foreman B, Linderoth B, Ardell J *et al.* Modulation of intrinsic cardiac neurons by spinal cord stimulation: implications for its therapeutic use in angina pectoris. *Cardiovasc Res* 2000; **47**: 367–75

36 Chaunan *et al.* Effect of transcutaneous electrical nerve stimulation on coronary blood flow *Circulation* 1994; **89**: 694–702

37 Sanderson J, Woo K, Chung H *et al.* The effect of transcutaneous electrical nerve stimulation on coronary and systemic haemodynamics in syndrome X. *Coron Artery Dis* 1996; **7**: 547–52

38 Jessurun G, Tio R, Dejonste M *et al.* Coronary flow dynamics during transcutaneous electrical nerve stimulation for stable angina pectoralis associated with severe narrowing of one coronary artery. *Am J Cardiol* 1998; **82**: 921–6

39 Norsell H, Eliasson T, Albertsson P *et al.* Effects of spinal cord stimulation on coronary blood flow velocity. *Coron Artery Dis* 1998; **9**; 273–8

40 Hauvast R, Blansma P, Dejonste M *et al.* Effects of spinal cord stimulation on regional myocardial blood flow assessed by positron emission tomography. *Am J Cardiol* 1996; **77**: 462–7

41 Chester M. Chronic refractory angina: time to sort out a neglected and growing problem. *Br J Cardiol* 2000; 7:108–11

# Index

*British Medical Bulletin* 2001;**59**

NEXT ISSUE          BRITISH MEDICAL BULLETIN     Volume 60  2001

# Type 2 diabetes: the thrifty phenotype

*Scientific Editor: D J P Barker*